Bioethics

Basic Bioethics
Glenn McGee and Arthur Caplan, editors

Pricing Life: Why It's Time for Health Care Rationing
Peter A. Ubel

Bioethics: Ancient Themes in Contemporary Issues
edited by Mark G. Kuczewski and Ronald Polansky

Bioethics

Ancient Themes in Contemporary Issues

edited by Mark G. Kuczewski and Ronald Polansky

A Bradford Book
The MIT Press
Cambridge, Massachusetts
London, England

This book was set in Sabon by Asco Typesetters, Hong Kong, in QuarkXPress. Printed and bound in the United States of America.

Library of Congress Cataloging-in-Publication Data

Bioethics : ancient themes in contemporary issues / edited by Mark G. Kuczewski and Ronald Polansky.
 p. cm. — (Basic bioethics)
 Includes bibliographical references and index.
 ISBN 0-262-11254-X (alk. paper)
 1. Medical ethics. 2. Philosophy, Ancient. 3. Medicine, Greek and Roman.
I. Kuczewski, Mark G. II. Polansky, Ronald M., 1948– III. Series.
 R724.B4585 2000
 174'.2—dc21   00-020815

Contents

Series Foreword   vii

Introduction   ix

I   The Character of Medical and Ethical Knowledge   1

1   Remembering the Hippocratics: Knowledge, Practice, and Ethos of
     Ancient Greek Physician-Healers   3
     Robert Bartz

2   Is Medicine Art, Science, or Practical Wisdom? Ancient and
     Contemporary Reflections   31
     Ronald Polansky

3   *Phronesis* and the Misdescription of Medicine: Against *The
     Medical School Commencement Speech*   57
     Kathryn Montgomery

4   Aristotle, *Phronesis*, and Postmodern Bioethics   67
     David Thomasma

5   Confessions of an Unrepentant Sophist   93
     Tod Chambers

6   Philosophical Therapy, Ancient and Modern   109
     Julia E. Annas

II   The Heuristic Value of Classical Approaches   129

7   Thrasymachus and Managed Care: How Not to Think about the
     Craft of Medicine   131
     Alex John London

8　Potentiality and Persons: An Aristotelian Perspective　155
Christopher Megone

9　Can Communitarianism End the Shrill and Interminable Public
Debates? Abortion as a Case-in-Point　179
Mark G. Kuczewski

10　Classical and Modern Reflections on Medical Ethics and the Best
Interests of the Sick Child　193
Daryl M. Tress

11　Facing Death Like a Stoic: Epictetus on Suicide in the Case of
Illness　229
Christopher E. Cosans

12　Euthanasia and the Physician's Role: Reflections on Some Views in
the Ancient Greek Tradition　251
Georgios Anagnastopoulos

Contributors　291
Index　293

Series Foreword

We are pleased to present the second volume in the series Basic Bioethics. The series presents innovative book-length manuscripts in bioethics to a broad audience and introduces seminal scholarly manuscripts, state-of-the-art reference works, and textbooks. Such broad areas as the philosophy of medicine, advancing genetics and biotechnology, end-of-life care, health and social policy, and the empirical study of biomedical life will be engaged.

Glenn McGee
Arthur Caplan

Introduction

This collection of essays explores themes from ancient Greek philosophy and medicine and their implications for contemporary medicine and biomedical ethics. Thus the work examines the relationship of two of the most popular areas in the current revival of ethics, namely, classical ethics and biomedical ethics—areas that have seldom been brought together in any serious or sustained way. The essays in this volume are written by established classical scholars and bioethicists. Each author works within the framework of his or her discipline while seeking to unearth the implications for the other. For example, classical scholars examine the import of the concept of practical wisdom (*phronesis*) for clinical medicine and bioethicists reinterpret *phronesis* based upon their observations of medical practice. In similar fashion, the issue of abortion is examined from within the theoretical framework of Aristotle's thought as well as from the perspective of the contemporary Aristotelian movement known as communitarianism.

This compilation of essays reflects a new and burgeoning dialogue between contemporary bioethicists and scholars of ancient Greek philosophy—an interchange begun by bioethicists, who have made copious use of classical themes in recent years. Everywhere one looks in current bioethics literature, references to Aristotle and remarks about the need for practical wisdom abound. This concern with classical ideas has roots in two focal needs of contemporary bioethics: (1) to characterize both ethical and medical knowledge in a way that avoids foundationalism and (2) to create a framework that can fruitfully elucidate particular ethical issues. In the quest for a way to think about issues that is both flexible and able to provide direction, bioethicists have turned to classical sources. In seeking help from ancient wisdom, bioethicists thus seek to engage those whose specialty is these original sources.

This book is divided into two parts. Each reflects one of the needs of contemporary bioethics and considers whether classical themes can offer a direction for alleviating current problems.

Part I.   The Character of Medical and Ethical Knowledge

Despite centuries of inconclusive debate among ethical theorists, philosophers have been prominent in the vibrant contemporary debate on bioethical issues. Many have left their offices in philosophy departments and headed for a variety of other venues. A few served on government commissions charged with making public policy recommendations; some were asked to provide consultations at the bedside; and a good number were invited to participate in the deliberations of institutional ethics committees in hospitals and nursing homes. Most of these endeavors have gone surprisingly well despite the fact that the "ethicists" failed to bring with them an established and confirmed ethical theory as a tool of their trade.

The success of bioethics has strengthened the conviction that such a thing as ethical knowledge exists. But because this knowledge has not been deduced from an abstract and universal ethical theory, new ways to characterize it have been sought. Knowledge in bioethics cannot be "applied" knowledge in the customary sense of application of universal theoretical propositions. Ethical knowledge is somehow tied to experience within the field and is confirmed by further experience. This kind of knowledge is "antifoundationalist" because it starts in media res rather than building on supposed indubitable starting points. Such a view of ethical knowledge, however, opens the door to skeptical challenges and raises a plethora of questions.

Moreover, once philosophers were in the clinic, they began to question the nature of medical knowledge itself. Medical science has often been characterized as an applied science and, as such, was expected to answer questions about particular patients by tracing their problems to their more general causes and treating those causes. Thus, medical science was held to be a science based upon chemistry, biology, and sometimes physics until these philosophers/bioethicists noted that physicians seldom possess the kind of diagnostic and prognostic certitude that should follow from such a scientific model. Also, some physicians seem to be better than others and to possess a great deal of skill of various sorts. An account of these phenomena is called for both as an ethical and an epistemic matter.

Classical philosophy has been recruited as an ally in the effort to cut a middle path between demands for scientific certitude and a lapse into skepticism regarding medical and ethical knowledge. The classical theme of a kind of practical wisdom that deals with a variable knowledge of particulars has proven especially appealing. However, the existence of such a faculty cannot simply be asserted. Its origin, how to develop it, how one knows when such wisdom is operative, and the kind of precision and certitude that can be expected from the body of knowledge produced must be explained.

We present three essays that directly address the nature of medicine as a kind of craft knowledge. Two, those by Robert Bartz and Ronald Polansky, consider the question from an historical perspective that takes the Hippocratic and Platonic-Aristotelian traditions as paradigmatic. Bartz examines the development of the Hippocratic art of medicine; Polansky considers whether medicine is actually an art (*techne*) or a kind of doing (*praxis*) directed by virtue—in particular, *phronesis*. Kathryn Montgomery considers the question of the status of medicine from a more contemporary perspective. She contrasts modern medicine's questionable self-understanding, as reflected in the typical medical school commencement speech, with her view of the art of medicine as practiced by the physician of *phronesis* whose virtue consists in a nuanced ability to draw upon a variety of narratives.

David Thomasma looks at the kind of knowledge that bioethics produces and directly confronts the skeptical challenge. He uses a neo-Aristotelian historicism in constructing an argument that ethical knowledge, despite having a provisional nature ("generally, for the most part, knowledge"), can acquire a privileged ontological status as it becomes part of a culture's or a society's way of being. Tod Chambers describes the reasoning of bioethicists as sophistry. He embraces this usually pejorative term to show how it can function as a metaphor of constructive engagement and consensus building. Both of these bioethicists mirror developments in classical scholarship in seeing Aristotle and the Sophists as more akin than earlier ages appreciated. Julia Annas brings together the reflections on the epistemological and ontological statuses of medicine and philosophy by considering the classical notion of philosophy as therapy.

Part II.   The Heuristic Value of Classical Approaches

Of course bioethicists want more than a way to understand and to reflect upon their reasoning activity. They hope that classical approaches can suggest fruitful ways to view contemporary problems—a challenge that is addressed regarding the issues of managed care, abortion, and suicide. Because classical approaches are not theories that can be applied in a deductive manner, there is much room for judgment and interpretation regarding how to use classical insights. These essays exemplify this fact.

Alex London examines the exchange between Socrates and Thrasymachus in Plato's *Republic* to show that understanding medicine as a kind of craft has implications for contemporary managed care arrangements. Christopher Megone examines Aristotle's notion of potentiality for the light it might shed upon the public policy abortion debate, concluding that, for Aristotle, the potentiality of the fetus is a relevant factor. Mark Kuczewski also considers the abortion question. Viewing the issue through the prism afforded by the contemporary Aristotelian approach known as communitarianism, he concludes that although this approach cannot end the public debate, it contains elements that can lead to a more fruitful approach to the issue. Daryl Tress explores how ancient Greek ethics has been used to reflect on contemporary issues, in particular medical decisions about young children. She challenges the largely secular and pluralistic assumptions of contemporary appropriations of classical views and their focus on case-by-case resolution of ethical problems. Finally, two scholars examine classical responses to the questions of suicide and euthanasia. Chris Cosans presents some of Epictetus's insights in relation to the contemporary suicide debate. This approach looks at suicide from the perspective of the sufferer and considers its effect on his or her virtue; Epictetus sees vice in focusing on suffering, and since killing oneself is a way of reacting to suffering. This approach provides an interesting contrast to current debates that focus on an individual's right to control his or her destiny by directly addressing suffering. Georgios Anagnostopoulos reflects on the art of medicine and describes how classical thinkers were concerned with the impact on the medical profession of aiding in dying. Anagnostopoulos's piece is a fitting conclusion to this volume because in raising the issue of the relationship of classical thought regarding the art of medicine to contemporary clinical medical practice, it brings our effort full circle.

I

The Character of Medical and Ethical Knowledge

1

Remembering the Hippocratics: Knowledge, Practice, and Ethos of Ancient Greek Physician-Healers

Robert Bartz

Most work on ancient Greek medical ethics written by bioethicists focuses on the Hippocratic Oath or selections from the Hippocratic corpus with explicit ethical content. This leads to the general conclusion that early Greek medical ethics began when codes of professional behavior were developed by Hippocrates or a group of physicians carrying the banner of Hippocrates.[1] Bioethicists derive ethical principles from these codes and present them as standards for comparison with later constructions of medical ethics. Absent from this characterization, however, is a sense of the complexity of the ethos of these early doctors as they interacted with the sick and attempted to understand and remedy affliction. Giving consideration merely to works with explicit ethical content fails to examine how ethical problems emerged out of the practices of ancient Greek physician-healers. Moreover, this approach fails to explore the tensions made both explicit and implicit in texts by the ancient Greek physicians as they struggled to apply their understanding of the body, disease, and the environment to the problems of the sick. In this discussion, I attempt to recover some of the Hippocratic writers' understanding of what it meant to be a physician-healer in Greece in the mid-to-late fifth century B.C. To describe the ethos of these ancient physicians and to explore the connections between clinical practice and ethical theory in the development of patient-physician relationships, I will discuss treatises other than those explicitly devoted to ethical topics.[2]

Although I refer to the works contained in the Hippocratic corpus as Hippocratic writings, it is important to refrain from firmly assigning Hippocrates as the author of any of these texts.[3] Very little is known about Hippocrates beyond some basic facts: he was born around 460 B.C., came from Cos, was a contemporary of Socrates, was famous in his time, and likely taught apprentices for a fee. The Hippocratic corpus is a collection of about sixty anonymous writings assembled in the third century B.C. I have selected texts deemed to be documents from the mid-fifth to the early fourth century B.C.[4]

Continuities between the Hippocratics and Other Healers

Calchas rose among them, Thestor's son, the clearest by far of all the seers who scan the flight of birds. He knew all things that are, all things that are past and all that are to come, the seer who had led the Argive ships to Troy with the second sight that god Apollo gave him. (Homer, *The Iliad* Book I: 68–72; Fagles trans. 1990, 79)

I hold that it is an excellent thing for a physician to practice forecasting. For if he discover and declare unaided by the side of his patients the present, past and the future, and fill in the gaps in the account given by the sick, he will be the more believed to understand the cases, so that men will confidently entrust themselves to him for treatment. (*Prognostic* LCL II, 7)

In ancient Greece between the eighth century B.C. and the writings of the Hippocratics in the fifth century B.C., many different healers were making claims to knowledge and skill in treating the sick, including seers, magicians, midwives, folk healers, and temple priests.[5] The earliest description of ancient Greek physicians comes from the *Iliad*, in which Machaon and Podalirius are shown fighting the Trojans and caring for soldiers injured in battle. While highly praised, their activities were limited to removing arrows and treating wounds;[6] they were not the healers called on to treat other forms of affliction. For example, when vast numbers of soldiers were dying from a plague, their leaders turned to the seer Calchas for help.[7] Seers traditionally went with soldiers in battle, worked in the courts of kings, and traveled from place to place attending to those, including the sick who wanted help interpreting and meeting their fate.[8] They practiced the ancient art of prognostics by deciphering omens such as the flight of birds or reading signs like the patterns of livers obtained from sacrificial animals (hepatoscopy).[9]

For the ancient Greeks, illness could be sent by an angry god or goddess who also had the power to heal when properly approached.[10] Religion was inseparable from the daily experiences of individuals.[11] When misery struck, the problem faced by the community was to ascertain whether the destruction was sent by a god or goddess, to determine which god brought on the danger, to find out why the god sent the misery, and to anticipate what the community could expect in the future. This was necessary knowledge for determining the ritual practices most likely to cast away the trouble and bring good fortune.

The Hippocratics themselves took up and applied the ancient art of prognostics in their healing activities in a manner that resembled seers.[12] Both the *iatros* and seer acting as prognosticators practiced telling the present, past, and future of the sick. For both the seers and the Hippocratic physicians, the establishment of a good reputation was a necessary dimension in the relationships of power and knowledge that structured particular healing situations.[13] The prognostic method was not simply part of a psychological strategy.[14] Application of the prognostic method produced knowledge. The challenge faced by the Hippocratics was to differentiate their practices from the activities of other healers and yet to remain engaged in healing in a way that was familiar to the sick and their attendants and that did not radically challenge the gods or the divine.[15]

Reading Bodies to Frame Judgments

The following were the circumstances attending the disease, from which I framed my judgments, learning from the common nature of all and the particular nature of the individual, from the disease, the patient, the regimen prescribed and the prescriber—for these make a diagnosis more favorable or less; from the constitution, both as a whole and with respect to the parts, of the weather and of each region; from the custom, mode of life, practices and ages of each patient; from talk, manner, silence, thoughts, sleep or absence of sleep, the nature and time of dreams, pluckings, scratchings, tears; from the exacerbations, stools, urine, sputa, vomit, the antecedents and consequence of each member in the successions of diseases, and the abscessions to a fatal issue or a crisis, sweat, rigor, chill, cough, sneezes, hiccoughs, breathing, belchings, flatulence, silent or noisy, hemorrhages, and hemorrhoids. From these things must we consider what their consequence also will be. (*Epidemics I*, LCL I, 181)

While prognostic concerns were of interest to many ancient healers, what varied among healers were the signs used to develop their interpretations and predictions. While some seers looked toward the flight of birds and other diviners examined entrails, the Hippocratic *iatros* examined signs on the surfaces of the human body, scrutinized material coming from inside the body, and studied the environment surrounding the body in order to make their prognosis. What differentiated the Hippocratic *iatros* from earlier healers was not principally a shift from the "magico-religious" to the "empirico-rational" but a focus on reading the body signs of the sick person before them.[16] Thus, the *iatros*, influenced by the writings and practices of the Hippocratic authors and intent on reading and interpreting bodily signs, looked at the sick in a distinctive manner. The Hippocratics concentrated upon the body that was to be carefully adjusted rather than the heavens, as did the seer-physician-philosopher Empedocles, who claimed to be able to alter the heavens in the interest of healing the body.[17]

Various views of the body and disease are expressed throughout the Hippocratic collection; they all appear, however, to be influenced by a humoral understanding of health and illness. Disease was due to an excess in some bodily fluid or humor that overcame the equilibrium of health. Bodies were considered to be in constant states of flux or potential flux, depending on climate, season, geographic location, individual constitution, diet, drink, and activity. Disease was understood as an unfolding process, reaching moments of crisis when the illness could turn toward recovery, move in an unfavorable direction, or be transformed into another disease with a new process of development. The Hippocratic physicians closely watched for temporal signs by carefully observing the pattern of fever in the sick.[18] They attended to the spatial unfolding of disease detected through direct examination of the surface of the body.[19] Marks on the body (for example abscesses, ulcers, joint swellings) were read as signs of what was to come as the disease process developed. Like the ripening of fruit, an abscess was thought to go through various changes in color and consistency in the process of becoming mature. As with fruit, however, the climate or other unfavorable constitutional elements could interfere with the process of ripening. Many of these were not under the control of either the patient or the physician. A breakdown in the ripening process produces immature abscesses, and immature abscesses, in turn, denote absence of crisis, pain, prolonged illness, return of symptoms, and death. To determine whether a favorable or unfavorable abscess was likely to form or a fever was likely to move in a harmful or helpful direction, the *iatros* took into account other signs.

The healthy body was thought to cook substances that were ingested. Heating of the substances in the proper manner was considered necessary for the mixture to be properly transformed. While this process was considered natural to the body, it could be affected by the seasons, the individual constitution, the types of matter taken in, and the actions of the patient or physician. The *iatros* examined materials coming from inside the diseased body—including urine, stool, vomitus, and sputum, noting location, color, texture, smell, and in some cases taste to aid in determining the direction of the disease. By taking all of the signs into consideration, the doctor was expected to determine whether the bodily cooking process was occurring properly and to take actions to support that process if it was going properly or modify it if it was misdirected.[20] Thus, the materials coming from inside the body were examined by the Hippocratic physicians both as signs of the unfolding of disease and as aids for determining what course of action to take to help the sick person. At the conclusion of *Prognostic*, we note: "You must take into account both the good signs and the bad that occur and from them make your predictions; for in this way you will prophesy aright" (*Prognostic* LCL II, 33).

Thus, the prognostic approach, explicitly described in various Hippocratic texts and implicit in the other writings in the corpus, was a complex method embedded in and informed by a polytheistic religious context in which many healers were engaged in practice.

If we had the written methods of priests and seers, their descriptions of the problems they encountered and the strategies they used for addressing them likely would be as rich and complex as the writings of the Hippocratics. Unfortunately, for this period we have no record of their activities, possibly because their practices remained part of an active oral tradition, either passed down through apprenticeship relationships or viewed as special gifts from the gods. Some Hippocratic writers emphasized the importance of reading and studying what had been written (e.g., *Epidemics III*, LCL I, section XVI, 257). Perhaps what is most significant about the practices of the physicians whose activities are represented in the Hippocratic writings is that they were written down.[21]

The Hippocratic physician tried to avoid a harmful action by paying careful attention to the timing and prediction of crisis. The wrong action, or an action taken at the wrong time, could prolong the disease, transform the disease into a more dangerous malady, or lead to the demise of the patient. But this approach did not prevent action. For example, in case 8 of *Epidemics III*, "Anaxion, who lay sick by the Thracian gate was seized with an acute fever" (case 8 of *Epidemics III*, LCL I, 269–271) the physician performed a venesection on the eighth day of his illness. "There was an abundant and proper flow of blood," and Anaxion's "pains were relieved, although the dry cough persisted." Suffering from empyema, Anaxion's fever went down on the eleventh day, he began to expectorate concocted sputa on the seventeenth day, had a minor crisis on the twentieth day, and a general crisis on the thirty-fourth day.

The stance taken by the Hippocratic *iatros* toward the afflicted was vigilant, requiring a keen mindfulness and an ability to read and interpret a vast array of signs. If the body was successful in warding off disease, the *iatros* recognized this, foretold the future, and did not interfere. If assistance was considered helpful, the physician intervened to direct or redirect the unfavorable disease process. Actions like venesection or administering purgatives or cathartics were performed from a topographical understanding of disease and the body. Efforts were made to shift humors from one site in the body to another, to bring the bad material to the surface, or to transform unconcocted matter into concocted matter or bad abscesses into good. Prognosis was crucial for treatment and much else in Hippocratic practice.

Defending the Art Against Critique: The Hippocratic *Iatros* as Craftsman

... those who blame physicians who do not undertake desperate cases, urge them to take in hand unsuitable patients just as much as suitable ones.... Those experienced in this craft have no need either of such foolish blame or of foolish praise; they need praise only from those who have considered where the operations of craftsmen reach their end and are complete, and likewise where they fall short; and have considered moreover which of the failures should be attributed to the craftsmen, and which to the objects on which they practise their craft. (*The Art* LCL II, 205)

Although the Hippocratics focused on the body of the afflicted to develop prognostic and therapeutic narratives about unseen disease, tensions emerged regarding their interactions with the sick. Critics claimed that the Hippocratics, to advance their popularity and defend their art and reputations, knowingly cared for those who would heal spontaneously while neglecting those who would die. To counter the notion of spontaneous recovery, the author of *The Art* (LCL II, 197) claimed that people who did not call in a physician inadvertently used in "self-treatment the same means as would have been employed had a physician actually been called in." By changing their regimen or through the administration of medicines and purgatives, the sick unknowingly did for themselves what a physician would have suggested in their particular situation. This was an important demonstration of the existence and the power of "the art" because it worked even in those who used it unknowingly and without belief (*The Art* LCL II, 197–201). To counter the more serious charge of mindful neglect, the Hippocratics claimed that they should be considered healing-craftsmen.

The author of *The Art* argues that like all other craftsmen, the quality of materials used by physicians determines the outcome of their practice. The materials or "objects on which [physician-craftsmen] practice their craft" include the power of the affection (disease), the substance and constitution of the body, and qualities of the patient; these are the elements to scrutinize when a sick person dies after a physician's visit (*The Art* LCL II, 203–205). While these objects of the craft can be distinguished, they combine to create special problems for physician-craftsmen.

The power of disease, particularly the length of time the affection has been hidden away in the afflicted, contributes to the possibility of cure. The Hippocratic physician could not change the fact that the disease may have existed for a long time prior to attending the patient. If called in early, the doctor might help; but if treatment was applied late, the disease would likely win the race. While some affections might be inherently more powerful than others, a major challenge to early treatment emerged out of difficulties related to "the constitution of human bodies" (*The Art* LCL II, 211).

The structure of the body creates problems for the Hippocratics. Although some diseases are readily visible, and considered potentially curable, most diseases were hidden away in the cavities of the body. The many cavities of the body included the limbs (space between muscles and also the veins), the trunk (liver, kidney, spleen, and bowels), the head (brain), the chest (heart), and the back (lungs). In sickness, these hollow organs of the body, normally "filled with air," became filled with deadly "juices" (*The Art* LCLII, 207). When facing someone suffering from hidden disease, attendants could not "see the trouble with their eyes nor learn it with their ears" (*The Art* LCLII, 211). In this context, "medicine while being prevented in cases of empyema, and of diseased liver, kidneys, and the cavities generally, from seeing with the sight with which all men see everything most perfectly, has nevertheless discovered other means to help it" (*The Art* LCLII, 213–215). The author of *The Art* writes that "their obscurity does not mean that they are our masters, but as far as is possible they have been mastered, a possibility limited only by the capacity of the sick to be examined" by educated and able physician-healers (*The Art* LCLII, 209). Observations on the quality of voice, the pace of respiration, the quality, timing, smell, color, and texture of bodily discharges gave practitioners of the art of medicine "the means of inferring" the condition the person suffered from and the parts of the body affected or likely to become affected (*The Art* LCL II, 215). This required special skill for "no man who sees only with his eyes can know anything of what [the author of *The Art*] has described. . . . More pains, in fact, and quite as much time are required to know them as if they were seen with the eye; for what escapes the eyesight is mastered by the eye of the mind" (*The Art* LCL II, 209–211). The author emphasizes that even experienced practitioners of the art face the problem that "both the methods to be employed and the signs produced differ from case to case. As a result the signs may be difficult for the physician to interpret and then cures are slow and mistrust in the power of the doctor persists."[22]

From the perspective of the author of *The Art*, the opinions and actions taken by the sick are a third form of material affecting the outcome of a physician-craftsman's healing practice. The sick struggle with difficulties created by their limited knowledge of the art of medicine, thus, "even the attempted reports of their illnesses made to their attendants by sufferers from obscure disease are the result of opinion, rather than of knowledge. If indeed they understood their diseases they would never have fallen into them" (*The Art* LCL II, 211). Combined with limitations in knowledge, the afflicted also face problems created by the "density of our bodies, in which disease lurk unseen. [Therefore], the careless neglect of patients [and the] advantage [this gives to disease], is not to be wondered at, as it is only when diseases have established themselves, not while they are doing so, that patients are ready to submit to treatment" (*The Art* LCL II, 211–213). Finally, the experience of being sick may create problems for patients in following the recommendations of a physician-craftsman. The author attacks those who criticize the art of medicine because some of the sick die after they are attended by physicians. These critics suggest that physicians may make mistakes, but patients never "disobey orders." However, this author believes the opposite is true. For, while the physician is healthy in mind and body as he carefully considers how the patient should be treated,

the patient knows neither what he is suffering from, nor the cause thereof; neither what will be the outcome of his present state, nor the usual results of like conditions. In this state he receives orders, suffering in the present and fearful of the future; full of the disease, and empty of food; wishful of treatment rather to enjoy immediate alleviation of his sickness than to recover his health; not in love with death, but powerless to endure (*The Art* LCL II, 201).

In this context, the author concludes, "surely it is much more likely that the physician gives proper orders, which the patient not unnaturally is unable to follow; and not following them he meets with death, the cause of which illogical reasoners attribute to the innocent, allowing the guilty to go free" (*The Art* LCL II, 203).

Demands for Rhetoric and Healing: The Hippocratic *Iatros* and Tensions in the Craft Analogy

The treatise *The Art* gives a glimpse of the concerns of physician-healers defending their practice against the criticisms of educated nonphysicians. Plato's dialogues provide insight into the views of educated nonphysicians about the concerns of both sick persons and physicians.[23] Plato's early dialogues contain several comparisons of the knowledge of physician-healers and the knowledge of craftsmen, along with a general working out of a craft analogy in relation to the healing arts. Plato used the analogies drawn from medicine not simply as descriptions of illness and healing but as part of his overall account of the nature of virtue.

In *Laches* 185e–186a, Plato noted that becoming an expert in a craft without having a teacher was possible; one who made this claim, however, would be expected to show "several well-made pieces of work as examples of their skill" (Lane trans.). While with other crafts the craftsmen could bring in products for people to judge, in the case of the healing crafts the product was more difficult to show prior to exercising the techniques of the craft. This problem was addressed in *Gorgias* 464 when Socrates discussed the difference between health and the appearance of health. "For example, many people appear to enjoy health in whom nobody but a doctor or trainer could detect the reverse" (Woodhead trans.). If health was considered the product of the medical craft and people could appear healthy when they were in fact sick, how could the physician-craftsmen convince people of the value of their remedies and demonstrate the outcome of their craft? It was here that the use of rhetoric was celebrated, as when Gorgias comments to Socrates, "I have often, along with my brother and with other physicians, visited one of their patients who refused to drink his medicine or submit to the surgeon's knife or cautery, and when the doctor was unable to persuade them, I did so, by no other art but rhetoric (*Gorgias* 456b)."

Although the doctor was likely to be more knowledgeable about health than the rhetorician, he might be less persuasive before a popular audience. From this observation, Socrates and Gorgias debate the general problem of the relationship between the rhetorician's claims and truth (*Gorgias* 459a–e). However, the fact that rhetoric was effective in the case of medicine, should not principally be viewed as rhetoricians working to convince the ignorant of something the rhetoricians knew to be false. Rather, the art of persuasion emerges in relationship to the art of medicine, because the product of the physician-craftsman is difficult to demonstrate prior to practice or outside of a verbal exchange. At the same time, the experiences of patients with some of the methods used by physician-craftsmen meant that some of the sick, even though they were suffering from serious ailments, would "avoid [giving] any account of [their] physical defects to doctors and undergoing treatment" because of fear of pain and suffering caused by cautery or surgery (*Gorgias* 479a–c). If this was true of someone obviously suffering from disease, it must have been over-whelmingly the case for those who felt healthy but were told that they were ill or would become ill from something that they could not yet observe.

A background of trust between the *iatros* and the patient was essential. In *Lysis* 209e–210d Socrates discussed the example of a King whose son had a problem with his eyes to show the interrelationships between knowledge, trust, friendship, and usefulness:

> If his son had something the matter with his eyes, would he allow him to touch them himself, if he thought him ignorant of the healing art, or rather hinder him. (Hinder him.) But, against us, on the other hand, if he conceived us to be skilled in the art, he would, I imagine, make no objection, even though we wished to force open the eyes, and sprinkle in ashes, as he would suppose us to be rightly advised. (True he would not.) And do with everything else whatsoever, he would entrust it to us rather than to himself or his son, if he believed that we knew more about it than either of them did... If you acquire knowledge my son all men will be friendly to you, for you will be useful and good. If not, you will have no friend in anyone, not even in your father or mother, or any of your family. (Plato, *Lysis* 209c–210d, Wright trans.)

The problem of trust is also addressed in *Protagoras* where Socrates asks Hippocrates to compare the danger of education for his soul: "If it were a case of putting your body into the hands of someone and risking the treatment turning out beneficial or the reverse, you would ponder deeply whether to entrust it to him or not, and would spend many days over the question, calling on the counsel of your friends and relations" (Plato, *Protagoras* 313a).[24]

The use of the craft analogy to define the aims and approach of Greek doctors did very little to differentiate them from other healers of the day. Thracian doctors, prophets, priests, and folk healers all aimed at reestab-lishing harmony, strength, and health in the people they treated.[25] Each examined disorder and gave an account of its nature and consequence and in many cases healing involved some degree of pain or sacrifice carried out because of the search for restoration and strength. When strangers came to town professing the ability to cure certain bodily ailments, the sick were faced with the difficult problem of determining whether they should fol-low the recommendations of the alleged healer. To entrust one's body to the actions of a physician-healer was an act requiring careful deliberation for educated Greeks. The difference between the Hippocratic *iatros* and all other healers turned on the latter's concentrated focus on the human body as affected by all that passed through it or surrounded it.

Integrating *Episteme, Techne, Ethos,* and Rhetoric in Reading the Hippocratic Corpus

In all dangerous cases you should be on the watch for all favorable coctions of the evacuations from all parts, or for fair and critical abscessions (abscesses). Coctions signify nearness of crisis and sure recovery of health, but crude and unconcocted evacuations, which change into bad abscessions (abscesses), denote absence of crisis, pain, prolonged illness, death, or a return of the same symptoms. But it is by a consideration of other signs that one must decide which of these results will be most likely. Declare the past, diagnose the present, foretell the future; practice these acts. As to diseases, make a habit of two things—to help, or at least to do no harm. The art has three factors, the disease, the patient, the physician. The physician is the servant of the art. The patient must co-operate with the physician in combating the disease. (*Epidemics I*, LCL I, 163–165)

In a time of increasing emphasis upon crafts and craftsmen, the Hippocratic practitioners adopted some practices of the marketplace surrounding their activity and, like some sophists and philosophers, looked to the work of craftsmen as models for what they were doing as healers.[26] Although the healing craft was generally viewed as involving three aspects—the *iatros*, the disease, and the patient—in the craft analogy, both patient and disease were considered materials worked upon by the craftsman. This meant that neither the *iatros* nor the healing craft could be criticized if a dying patient was refused treatment, for a craftsman would not knowingly use defective materials. If he did and the outcome was poor, this would be blamed on the materials and not on the craft or the craftsman.

The ethical orientation of the Hippocratic *iatros* developed out of practices based on personal encounters with the sick and other members of their household. Shifting attention to the body of the sick, the Hippocratic *iatros* needed to make an effort to personalize this encounter in order to read the signs necessary for correctly interpreting the direction of the illness and to determine what was needed to help and not to harm the afflicted. Since Hippocratic prognostic involved so much attention to bodily signs, the need to establish trust, maintain confidentiality, and develop a good reputation were cast differently by the Hippocratics than by traditional healers. The physician had either to observe the bodily materials closely or have them described carefully and in sequence by the sick person or his/her attendant. In order to obtain access, the physician needed to gain the trust of the patient so that personal or bodily secrets would be revealed. Coercion might work for momentary observations but would not be compatible with the detailed observations recorded in the *Epidemics I* and *III*.[27]

These case histories document the ongoing interaction with and observation of the sick. The establishment of some basic level of trust sprang from the needs of the practice of the Hippocratic art and, in turn, made the practice of the art possible. Physicians had to clarify their interest in the bodies of the sick while reassuring the patients and their attendants that they were not going to make any sexual advances or in any other way take advantage of the afflicted or their household members. They also needed to teach the ill and their attendants how to conduct and report their own bodily observations that were required for appropriate application of the art. Thus, establishing trust was not merely an outcome or product of the Hippocratic prognostic art but also a means to proper prognostic. Trust and reputation were not simply goals of the Hippocratic practitioner competing in the medical marketplace.[28] Instead, trust and reputation were essential to practice, emerging from the demands of a transforming *episteme* focused on reading and interpreting bodily signs and a changing ethos reflecting the problems inherent in craftsmen's relationships.

While the changing *episteme* required close interactions they frequently occurred between strangers at a time when the traditional ethic of helping friends and harming enemies was prevalent but undergoing revision. Differentiating friends from enemies was not a simple process as traditional family-based ethics were challenged by debates over polis or citizen-based ethics.[29]

Many of the writings in the Hippocratic corpus reflect the concerns of physicians traveling from place to place throughout Greece and Asia Minor.[30] This meant that in their interactions with the sick they frequently began from the position of stranger. They had to demonstrate through practice and rhetoric that they would approach the concerns of the sick from the position of a friend. Thus when the author of *Diseases I*

(LCL V, 119) argues that "we start out in medicine sometimes by speaking, at other times by acting," the claim emerges simultaneously out of concerns for caring appropriately for the sick (through correct application of prognosis and *techne*) and for the appropriate manner of approaching the sick (through correct character and rhetoric).[31] Therefore, "To help or at least to do no harm" must first be understood as part of a strategy of healing that is necessarily embedded in close personal encounters and interactions.

Forgetting Hippocrates and Remembering the Hippocratics

In this constitution there were four symptoms especially which denoted recovery:—a proper hemorrhage through the nostrils; copious discharges by the bladder of urine with much sediment of a proper character; disordered bowels with bilious evacuations at the right time; the appearance of dysenteric characteristics.... Women and maidens experienced all the above symptoms ... in fact I know of no woman who died when any of these symptoms took place properly. For the daughter of Philo, who died, though she had violent epistaxis, dined rather unseasonably on the seventh day. (*Epidemics I*, LCL I, 175)

Several examples clearly illustrate that establishing this kind of personal contact was challenging and at times frustrating for the Hippocratic *iatros*. Both *Diseases I* and *Affections*, which are primarily detailed texts about diseases and their treatments, begin with descriptions of what laymen needed to know and the complexity of interacting with patients.[32] The forty-two case narratives presented in *Epidemics I* and *Epidemics III* illustrate the difficult decisions faced by the Hippocratic *iatros*.[33] The cases frequently display rather detailed daily observations made of the sick person followed by gaps in observations that may last days, only to be followed by more detailed and complete narrative.[34] This pattern suggests that the *iatros* either was required to leave the presence of one sick person to attend to another person or was not called back with any regularity. In order to prevent inappropriate administration of regimen at a time of crisis, to be called at a critical moment in the illness, and to be assured of an accurate description of what went on in their absence, the *iatros* needed to involve others in both the prognostic and therapeutic process.

It is likely that from the author's perspective, the daughter of Philo in *Epidemics I*, died needlessly because she "dined unseasonably" on a criti-

cal day during her illness (*Epidemics I*, LCL I, 175). The author emphasizes the point that all others who bled recovered. She bled but did *not*
recover. Given the central place of regimen in the theory of disease (and
the fact that this author mentions this case) suggests to him that a season-
able regimen had been described to this patient and she did not follow the
recommendations. Or perhaps the doctor was called in late after the crisis
occurred and the mistake in regimen had already been made. In either
case, a needless death by their own criteria must have been disturbing for
the Hippocratics.[35] Cases like Philo's daughter point to a need to educate
the public generally about the nature of health and illness, but they also
underscore the difficulties the Hippocratics faced in their daily clinical
interactions.[36]

It was important for the *iatros* to establish a good and trusting relationship not only with the sick person but also with other members of the
household. Both family members and servants could provide critical observations of the sick and often decided when another visit would take
place. *The Art* detailed some of the frustrations faced by the *iatros* in
interacting with household members. However, they were clearly necessary to a healing practice focused on the body of the sick person and often
carried on in the dwelling of the sick. All of these relationships required a
fair measure of trust and it is out of these personal interactions that
documents like the Hippocratic Oath likely emerged.

Thus ethical statements contained in writings like the Hippocratic Oath
developed out of a pattern of healing practices that required close attention to a sick person's body by the physician-healer. The terms in the Oath
presuppose a model of care based on selected household visits in a competitive healing environment populated by other healers. This situation
required close collaboration between the Hippocratic *iatros*, his apprentices, the sick person, family and other members of the household. The
Hippocratic *iatros* needed assurance that any of his apprentices could be
trusted and thus demanded a pledge or oath from them modeled after the
traditional concerns of family relationships. At the same time, patients
needed to be reassured that they and their household members would
be handled with dignity in their interactions with the *iatros*. This is the
background to the statements proscribing sexual acts and emphasizing
confidentiality.[37]

If we focus on "to help, or at least to do no harm," it should not be read simply as attempting to maximize benefit or minimize pain. The *Epidemics I* and *III* give us the opportunity to garner information within a clinical context and find that this ethic is process-based rather than outcome-based. The content of the actions to be taken was highly contextual, involving a complex reading of bodily signs and the establishment of a relationship with the patient that sought friendship between strangers. This stance would make disease the common enemy of the afflicted and physician-craftsman. Taking all of this together, the *iatros* was to act to help and at least to do no harm.

I have tried to show how the ethical treatises likely emerged out of a practice of healing focused on the body and requiring personal interactions between the *iatros*, the sick, and friends or household members of the sick. Much of what we now take to be the classical basis of Western ethics was developed only *after* the early Hippocratic writings. Thus, the ethical considerations raised in the Hippocratic treatises should be read as concerns deriving directly from the practice of medicine, and preceding and influencing the more structured subsequent philosophies of Plato and Aristotle. The Hippocratic writings tell us about the social structures and ethical assumptions that provided the background for the development of philosophical ethics that followed.

The Hippocratic writings do not present us so much with overarching ethical principles as with insights gained from grappling with the clinical problems faced and described. While it is obviously true that the Hippocratics could not anticipate our specific ethical challenges, study of the activities of the ancient Greek *iatros* may cast important light on the general problems faced by healers and patients that included hopelessness, suffering, uncertainty, and competitive healing environments— all of which continue to be of concern in patient-physician relations.[38] Rather than focusing narrowly on the Hippocratic Oath, by extending our reading we may appreciate how the ethical documents were produced out of the concerns of both the ancient physician-healers and the afflicted as they interacted in changing healing relationships. In this sense the ethos of healing for the Hippocratics is co-constructed from the concerns of the *iatros* and the sick during the final decades of the fifth century B.C.[39]

Notes

1. There is an extensive literature in contemporary bioethics that makes reference to Hippocrates and Hippocratic ethics. A comprehensive review of this literature is beyond the scope of this paper. Some exemplary work in this area includes Beauchamp and Childress 1989, Bulger 1987, Pellegrino 1987, 1988, Pellegrino and Thomasma 1988, and Veatch 1981. For a more detailed discussion of previous work on Hippocratic ethics as well as issues involved in the historiography of Hippocratic scholarship, see Bartz 1998. I use the terms *physician, physician-healers, physician-craftsmen,* or the Greek word *iatros* to refer to the healers whose writings are presented in the Hippocratic corpus. During this era (mid-to-late fifth century B.C.) these healers were trying to differentiate their activities from that of many other healers.

2. This project is based on my reading of English translations of the Hippocratic Collection. Within the field of medical ethics, very little attention has been paid to reading texts other than those that are clearly focused on ethics, even though they are available in English translations.

3. For general discussions of Hippocrates and Hippocratic scholarship, see Lloyd 1978/1983, Smith 1979, and Jouanna 1998. For two important opposing views on the problem of the "authentic Hippocrates" or the "Hippocratic School," see Joly 1983 and Mansfeld 1983.

4. This includes the following treatises: *Ancient Medicine, Epidemics I, Epidemics III, Airs Waters Places, Prognostic, Sacred Disease, The Art, Regimen in Acute Disease, Regimen I–IV, Affections, and Diseases I.* I have chosen to work primarily with the editions and translations of W. H. S. Jones and Paul Potter available in the Loeb Classical Library (LCL) because they comprise the most extended and complete set of translations available in English. In a few cases I use (and note) the Chadwick and Mann translations collected in Lloyd 1978/1983. The citations for the Loeb Classical Library (LCL) will occur as follows: Name of Hippocratic treatise, volume of Book in the Loeb Series, page of English translation. For example the commonly cited phrase "to help, or at least do no harm" would be cited: *Epidemics I* LCL I, 165.

5. On the range of healers and healing practices in ancient Greece, see Nutton 1992. Women played an important role in the development of much of this knowledge and practice, and although this had been a neglected history, it has received considerable attention recently. For examples on the relationships between women's knowledge and the development of knowledge represented in the Hippocratic corpus, see Hanson 1991, Dean-Jones 1995, and King 1998. For further discussion of folk beliefs and practices and magical traditions, see Lloyd 1983, Parker 1983, Riddle 1987, and Scarborough 1991. On temple healing and religious practices, see Edelstein and Edelstein 1945 and 1998, Burkert 1988, Aleshire 1989, and Garland 1992.

6. During the conflict, Machaon was struck with an arrow and the Acheans feared that the tide of the battle would turn against them, since "a man who

[could] cut out shafts and dress wounds—a good healer [was] worth a troop of other men" (Homer, *Iliad*, Book 11: 514–515, Fagles 1990, 606–607). For the broader context of social practices in Homeric Greece, see Finley 1978/1988 and Bye 1987.

7. See Homer, *Iliad*, Book 1. Burkert 1992, 41 comments that "seers and doctors are the first enumerated by Homer as migrant 'craftsmen,' individuals whom a community would be concerned to attract. They [were] specialists of a particular kind, having their art—*techne*—which no one else [could] master." For a discussion of the knowledge of seers and the epistemological assumptions in the Homeric poems, see Hussey 1990.

8. Fridolf Kudlien traces the activities of seers through the work of Aeschylus, thereby situating their practices in the decades before the earliest Hippocratic writings (Kudlien 1968). Their approach, patterned after the description of Apollo in the *Eumenides* that follows here, involved the interpretation of signs for purposes of conducting healing rituals and clearly linked *iatros* (physician-healer) and *mantis* (seer/prophet/diviner). "Apollo the master of this house, the mighty power. Healer, prophet, diviner of signs, he purges the halls of others" (Aeschylus, *The Eumenides*, 64–66, trans. Fagles, 1977, 233).

9. For further discussion of hepatoscopy, see Burkert 1992, 46–53.

10. This is depicted in the opening of the *Iliad* when Apollo, "incensed at the king [Agamemnon] swept a fatal plague through the army—men were dying and all because Agamemnon spurned Apollo's priest" (Homer, *Iliad*, Book 1: 10–12, trans. Fagles, 1990). For an overview of popular beliefs and practices, see Parker 1983.

11. See Dodds 1951, Burkert 1987, Zaidman and Pantel 1992, and Sourvinou-Inwood 1991.

12. The connections between magic, religion, and folk practices and the emergence of "science" have been studied extensively by Lloyd 1979, 1987, 1991.

13. In the *Iliad*, when Calchas was called upon to find a solution to the problem, he knew that his vision of the cause and his subsequent recommendations would challenge the honor of Agamemnon. In a public display, he asked for protection from Achilles before he spoke out. This scene shows both the possibilities and the dangers present in the application of prognosis by the seer. The gift from Apollo of second sight allowed Calchas to provide diagnostic and prognostic knowledge that confronted the power of Agamemnon. This knowledge was necessary to aid the Achaeans but threatened the king and thereby placed the safety of the seer at risk. Reputation allowed Calchas to come forward and gain the protection of Achilles in order to provide the Achaeans with the approach they needed to address the scourge. Calchas linked prognostic knowledge to a ceremonial remedy that, once properly performed, appeased Apollo, who ended the plague. The knowledge necessary for understanding the etiology of the plague emerged from existing power relations between the gods and humans. Through both telling and performance this knowledge was embedded in new power relationships involving humans and the gods.

14. Edelstein 1967, 70 claims that application of the art of prognosis helped the Hippocratic physicians build and maintain reputations. He concludes that "prognosis and prediction [were] consequently of significance for *people*, for the physician and for the patient, and only thereby for the curing of the disease itself. In the therapeutic procedure prognosis [was] therefore *important not as knowledge from which to derive other knowledge; its importance [was] psychological*" (author's italics).

15. Although certain Hippocratic writers criticized magical practices in general and some particular religious activities, nothing in the Hippocratic corpus suggests that the writers were criticizing the general belief in gods; see *The Sacred Disease* (LCL vol. 2). For the problem of differentiating Hippocratic practice from divination, see *Regimen in Acute Diseases*, LCL II, section VIII, 69 and also Van der Eijyk 1990 and 1991.

16. The categories "magico-religious" and "empirico-rational" were used by Henry Sigerist in his classic work *History of Medicine, Volumes I and II* (1951, 1961). For a discussion of the epistemological significance of reading bodies for purposes of distinguishing between the Hippocratics and other healers, see Bartz 1998. King 1998 discusses Hippocratic interpretations of female bodies.

17. For further discussion of Empedocles, see Kirk, Raven, and Schofield 1983, 280–321 and Kingsley 1995.

18. Several discussions throughout the corpus provide detailed observations of the pattern of fevers where the authors attempt to differentiate predictable fevers from the unpredictable, as well as the endemic and less dangerous fevers from the acute and dangerous; see, for example, *Epidemics I*, LCL I, section VI, 157–159. To make this differentiation, the physician needed to learn the pattern of illness specific to certain places and corresponding to particular seasons. Although the approach of seers directly influenced the development of the prognostic method used by the Hippocratic physician-healers, the pattern of disease present in Greece in the fifth century B.C. also influenced the development of the method and the possibilities for knowledge of the body that would be attained through that method. Malaria is suspected to have been prevalent in particular regions of Greece at the time of the Hippocratics and likely influenced the pattern of fevers the Hippocratic writers described; see Sallares 1991, 221–293, Grmek 1991 on the ecology of disease in ancient Greece, and Risse 1979 for further discussion of the relationship of disease to medical thought and practice.

19. The treatise *Prognostic* gives detailed descriptions of how to conduct both an inquiry and an examination of a person suffering from an acute disease. See especially *Prognostic* LCL II, 9–11.

20. *Prognostic* LCL II, 19–31 and for a general discussion of this approach, see *Regimen in Acute Disease* LCL II.

21. For a review of many of the scholarly debates regarding oral and written communication in ancient Greece, see Thomas 1992.

22. *The Science of Medicine*, in *Hippocratic Writings*, ed. G. E. R. Lloyd, trans. J. Chadwick and W. N. Mann 1978, 147. For these lines the translation from

Jones is overly clumsy and confusing, so in this case I have selected the translation from Chadwick and Mann. The section from the Jones translation reads as follows: "Now as the relation between excretions and the information they give is variable, and depends upon a variety of conditions, it is accordingly not surprising that disbelief in this information is prolonged, but treatment is curtailed, for extraneous factors must be used in interpreting the information before it can be utilized by medical intelligence" (*The Art* LCL II, 217). Additional sections in the corpus link knowledge and trust. For example, in *Prognostic* (LCL II, 7) the author connects the prognostic method to the problems of being believed and establishing trust with the sick person:

I hold that it is an excellent thing for a physician to practice forecasting. For if he discover and declare unaided by the side of his patients the present, the past, and the future, and fill in the gaps in the account given by the sick, he will be the more believed to understand the cases, so that men will confidently entrust themselves to him for treatment.

23. My reading of Plato's early dialogues moves beyond the approach taken by writers such as Edelstein in discussing the relationships between philosophy and medicine. Edelstein argues that philosophy laid the intellectual groundwork for medicine (1967, 349–366). We should look instead at the close interactive relationship that must have existed between the writing and practices of the Hippocratics and that of their philosopher contemporaries. I am experimenting with a double reading of texts to eliminate both dichotomies: physician versus patient and philosopher versus physician. In addition to the outlook of the writer as physician, my aim is to glean from the Hippocratic writings what is revealed about the concerns of the sick person. My reading of Plato's early dialogues focuses on them not only as works of philosophy but also as a way of reconstructing educated nonphysicians' views about interactions between physicians and patients. We need to break down the boundaries between science, medicine, literature, and philosophy if we want to piece together the fragments of ethical understanding in premodern societies. This has also been recognized by philosophers who have turned to the Hippocratic writings to help understand the context for the philosophical concerns in Plato and Aristotle, the best example of which is perhaps Nussbaum 1986, 89–121, and 1994.

24. *Protagoras* (Guthrie trans.). Hippocrates here is not the physician Hippocrates although earlier in the dialogue Plato alludes to the physician Hippocrates in order to strengthen the point that is being made here.

25. On the range of accepted healers at the time of the Hippocratics, Lloyd 1992, 130 writes:

In antiquity there was not just the one image of the ideal physician, but a great variety of images, some overlapping, some mutually exclusive. some people were for assimilating the doctor to the diviner or the seer, or otherwise for bringing medical practice under the aegis of the gods. But others saw doctors as craftsmen, where what counted was skill built up from long experience, and more especially a trained eye.

26. For discussion of ancient Greek economy relevant to this discussion, see Finley 1985/1999 and Starr 1977. For discussions of the craft analogy in Plato and Protagoras, see Irwin 1991, and for a general overview of Sophist perspectives see Kerferd 1989.

27. See, for example, *Epidemics III*, Case 2, LCL I, 261:

In Thasos the woman who lay sick by the Cold Water, on the third day after giving birth to a daughter without lochial discharge, was seized with acute fever accompanied by shivering. For a long time before her delivery she had suffered from fever, being confined to bed and averse to food. After the rigor that took place, the fevers were continuous, acute, and attended with shivering. Eighth and following days. Much delirium, quickly followed by recovery of reason; bowels disturbed with copious, thin, watery and bilious stools; no thirst. . . .

It seems very likely that to get the history of what happened before the delivery of the infant, the *iatros* had to carry on a discussion with a member of the household, given that the woman was acutely ill and delirious during much of her illness. This was a very protracted illness, and death occurred on the eightieth day. The *iatros* records entries on days 8, 11, 20, 27, 40, 60, and 80. On the sixtieth day, he wrote, "on the succeeding days she lost power of speech, but would afterwards con- verse." However, the next entry is not until the 80th day and is simply written: "Death." This suggests that the description afterward was gathered again from someone close to this woman.

28. Edelstein 1967, 87–88 considered the competitive marketplace the driving force behind the interrelationships among ancient Greek medical knowledge, practice, ethics, and interactions between physicians and patients. He wrote that, "For the patient, the physician is not the doctor, the educated man to whose knowledge he defers and whom he recognizes as an authority in his field. . . The authority that is essential in every treatment must first be established and this means the physician's behavior was dictated by nonmedical considerations to a much greater extent than are the actions of today's physician in his relations with his patient."

29. See, in particular, Blundell 1989 for discussion of the traditional ethic of "helping friends and harming enemies" and tensions in that ethic present in the work of Sophocles, an important contemporary of the Hippocratic authors. For a discussion of emerging tensions between the household (*oikos*) and the city (*polis*) in classical Greece, see Humphreys 1993 and Pomeroy 1995. For a history of friendship, see Konstan 1997.

30. *Airs Waters Places*, LCL I and *Epidemics I* and *III*, LCL I are particularly good examples.

31. The author of *Diseases I* makes clear that the process of interacting with the sick is complex and requires careful attention to rhetoric:

Anyone who wishes to ask correctly about healing, and, on being asked, to reply and rebut correctly, must consider the following: . . . What physicians treating patients achieve by luck. What good or bad things patients suffer in diseases. What is said or done on conjecture by the physician to the patient, or by the patient to the physician. What is said and done with precision in medicine" (*Diseases I*, LCL V, 99).

32. "Any man who is intelligent must, on considering that health is of the utmost value to human beings, have the personal understanding necessary to help himself in diseases, and be able to understand and to judge what physicians say and what they administer to his body, being versed in each of these matters to a degree reasonable for a layman" (*Affections*, LCL V, 7). Potter, the translator of *Affections*, convincingly argues against the view that this was a book on popular medicine. Whether the treatise was directed at a popular audience or not it clearly shows a concern for the "lay view" and demonstrates what it is necessary for an *iatros* to know to be able to communicate with educated patients.

33. "Epidemic" should not be translated in our modern sense of a disease spreading to affect an entire population (e.g., an influenza epidemic) or, more generally as the study of disease incidence and prevalence (as in epidemiology). As Burkert 1992, 43 notes, it is instead "the term for a temporary sojourn, *epidemia*, typically used of migrant physicians [that] can equally be applied to seers."

34. A good example is *Epidemics III*, Case 2, LCL I discussed above.

35. A reader today may identify individuals scattered throughout the Hippocratic cases that should have lived if they had the treatments "we have now." That is not what is at stake in this case. It is clear that the author of the treatise believes that Philo's daughter would have lived if she had not eaten unseasonably on a critical day. By their own standards, this was a preventable death.

36. Examples of a series of treatises that seem to have been directed at the public are: *Regimen I*, *Regimen II*, and *Regimen III* (LCL IV). These writings offer very detailed instructions on regimen in daily life, suggesting that if they were followed, the individual could come closer to achieving health and harmony in life and warding off disease early if stricken.

37. For further discussion of the interrelationships between the personal and the professional in the construction of the Hippocratic Oath, see Von Staden 1996. Henrich von Staden provides a new translation of the Oath and the sections relevant here are as follows:

Into as many houses as I may enter, I will go for the benefit of the ill, while being far from all voluntary and destructive injustice, especially from sexual acts both upon women's bodies and upon men's, both of the free and of the slaves.... And about whatever I may see or hear in treatment, or even without treatment, in the life of human beings—things that should not ever be blurted out outside—I will remain silent, holding such things to be unutterably [sacred, not to be divulged].... And in a pure and holy way I will guard my life and my *techne*.

He has also seriously called into question the more narrow reading of the Oath offered by L. Edelstein who considered the Oath to be a product of a Pythagorean sect. For von Staden, the religious elements of the Oath reflect more mainstream religious views. He concludes by arguing that

The prayed-for reputation stands in direct relations to the sworn moral and religious commitment to live one's life, and to practice one's profession, in a way that will not offend any of the gods witnessing the oath. These reciprocal divine-human dynamics ensure that the Oath's conception of reputation does not tolerate a discrepancy between seeming and being, between appearance and reality, between opinion and truth. The oath-taker's 'holy and pure' life and practice will bind the gods to grant him an eternal, universal good reputation, just as his solemn oath, sworn before all the gods, binds him both to live such a life and to practice his profession 'in a pure and holy way' (von Staden, 437).

38. Some bioethicists argue that the Hippocratics have little relevance because they could not anticipate the specific ethical dilemmas that would emerge in patient-physician relationships in the late-twentieth century as a result of "life-sustaining treatments, AIDS, or managed care"; see, for example, Lo 1995, 12.

39. An earlier version of this chapter was presented at a meeting of the Society for Health and Human Values Conference—Whose Ethics? Which Medicine?: The Tacit and Explicit Development of a Medical Ethic, April 17–19, 1998, Youngstown Ohio. I gratefully acknowledge the very constructive comments from Vivian Nutton and Guenter Risse on previous drafts.

References

Aleshire, S. 1989. *The Athenian Asklepieion: The People, Their Dedications, and the Inventories*. Amsterdam: Gieben.

Bartz, R. 1998. *Hippocratic Practice: Context and Ethos, Lessons for Contemporary Patient-Physician Relations*. M.A. Thesis, History of Health Sciences, University of California, San Francisco.

Beauchamp, T., and J. Childress. 1989. *Principles of Biomedical Ethics*. New York: Oxford University Press.

Blundell, M. W. 1989. *Helping Friends and Harming Enemies: A Study in Sophocles and Greek Ethics*. Cambridge: Cambridge University Press.

Bulger, R. 1987. "The Search for a New Ideal," 9–21 in *In Search of the Modern Hippocrates*, ed. R. J. Bulger. Iowa City: University of Iowa Press.

Burkert, W. 1987. *Greek Religion*, trans. J. Raffan. Cambridge, MA: Blackwell and Harvard University Press.

Burkert, W. 1988. "The Meaning and Function of the Temple in Classical Greece," 27–47 in *Temple in Society*, ed. M. V. Fox. Winona Lake, Ind.: Eisenbrauns.

Burkert, W. 1992. "'A Seer or a Healer': Magic and Medicine from East to West," 41–87 in *The Orientalizing Revolution: Near Eastern Influence on Greek Culture in the Early Archaic Age*, trans. M. Pinder and W. Burkert. Cambridge, Mass.: Harvard University Press.

Bye, C. R. 1987. *Ancient Greek Literature and Society*. Ithaca, N.Y.: Cornell University Press.

Dean-Jones, L. 1995. "*Autopsia, Historia and* What Women Know: the Authority of Women in Hippocratic Gynaecology," 41–59 in *Knowledge and Scholarly Medical Traditions*, ed. D. Bates. Cambridge: Cambridge University Press.

Dodds, E. R. 1951. *The Greeks and the Irrational*. Berkeley: University of California Press.

Edelstein, E., and L. Edelstein. 1945/1998. *Asclepius: Collection and Interpretation of Testimonies*. Baltimore: Johns Hopkins University.

Edelstein, L. 1967a. "The Hippocratic Oath: Text, Translation and Interpretation," 3–63 in *Ancient Medicine: Selected Papers of Ludwig Edelstein*, eds. O. Temkin and C. Temkin. Baltimore: Johns Hopkins University Press.

Edelstein, L. 1967b. "Hippocratic Prognosis," 65–86 in *Ancient Medicine: Selected Papers of Ludwig Edelstein*, eds. O. Temkin and C. Temkin. Baltimore: Johns Hopkins Press.

Edelstein, L. 1967c. "The Hippocratic Physician," 87–110 in *Ancient Medicine: Selected Papers of Ludwig Edelstein*, eds. O. Temkin and C. Temkin. Baltimore: Johns Hopkins Press.

Edelstein, L. 1967d. "The Relation of Ancient Philosophy to Medicine," 349–366 in *Ancient Medicine: Selected Papers of Ludwig Edelstein*, eds. O. Temkin and C. Temkin. Baltimore: Johns Hopkins Press.

Fagles, R., trans. 1977. Aeschylus, *The Eumenides* in *The Oresteia*. New York: Penguin Books.

Fagles, R., trans. 1990. Homer, *The Iliad*. New York: Penguin Books.

Finley, M. I. 1978/1988. *The World of Odysseus*. New York: Penguin Books.

Finley, M. I. 1985/1999. *The Ancient Economy*. Berkeley and Los Angeles: University of California Press.

Garland, R. 1992. *Introducing New Gods: The Politics of Athenian Religion*. Ithaca, N.Y.: Cornell University Press.

Grmek, M. 1991. *Diseases in the Ancient Greek World*. trans. M. Muellner and L. Muellner. Baltimore: Johns Hopkins University Press.

Hamilton, W., and Cairns, H., eds. 1972. *Collected Dialogues of Plato*. Princeton, NJ: Princeton University Press and the Bollingen Foundation.

Hanson, A. E. 1991. "Continuity and Change: Three Case Studies in Hippocratic Gynecological Therapy and Theory," 71–110 in *Women's History and Ancient History*, ed. S. Pomeroy. Chapel Hill: University of North Carolina Press.

Humphreys, S. C. 1993. "*Oikos* and *Polis*," 1–21 in *The Family, Women and Death: Comparative Studies*. 2d ed. ed. S. C. Humphreys. Ann Arbor: University of Michigan Press.

Hussey, E. 1990. "The Beginnings of Epistemology: From Homer to Philolaus," 11–38 in *Companions to Ancient Thought 1: Epistemology*, ed. S. Everson. Cambridge: Cambridge University Press.

Irwin, T. 1991. *Plato's Moral Theory: The Early and Middle Dialogues*. Oxford: Oxford University Press.

Joly, R. 1983. "Hippocrates and the School of Cos," 29–47 in *Nature Animated*, ed. M. Ruse. Dordrecht, Holland: D. Reidel.

Jones, W. H. S. ed. and trans. 1923. *Hippocrates*, vols. 1, 2, 4, Loeb Classical Library. Cambridge, Mass.: Harvard University Press.

Jouanna, J. 1999. *Hippocrates*, trans. M. B. DeBevoise. Baltimore: Johns Hopkins University Press.

Kerferd, G. B. 1989. *The Sophistic Movement*. Cambridge: Cambridge University Press.

King, H. 1998. *Hippocrates's Woman: Reading the Female Body in Ancient Greece*. London/New York: Routledge.

Kingsley, P. 1995. *Ancient Philosophy, Mystery, and Magic: Empedocles and Pythagorean Tradition*. Oxford: Oxford University Press.

Kirk, G. S., J. E. Raven and M. Schofield. 1983. *The Presocratic Philosophers*. 2d ed. Cambridge: Cambridge University Press.

Konstan, D. 1997. *Friendship in the Classical World*. Cambridge: Cambridge University Press.

Kudlien, F. 1968. "Early Greek Primitive Medicine." *Clio Medica* 3: 305–336.

Kudlien, F. 1970. "Medical Ethics and Popular Ethics in Greece and Rome." *Clio Medica* 5: 91–121.

Lloyd, G. E. R. ed. 1978/1983. *Hippocratic Writings*, trans. J. Chadwick and W. N. Mann. Harmondsworth, England: Penguin Books, Ltd.

Lloyd, G. E. R. 1979. *Magic, Reason and Experience: Studies in the Origins and Development of Greek Science*. Cambridge: Cambridge University Press.

Lloyd, G. E. R. 1983. "Developments in Pharmacology, Anatomy, and Gynaecology," 112–200 in *Science, Folklore and Ideology: Studies in the Life Sciences in Ancient Greece*, ed. G. E. R. Lloyd. Cambridge: Cambridge University Press.

Lloyd, G. E. R. 1987. *The Revolutions of Wisdom: Studies in the Claims and Practice of Ancient Greek Science*. Berkeley: University of California Press.

Lloyd, G. E. R. 1991. "Who Is Attacked in 'On Ancient Medicine,'" 49–69 in *Methods and Problems in Greek Science*, ed. G. E. R. Lloyd. Cambridge: Cambridge University Press.

Lloyd, G. E. R. 1992. The Fielding H. Garrison Lecture. "The Transformations of Ancient Medicine." *Bulletin of the History of Medicine* 66: 114–132.

Lo, B. 1995. *Resolving Ethical Dilemmas: A Guide for Clinicians*. Baltimore: Williams and Wilkins.

Mansfeld, J. 1983. "The Historical Hippocrates and the Origins of Scientific Medicine," 49–76 in *Nature Animated*, ed. M. Ruse. Dordrecht, Holland: D. Reidel.

Nussbaum, M. 1986. *The Fragility of Goodness: Luck and Ethics in Greek Tragedy and Philosophy*. Cambridge: Cambridge University Press.

Nussbaum, M. 1994. *The Therapy of Desire: Theory and Practice in Hellenistic Ethics*. Princeton: Princeton University Press.

Nutton, V. 1992. "Healers in the Medical Market Place: Towards a Social History of Graeco-Roman Medicine," 15–58 in *Medicine in Society: Historical Essays*, ed. A. Wear. Cambridge: Cambridge University Press.

Parker, R. 1983. *Miasma: Pollution and Purification in Early Greek Religion.* Oxford: Clarendon Press.

Pellegrino, E. 1987. "Toward an Expanded Medical Ethics: The Hippocratic Ethic Revisited," 45–64 in *In Search of The Modern Hippocrates*, ed. R. J. Bulger. Iowa City: University of Iowa Press.

Pellegrino, E., and D. Thomasma. 1988. *For the Patient's Good: Restoration of Beneficence in Health Care.* New York: Oxford University Press.

Pellegrino, E. 1988. "Medical Ethics: Entering the Post-Hippocratic Era." *Journal of the American Board of Family Practice* 1: 230–237.

Pomeroy, S. 1995. *Xenophon Oeconomicus: A Social and Historical Commentary.* Oxford: Clarendon Press.

Potter, P., ed. and trans. 1927/1988. *Hippocrates*, vol. 5, in Loeb Classical Library. Cambridge, MA: Harvard University Press.

Riddle, J. 1987. "Folk Tradition and Folk Medicine: Recognition of Drugs in Classical Antiquity," 33–61 in *Folklore and Folk Medicine*, ed. J. Scarborough. Madison, WI: American Institute of History of Pharmacy.

Risse, G. 1979. "Epidemics and Medicine: The Influence of Disease on Medical Thought and Practice." *Bulletin of the History of Medicine* 53: 505–519.

Sallares, R. 1991. *The Ecology of the Ancient Greek World.* London: Duckworth Press.

Saunders, T. J., ed. 1987. Plato, *Laches*, trans. I. Lane, in *Early Socratic Dialogues.* New York: Penguin Books.

Scarborough, J. 1991. "The Pharmacology of Sacred Plants, Herbs, and Roots," 138–174 in *Magika Hiera: Ancient Greek Magic and Religion*, ed. C. Faraone and D. Obbink. Oxford: Oxford University Press.

Sigerist, H. 1951. *A History of Medicine*, Vol. I, *Primitive and Archaic Medicine.* New York: Oxford University Press.

Sigerist, H. 1961. *A History of Medicine*, Volume II, *Early Greek, Hindu and Persian Medicine.* New York: Oxford University Press.

Smith, W. 1979. *The Hippocratic Tradition.* Ithaca, N.Y.: Cornell University Press.

Sourvinou-Inwood, C. 1991. "What Is Polis Religion?" 295–322, in *The Greek City: From Homer to Alexander*, eds. O. Murray and S. Price. Oxford: Clarendon Press.

Starr, C. G. 1977. *The Economic and Social Growth of Early Greece 800–500* B.C. New York: Oxford University Press.

Thomas, R. 1992. *Literacy and Orality in Ancient Greece.* Cambridge: Cambridge University Press.

Van der Eijyk, P. J. 1990. "The Theology of the Hippocratic Treatise 'On the Sacred Disease.' " *Apeiron* 23: 87–119.

Van der Eijyk, P. J. 1991. " 'Airs, Waters, Places' and 'On the Sacred Disease': Two Different Religiosities?" *Hermes* 119: 168–176.

Veatch, R. 1981. *A Theory of Medical Ethics*. New York: Basic Books.

Von Staden, H. 1996. " 'In a pure and holy way': Personal and Professional Conduct in the Hippocratic Oath?" *Journal of the History of Medicine and Allied Sciences* 51: 404–437.

Zaidman, L. B., and P. S. Pantel. 1992. *Religion in the Ancient Greek City*, trans. Paul Cartledge. Cambridge: Cambridge University Press.

2

Is Medicine Art, Science, or Practical Wisdom? Ancient and Contemporary Reflections

Ronald Polansky

Classical philosophy devoted considerable energy to the division and demarcation of sciences. For anyone responsibly working in or learning a science, recognizing its position among the various sciences seems vital. The type of science affects the aim, method, and exactness of the enterprise. For the ancient Greeks, medicine was an important undertaking, provoking questions about its place within the divisions of the sciences.[1] Reflecting today upon medicine, we may also wonder how to formulate its study and practice in relation to the various sciences. Is it a natural science, practical intelligence, or an art? Will traditional thought support any such assignment?[2] We begin with a sketch of the traditional articulation of the sciences and then consider the relationship of medicine to it.

The ancients primarily conceived of medicine as an art—an exceptional art closely related to natural science and to practical wisdom—a conception of medicine that still seems applicable. In both the past and present, medicine, for better or worse, inevitably has complex relationships with the other sciences. The vast expansion of today's medical knowledge and range of treatments tends to join medicine even more closely to other fields.

Aristotle's Division of the Sciences

The classic division of the sciences is found in the works of Aristotle. His divisions were prepared by his predecessors, especially Plato, but Aristotle seems the first to have set up a scholastic scheme that he largely adheres to throughout his corpus.[3] Aristotle carries over from Plato the premise that *knowing* involves the ability to state causes or principles.[4] Different sorts of sciences presumably require different sorts of principles or a different relationship to principles. Aristotle can distinguish the sciences based on: (1) the status of their principles, (2) the aim or result or work (*ergon*) of the science, (3) the subject matter of the science, (4) the method or approach taken in the science, (5) the exactitude achievable by the science, and (6) the way in which the science is imparted. We shall examine how these criteria enter into the main branches of the sciences.

An important text for distinguishing theoretical, practical, and productive sciences, based primarily on the status of the principles, is found in *Metaphysics* vi 1. Discussing the place of physics or natural science in particular, Aristotle says:

> And since natural science, like other sciences, confines itself to one class of beings, i.e. to that sort of substance which has the principle of its movement and rest present in itself, evidently it is neither practical nor productive. For the principle of production is in the producer—it is either reason or art or some capacity, while the principle of action is in the doer—viz. choice, for that which is done and that which is chosen are the same. Therefore, if all thought is either practical or productive or theoretical, natural science must be theoretical, but it will theorize about such being as admits of being moved, and only about that kind of substance which in respect of its formula is for the most part not separable from matter. (1025b18–28)

Aristotle here constructs a three-part division of scientific thought—theoretical, practical, and productive—based on the location of the pertinent principles.[5] Natural science is theoretical because its principle, that which causes the rest and motion of natural beings, is in the natural beings themselves. In contrast, practical and productive sciences have their principles in the humans who engage in them.

Features of the Theoretical Sciences
In the case of theoretical sciences—first philosophy (metaphysics or theology), physics (natural science), and mathematics (see *Metaphysics* vi 1.1026a18–19)—the principles, as noted, are in the subject matters themselves. That the principles are *in* the subject matters, separate from human intervention, gives the principles stability so that they can be approached theoretically with relative precision. Though first philosophy, natural science, and mathematics are elaborated as sciences *by us*, the principles we employ have firm grounding in the matters under investigation. Unlike other philosophical positions, such as nominalism, subjectivism, idealism,

historicism, and so on, which attribute the principles even of the theoretical sciences to the knower, who in some way constitutes what is to be known, the Aristotelian position emphasizes the independent nature of the theoretical object. Aristotle agrees with Plato that changeable things as such are not fully knowable, since what is changeable will come to differ from what it was and so could not be known to be any definite way (see *Posterior Analytics* i 2.71b15–16 and *Metaphysics* i 6.987a32–b1). Yet because for Aristotle unchanging principles are *within* even changeable things, the changeable things can be known in their essence and essential relationships—that is, in terms of the principles (or kinds) they instantiate. Thus, that principles are in the subject matters rather than in us suggests that these sciences do not depend for their possibility upon us.[6]

The aim of theoretical science as such is truth or knowledge. The very word "theoretical" (θεωρητική)—from *theoreo* (θεωρέω), meaning to look at, to behold ("speculative," the Latin-based equivalent, similarly connects with sight)—suggests that such science is for the sake of seeing or knowing. Such sciences are not primarily utilitarian, as are other sciences. For Aristotle, "the end of theoretical knowledge is truth, while that of practical knowledge is action" (*Metaphysics* ii 1.993b20–21). Speaking of the first philosophers, he says:

... since they philosophized in order to escape from ignorance, evidently they were pursuing science in order to know, and not for any utilitarian end. And this is confirmed by the facts; for it was when almost all the necessities of life and the things that make for comfort and recreation had been secured, that such knowledge began to be sought. Evidently then we do not seek it for the sake of any other advantage; but as the man is free, we say, who exists for his own sake and not for another's, so we pursue this as the only free science, for it alone exists for its own sake. (*Metaphysics* i 2.982b19–28)

Clearly Aristotle does not suppose that theoretical science initiates technological development or aims for further objectives.[7]

The different theoretical sciences are distinguished mainly by their subject matters: mathematics is about being insofar as it is quantified, physics about being as movable, and first philosophy about being as being. The methodical presentation of theoretical science, once the principles are ascertained, should be through demonstration (*apodeixis*). Rigorously axiomatic presentation of theoretical results is at least possible; geometry in the form it takes in Euclid might be exemplary. The exactitude or precision of theoretical science surpasses that of any other sort of science. Precision depends upon at least two factors, the assumption of fewer sorts of principles and decreased variation in the working out of results (due to the stability of principles).[8] Consider how fewer principles may be needed. Arithmetic will be more precise for Aristotle than geometry because arithmetic only assumes numbers of things whereas geometry must also assume continuous quantity for geometrical figures (*Metaphysics* i 2.982a25–28 and xiii 3.1078a9–13). Theoretical sciences depend on fewer principles than any of the practical or productive sciences. Variation in results concerns the extent to which the subject of the science is involved with matter. Matter, for Aristotle, is what has the potentiality to be or not to be, i.e., to be in various ways. Hence, greater involvement with matter, i.e., matter as a principle of the science, means greater variability. Mathematics can be so precise because mathematical entities are so removed from perceptible matter. For the same reason, metaphysics is quite precise. But natural sciences, which involve movable objects, have less precision because these objects are enmattered.

How is theoretical science supposed to affect the life of the person engaged in it? The traditions of Presocratic thought and particularly of Plato and Aristotle link theoretical science with human happiness.[9] Theorizing seems the highest sort of activity to which humans can aspire—the most godlike of activities. Whether those spending considerable time engaged in it must also be completely morally virtuous is an open question. Surely those most occupied with eternal things seem to have less energy and concern for mortal things (see Plato *Republic* vi 485d), and hence less likelihood of indulging in conventional injustices. Further, those devoted to investigating eternal things tend to imitate them, employing them as paradigms for their life (see, e.g., *Phaedo* 82d–84b).

Theoretical science is generally imparted through teaching. Since such science may be demonstrative and even have an axiomatic presentation, ready textbook treatment of the science could be possible. Yet first principles cannot be demonstrated in this manner since an infinite regress of principles must not occur. A dialectical sifting of the *endoxa*—the prominent, plausible views—serves both to gain and to teach principles. Allowing that humans are intelligent, Aristotle supposes that widely held thoughts, based upon a wealth of experience, guide us to understanding the required principles of a field.[10]

Features of the Productive Sciences

The productive sciences—including crafts or arts (τέχναι, *technai*) such as carpentry, shoemaking, poetry, dance, rhetoric—have their principles in the maker himself or herself.[11] In Aristotle's understanding of production, we first have the form or conception of the product that is to be made in our souls; we then make it by progressively realizing it in some external matter (see, e.g., *Metaphysics* vii 7–8). Because the form has some generality, we may be capable of producing various sorts of particular things. For example, housebuilders can make various sorts of houses. Although to speak of all the arts as productive is appropriate, Aristotle distinguishes between arts that *make* things and arts that *use* things (see *Physics* ii 2.194a36–b7). For example, the shipbuilder makes the ship that the art of the pilot knows how to use and steer. Using arts may approach practical sciences more closely. Characteristic of all arts is that each has an end or aim beyond itself. Since this end is brought about by the artist and in accordance with the form in the artist's soul, the principles of art especially reside in the artist.

The form that productive art generates in the matter may be more or less easy to apprehend inasmuch as that form may be more or less evident to the senses. In *Parts of Animals* Aristotle says, "For the doctor and the builder define health or house, either by the intellect or by perception, and then proceed to give the accounts and the causes of each of the things they do and of why they should do it thus" (i 1.639b17–19). Health seems less obvious to the senses than the order and structure of a house and, consequently, the principles of medicine more difficult to learn. Moreover, the principles of art seem to be in the maker to a different extent for different arts. The form of house is more our conception than is health, insofar as health is a state natural to living things. Nevertheless, an art of medicine, much like house building, may devise a sequence of human interventions to attempt to bring about the realization of the end aimed at. Though the principle or conception of what is to be made is somehow "in us," art or science is possible because making has definite standards. Standards for good products, the standard of the art, always obtain even if these standards may be modified as the arts develop. In the ultimate defense of the existence of real standards, Aristotle can insist that "art imitates nature" (see, e.g., *Physics* ii 2.194a21–27). Art is understood to supplement nature and to fill in what nature failed to provide or only provided insufficiently.

In its various sorts of connection with nature, art more or less seems under the control of human design. Aristotle has to admit that "art loves chance." In the case of the medical art, since nature aims for the health of the organism just as the art does, many cures may seem to be spontaneous as well as the result of the art (see *Parts of Animals* i 1.640a28–30). Many developments in the arts likely result from the appreciation of chance outcomes and the subsequent deliberate pursuit of such outcomes. But the practice of the arts is always more or less under human control, with chance or factors outside human control merely having some impact.

A real test of art seems to be nonaccidental success. The more the complex nature of the material worked upon is simplified and only a small portion of its natural capacity is used, the more reliably we should expect that the artist can work upon it. The potter, housebuilder, shoemaker deal with nonliving materials that resist the work of the artisan minimally, though of course the matter may always be recalcitrant to some extent. Arts concerned with living things and nature more generally—farming, medicine, and dance—seem much less certain of success because the art must interact with other powerful forces.

We touch here upon one factor in the precision and reliability of the practice of the arts: the greater the involvement with more complex matter, the less the precision and the less predictable the success. Another factor regarding the precision and reliability of art is that the closer the practice of the art approaches what occurs in theoretical science, the greater the precision and reliability. Hence surveying, depending so much upon mathematics, will be a quite precise art.

Because art depends upon apprehension of principles and a fairly comprehensive subject matter, the term "art" is generally reserved for relatively high-level abilities. Shoemaking, carpentry, navigation, poetry, rhetoric, flute-playing, and so on are called arts, but trivial skills as how to put on a cloak or to drive in a nail would each not normally be called arts. The expectation, perhaps, is that a person typically devotes his or her life, or a significant portion of it, to real proficiency in an art (the scheme in Plato's *Republic* urges "one person one art"; and see *Rival Lovers* 135c–d). The various genuine arts seem distinguishable from each other in terms of their different subject matters, their aims, and their methodologies. We may also need to introduce aims and methods together with subject matters because different arts could work in closely related subject fields; for example, horse trainers and horse racers are both involved with horses.

The artist, who has the form of the product in the soul, also thereby has the privation or opposite of the form in soul, i.e., the good artist is also the best at deliberately wrecking the product. The best doctor will also be the best poisoner (see Plato *Republic* i 333e–334b, *Lesser Hippias* 366e–369a, and Aristotle *Metaphysics* ix 2, 5 and *Nicomachean Ethics* vi 5.1140b22–24). Knowledge provides understanding of contraries so that insofar as art is knowledge and technical skill, it permits its possessor to make the product well or poorly. What determines whether the art produces the good result or its opposite is the choice of the practitioner. But choice and what determines the choice seem something outside and beyond the art or technical skill itself. Hence, arts may be considered morally neutral and in need of regulatory oversight.

Moreover, the arts offer expertise merely in a rather determinate field and cannot themselves ascertain when and where the art should be practiced. Shoemaking knows good shoes and medicine good health, but because they do not understand the complete human good, they do not themselves determine when shoes should be made or which patient should be treated and to what extent (see Plato *Laches* 195c–d; *Gorgias* 512a–b). Similarly, the engineer knows how to build a bridge but whether a bridge should be built and where is not solely a technical question. Not only, then, may the practice of the arts require oversight to keep the practitioners exercising their skill to produce good results—rather than using the expertise to produce the contraries—but also some overall direction may be needed regarding when and where the arts operate. Ancient thought tended to posit a hierarchy of arts that produce things subserving higher and higher ends, and that, ultimately, political understanding should be ordering all the subservient arts.[12]

Little effort is required to imagine skilled artists using their expertise selfishly and not producing the best results. Yet art as such aims more fundamentally toward the positive result than its opposite (see *Metaphysics* ix 2.1046b10–15). And, since practice of the arts requires numerous choices on the part of the practitioner and acquiring artistic skill requires the discipline of the proper standard of the art, real competence in the arts can be expected to make an important contribution to the life of the practitioner as well as to the recipients of the artist's work. The attainment of excellence in art and the proper practice of the arts may bring orderliness, aspiration for achievement, and satisfaction in achievement to the lives of the practitioners. Hence, art as such is not morally neutral inasmuch as its practice bestows order (cf. Aristotle *Topics* vi 5.143a1–8).

Art is imparted not merely by teaching but also by engaging in the productive work itself. Textbook learning must be combined with direct practice, typically under the watchful eye of those more skilled (see Aristotle *Metaphysics* i 1.981a12–28).

Features of Practical Science
The practical sciences—including ethics, politics, and most likely economics (household management [*oikonomia*])—also have their principles or causes in the actor himself or herself. The principle here is the very choice of the agent, however, rather than any external end. Choice (*proairesis*) is what initiates action. The artist, too, must choose what to make, but the choice is not itself part of the art, which is technical skill for realizing certain kinds of ends that go beyond the art itself. In the practical sciences, the choice itself is the exercise of the practical science. What is aimed at is a certain kind of action or manner of choosing, i.e., morally virtuous action, since there is no end beyond the very exercise of the practical science. Action itself is the primary subject of the practical sciences and the principles of action are to be found in those choosing and acting. The distinction of making (*poiesis*) and doing (*praxis*) divides the productive from the strictly practical sciences. Production is concerned with making a product, or at least with some result of the process that goes beyond it, whereas practical science concerns itself mainly with the choice of the action itself, with the quality of the doing.[13]

Because practical wisdom principally concerns choice and action, it inevitably has the welfare of its possessor and of the associations to which its possessor belongs as its primary concern. In contrast, art makes a product that will serve humans in some way—otherwise humans would have little interest in the product. However, art as knowledge capable of developing a good result, which is then of some use to humans, need not much serve the practitioner of the art. In book 1 of the *Republic*, Plato describes the shepherd's looking out for the welfare of the sheep and thereby also for that of the master who will use the wool of the sheep or eat the sheep. The *art* of the shepherd does not much concern itself with the shepherd, though of course the shepherd also looks out for his own welfare through some compensation for keeping the sheep (*Republic* i 345b–d). But the art of shepherding, while leading indirectly to benefit for the shepherd, is not a knowledge primarily benefiting the shepherd: it is expertise at looking out for the good condition of the sheep, a condition benefiting users of the sheep. Art as such, therefore, while serving humans who use the result of the art, does not directly or especially serve the practitioner of the art (see London's discussion in this volume pp. 137–141). Practical wisdom, however, is the intelligence to do what is in one's own interest and to guide others and associations of others in what is to their genuine interest and good. Practical wisdom concerns both public and private good. By its direct concern with choice and action it itself deals with ultimate human ends rather than with products or results that can further be used in the service of human ends, as do the arts.

Choice is unique to humans, resulting from a conjunction of thought and desire. Thought is deliberation that weighs the respective advantages of various alternatives and calculates what means may achieve a desired end. The sort of desire involved in choice tends to go beyond mere appetite (*epithumia*) for immediate pleasures; rather, it is wish (*boulesis*) directed toward ends. Hence, our choices reflect and are based upon our character as persons, which gives shape to our wishes. Our moral virtues, vices, or states in between, developed from our previous choices of actions, affect our present choices and so tend to be reinforced and to affirm our character further.[14] Unlike the productive arts, which may not thus involve character fully but pertain mainly to technical knowledge (and hence bestow the capacity for contraries), practical science has implications for full development of character. Excellence at practical science, which is called practical wisdom (*phronesis*) or political wisdom, can only, Aristotle suggests, be combined with a virtuous moral character (*Nicomachean Ethics* vi 12.1144a36–b1). Hence, the practically wise person not only knows what to do but chooses to do it. The practically wise and good person could not deliberately choose evil, and hence is a law unto himself or herself and not in need of regulation.[15] Such a person discerns what should be done in his or her own life and can aid others and the political community in determining what is most likely to be the best choice. The aim for practical science is happy life, but unlike the aim for art—making a product or fostering some external result—choosing appropriate things to do itself constitutes the happy life that is the aim of practical science. The practically wise person is not technically proficient in a narrow, determinate sphere, as in the arts, but is aware of the whole human good. Therefore, when and where things should be chosen fits within practical science and no further science orders it, in contrast to the arts, which need some expertise to arrange them.[16]

Though the principles are in humans, science is possible in the realm of practical action because it requires knowledge of causes and principles. The practically wise person is the standard of practical science. Practical science for Aristotle (surprisingly, given its scope) is, in a sense, more precise than any of the arts (see *Nicomachean Ethics* ii 6.1106b14–16) because moral virtue, which is intimately tied to practical wisdom, is more precise than art. Moral virtue has qualities analogous to those of the arts inasmuch as excess and deficiency detract from the outcome in both realms. This gives rise to the doctrine of the mean, which pervades moral virtue even more than the arts. Virtue itself is a state of character that lies in a mean between vicious states of character (e.g., courage is between rashness and cowardice), and this state of character tends toward the intermediate—what is appropriate in actions and passions. The arts are merely capacities to produce things that are intermediate and by techniques that are intermediate but they are not themselves states between extremes.[17] Aristotle also holds that other sciences are more capable of being forgotten than the practical sciences. We may forget theoretical science and lose our skill in the arts, but practical science has the strongest hold upon us (*Nicomachean Ethics* vi 5.1140b25–30). Regarding virtue and character, it has hold not only on our intellects but on the configuration of our desires.

Imparting practical science mainly involves habituation and practical action: We become certain kinds of persons by our choice of actions. The role of teaching is secondary (ethical treatises such as Aristotle's are for fine tuning those persons already well brought up and for giving them more confidence in their better inclinations). The practice for practical wisdom and moral virtue is character training and reflection upon it, which leads us to enjoy what we should and be pained by what we should (*Nicomachean Ethics* ii 3). Whereas practice of the art is guided by the success of the product or result, practice in the moral sphere concentrates on the way action is undertaken. It is doubtful that virtue can be taught readily because so much more than technical skill is needed.

Having considered these rich, basic reflections of the ancients upon the division of the sciences, we may turn more particularly to how medical science and medical practice enter into the scheme of the sciences.[18]

The Place of Medicine within the Sciences

Medicine's Connection with Theoretical Science

The ancient Greeks routinely speak of medicine as an art (τέχνη). Since "art" is sometimes used very broadly, especially in Plato, this might mean little. Yet the ancients also, as we have seen, demarcate art from other intellectual disciplines as knowledge directed at making a product or securing a result external to the practice of the art itself. Even taking art in this more restricted way, they still tend to include medicine among arts, such as shoemaking, carpentry, farming, rhetoric, and poetry, inasmuch as medicine engenders health. Since it generates health, though by assisting nature and using various instruments, medicine seems both a making and a using art.

Classical philosophers find reasons for giving medicine a peculiar place among the arts.[19] In *Sense and Sensibilia*, Aristotle states:

It behooves the natural scientist to obtain also a clear view of the first principles of health and disease, inasmuch as neither health nor disease can exist in lifeless things. Indeed we may say of most physical inquirers, and of those physicians who study their art more philosophically, that while the former complete their works with a disquisition on medicine, the latter start from a consideration of nature. (436a17–b1; see also *On Youth, Old Age, Life and Death, and Respiration* 480b28–30)

This acknowledges that the study of natural science leads to medicine and that those giving an intellectual treatment of the medical art begin with principles from natural science.[20]

Could the same be said for all the other arts, or does medicine have an unusual standing? Since every art aims to produce some product or to foster some end, and this requires motion by the practitioner through which some change is effected, all the arts will have some connection with natural science, which is the science of movable or changeable things. Also, the materials worked upon by the arts are, at least originally, natural beings. Yet medicine approaches natural science more closely than other arts because it aims for its result, health, which is itself a natural condition, in a living, natural being, the human being, that continues subsequently as a natural being. Though arts such as shoemaking and carpentry work on natural materials (leather and wood, for example), these materials are removed quite far from their natural condition by the productive process. The securing of health, by contrast, restores the natural state of the living organism; the doctor is in the service of health (see *Nicomachean Ethics* vi 13.1145a7–9). Since the very aim of the art is a natural condition, the principles of medicine are largely natural principles. No art that greatly reconfigures natural materials or utilizes them to achieve an end quite removed from nature would require so much knowledge of nature. Other arts working closely with nature, such as gymnastics, farming, gardening, and animal husbandry, may be less deeply involved in natural science because the aim is less natural, the need for natural science for its success is less, or humans ultimately have less interest in plant or animal health than human health.[21]

That medicine has inescapable connection with natural science should be evident.[22] This is truer today than in antiquity. Our greater sense of progress in natural science makes medicine seem more intimately tied to its own development. We believe that the efficacy of treatment grows apace with our knowledge of the relevant natural sciences. Since modern science is experimental in a more embracing way than ancient science, medical practice and scientific research are linked even more closely than they were in the past.[23]

Medicine's Connection with Practical Science

However much medical science depends upon physical principles and treatments are considered experimental, medical practice can hardly simply be theoretical science. Medicine applies its knowledge in practice to generate health in particular individuals and populations rather than merely to gain understanding. There should be great interest, then, in exploring whether medicine is not only an art especially akin to natural science but also an art associated closely with ethics and politics, i.e., the practical sciences.

Is medical practice concerned quite exclusively with bodily health, whether its maintenance or restoration? The more medicine concentrates upon the body, the more it may resemble other arts focused upon bodies. For the ancients, health is some sort of order or balance of the components of the body. The Presocratic philosopher Alcmaeon compared health to *isonomia* (equality before the law in a political community) and disease to *monarchia* (the undue aggrandizement of one component at the expense of the rest).[24] Plato adheres to this line of thought when he views health as analogous to justice: health is the good condition of the body when each component has its rightful position as justice is the good condition of the soul (see *Republic* iv, especially 444c–445b). Although health and medicine are thus seen as analogous, respectively, to justice and statesmanship, medicine nevertheless remains an art. Whereas justice is the very aim of the understanding of justice (i.e., the soul aims to perfect itself), medical art generates health in something other than itself, the body. (Even medical education, which produces more doctors, has the health of patients as its ultimate aim.)

Need medical practice have the limitation that this suggests so that it is simply an art? Is medicine only analogous to statesmanship, and loosely analogous at best? The more medicine is restricted to the body's condition and the more the human body seems solely a tool or instrument, as a hammer or a wagon is a tool, the more medicine seems strictly an art. But treatment of the human body appears rather unlike treatment of other bodies. In Plato's *Charmides* we find these striking statements:

You [Charmides] have probably heard this about good doctors, that if you go to them with a pain in the eyes, they are likely to say that they cannot undertake to cure the eyes by themselves, but that it will be necessary to treat the head at the same time if things are also to go well with the eyes. And again it would be very foolish to suppose that one could ever treat the head by itself without treating the whole body. In keeping with this principle, they plan a regime for the whole body with the idea of treating and curing the part along with the whole... Well Charmides, it is just the same with this charm. I learned it while I was with the army, from one of the Thracian doctors of Zalmoxis, who are also said to make men immortal. And this Thracian said that the Greek doctors were right to say what I told you just now. "But our king Zalmoxis," he said, "who is a god, says that just as one should not attempt to cure the eyes apart from the head, nor the head apart from the body, so one should not attempt to cure the body apart from the soul. And this, he says, is the very reason why most diseases are beyond the Greek doctors, that they do not pay attention to the whole as they ought to do, since if the whole is not in good condition, it is impossible that the part should be. Because," he said, "the soul is the source both of bodily health and bodily disease for the whole man, and these flow from the soul in the same way that the eyes are affected by the head. So it is necessary first and foremost to cure the soul if the parts of the head and of the rest of the body are to be healthy. And the soul," he said, "my dear friend, is cured by means of certain charms, and these charms consist of beautiful words. It is a result of such words that temperance arises in the soul, and when the soul acquires and possesses temperance, it is easy to provide health both for the head and for the rest of the body." So when he taught me the remedy and the charms, he also said, "Don't let any one persuade you to treat his head with this remedy who does not first submit his soul to you for treatment with the charm. Because nowadays," he said, "this is the mistake some doctors make with their patients. They try to produce health of body apart from health of soul." (156b–157b)

Observe that good medical practice is said to treat parts of the body with attention to the good condition of the whole body.[25] The Thracian god of healing Zalmoxis urges more than this. While ordinary Greek doctors principally treat the body, the god holds that health of the body must be based upon virtue or temperance of the soul. Although this passage might be less a serious recommendation for medical practice than a Socratic device by which he entices the young Charmides to speak with him to achieve some kind of cure for his headache, it is more plausible that these lines convey that the more medicine goes beyond being merely an ordinary art, the more it should aim at a good condition of the soul and a proper way of life.[26]

Have not many fields of medicine concerned themselves with how we should live? The *Charmides* links medicine with the virtue of temperance (*sophrosune*), i.e., sensible living generally, since the medication for headache will be ineffective unless the patient is prepared to live a temperate life. It seems likely that ancient and modern doctors make recommendations about diet, exercise, and so on that serve both the body and the soul. Clearly, the treatment of heart-related ailments and other systemic ailments frequently raises issues about patterns of living, personal relationships, work satisfaction, and so on, that go beyond diet and exercise. Obviously psychiatry, pediatric medicine, gynecology, and so on have such concerns. The notions that our patterns of living contribute to loss or maintenance of health and even that moral virtue may foster physical health are compelling. Doctors' concern for the health of patients may often, then, take on aspects of counseling virtuous living inasmuch as soul affects body importantly.

As significant as proper living may be for a happy life and a life as healthy as it can be, such patterns of living only aid in reducing the incidence of disease and injury. Good patterns of living cannot ensure that we shall not become sick or be injured. Humans may themselves be responsible for some diseases and injuries, and partly responsible for others, though not at all responsible for some. They are, however, responsible for how they respond to them (see Cosans' discussion in this volume).[27] There will be a need for doctors even in the just community depicted in Plato's *Republic* (see iii, especially 408c–410a). Good habits only improve the odds of health and the efficacy of medical treatment.[28] Therefore, medical practice, though intimately related to practical wisdom, cannot be just the same as ethics inasmuch as the doctor primarily considers health rather than the moral life.

We have been suggesting that the more care is given soul along with body, the closer medicine approaches practical wisdom. Yet medicine must be an unusual art, even beyond the possibly of its prescribing moral ways of life. Human health is a most extraordinary subject matter and aim of art, and the doctor must intervene carefully. Medicine cooperates with nature, hopefully, to return the patient to a condition of balance and equilibrium so that he or she can return to ordinary (or improved?) life. As Gadamer 1996 points out:

the doctor's contribution consummates itself by disappearing as soon as the equilibrium of health is restored. (37)

[medicine] is not an art that involves the invention or planning of something new ... it is from the beginning a particular kind of doing and making which produces nothing of its own ... this art inserts itself entirely within the process of nature in so far as it seeks to restore this process when it is disturbed, and to do so in such a way that the art can allow itself to disappear once the natural equilibrium of health has returned. (34)

In seeking health and equilibrium so that the person can return to his or her way of life, the doctor inevitably deals with human life generally and not solely the condition of the body. The living human body and its health is not merely an instrument of the soul much as any nonliving tool. Our body and its condition enters into all our actions and choices.[29] Most actions and occupations presuppose rather good health. Incapacity, pain, and worry prevent us from functioning as we wish. The doctor is assisting nature and doing what the patient would do for himself or herself.[30]

In intervening to assist nature, the doctor must avoid doing too little or too much—only what is appropriate for reestablishing equilibrium. Medical practice in seeking the appropriate seeks the intermediate. Methodologically, it thus closely resembles the use of practical wisdom in moral and political life. As the statesman must have an intelligent assessment of the condition of the community and what is possible for it, the doctor must weigh the evidence testifying to the condition of the patient— some of which comes from conversation with the patient—and consider the prospects for treatment. The character of the patient may enter into the assessment. While it might be optimal that humans live in prescribed ways, the doctor must also appreciate the likelihood that habits are hard to change: the doctor may need to use some practical wisdom about the forming and maintaining of habits if he or she seeks to enable the sick or injured person to resume, if possible, an acceptable sort of life.

Methodologically, medicine thus resembles politics in its use of practical wisdom inasmuch as it takes account of ways of life and may require assessment of the character of those who are to be treated, and also because the medical treatments that are possible may vary considerably. The difficulty of correct diagnosis and the plenitude of treatment options call for considerable discernment regarding how to think of the case and which approach to employ. The more an art must size up a situation and select from a variety of options under pressure of time and with much riding on the decision, the more it resembles practical political decision making and action with its need of practical wisdom. Consider these comments by Aristotle about moral life and deliberation:

This must be agreed upon beforehand, that the whole account of matters of conduct must be given in outline and not precisely, as we said at the very beginning that the accounts we demand must be in accordance with the subject-matter;[31] matters concerned with conduct and questions of what is good for us have no fixity, any more than matters of health. The general account being of this nature, the account of particular cases is yet more lacking in exactness; for they do not fall under any art or set of precepts, but the agents themselves must in each case consider what is appropriate to the occasion, as happens also in the art of medicine or of navigation.[32] (*Nicomachean Ethics* ii 2.1103b34–1104a10)

in the case of exact and self-contained sciences there is no deliberation, e.g. about the letters of the alphabet (for we have no doubt how they should be written); but the things that are brought about by our own efforts, but not always in the same way, are the things about which we deliberate, e.g. questions of medical treatment or of money-making. And we do so more in the case of the art of navigation than in that of gymnastics, inasmuch as it has been less exactly worked out. (iii 3.1112a34–b6)

Hence, the art of medicine in its demands approaches the case of the moral agent. Medicine similarly involves imprecision and deliberation. The similarity seems to go beyond mere analogy with practical science. Because medicine often has the urgency and importance of moral deliberation, the practice of the art is often emotion laden for those who are the agents or the patients. The art thus becomes surrounded by the sorts of desiderative and emotional accompaniments of moral reflection. Moreover, the recipient of the art may become involved in a kind of intimacy and friendship with the practitioner, which again makes moral demands.[33] Such arts that force those involved to bring the character of agent and patient into play take on many of the features of practical wisdom.[34]

Medical practice also resembles practical wisdom because of the particular relation of the doctor to his or her own self. Most arts involve knowledge by which their work is accomplished. The art as such aims to engender this work, but it does not do this especially for the practitioner of the art. Typically, the artist requires some compensation for doing the service of performing the art expertly. Unlike these arts, practical wisdom enables one to act well publicly and privately. The practically wise person assists the community and other persons in living well, while the practically wise person has his or her life own in order as well. The doctor aids others to be healthy and to live their lives soundly. But the doctor also has body and soul. The doctor's capacity to assist others should apply as well to the doctor's own life. The closer connection of medicine than other arts to a generally good life may facilitate the doctor's care for self and others.

Medicine may perhaps fail to benefit the patient and the doctor. The doctor may be tempted by money to perform unneeded medical procedures or in some other way to allow medical practice to become perverted. Or the doctor may be indifferent to his or her own health. Medical skill may be used in contrary ways: it can heal or deliberately cause sickness and death. It may always, then, require some oversight. But much of this oversight is not simply external to the medical field in the form of laws, lawsuits, and market forces. The expectations of the community and the standards of medicine itself tend to keep practitioners using their skills to benefit people. The internalization of the demand that medicine be beneficial again contributes to making its practice more like moral action.

Any art with a fairly narrow field must be guided by some greater insight into human good regarding when it should be put into practice and how. Questions of justice involved in medicine need some resolution. As medicine has become more expensive and used increasing amounts of community resources, issues of the allocation of means of treatment have become pressing.[35] Additional issues arise regarding when, where, for whom, and to what extent care should be administered. But again, such political and moral questions are not raised totally outside the sphere of practicing physicians; for example, questions about public allocation of research funds are not made without input from medical researchers and practitioners. Hence medicine itself seems to enter into questions of justice and thus to move beyond the strict confines of art.

Finally, medical education directed toward practice requires a combination of experience and reflection rather like moral education. Training that is too exclusively intellectual or experiential limits the capacity for good practice. Consequently, medical training, much as moral preparation, should not shortchange either focus. For both fields, experience contributes to illumination of the intellect. The two required components thus may not be separable.

Conclusion

I have traced how many factors that affect demarcation of the sciences blur the position of medicine. Clearly medicine is fundamentally an art—yet a most extraordinary art in that it goes beyond art in its connections with theoretical and practical sciences. This was true in antiquity and is even more so today. Understanding these tendencies aids our appreciation of the place of medicine within both the arts and the sciences, as well as our comprehension of many issues surrounding medicine and its practice.

Notes

1. About Greek medicine, Porter 1997, 51 says, "The contrasts between old Egyptian and new Greek medicine are striking.... Greek medicine as known from written sources is highly distinctive, for from the beginning Greek medical texts were essentially secular." Further, he states:

Hippocratic medicine, the foundation of Greek written medicine, explicitly grounds the art upon a quite different basis: a healing system independent of the supernatural and built upon natural philosophy.... This separation of medicine from religion points to another distinctive feature of Greek healing: its openness ... which it owed to political diversity and cultural pluralism.... Unlike healing in the Near East, elite Greek medicine was not a closed priestly system: it was open to varied influences and accessible to outsiders, guaranteeing its flexibility and vitality. (pp. 53–55)

2. A reason for considering ancient Greek divisions is that modern divisions—natural sciences, social sciences, humanities, and pure and applied sciences—seem no more promising for assessing the position of medicine than the traditional ones. The aim of this discussion may be compared with that of some of the essays in Gadamer 1996, especially ch. 2.

3. Even Aristotle, however, does not have a sustained discussion of the division of the sciences, although scattered passages make clear his basic position. He fairly often uses the scheme of the sciences to locate a science being considered or to ensure comprehensiveness in some discussion. Perhaps a reason that division of the sciences never becomes a central topic in itself is that such division does not obviously fall within any of the major sciences. Surprisingly, the fullest discussion of the various intellectual capacities utilized by the sciences is provided in the *Nicomachean Ethics* vi, because first, the happy life may depend upon the proper estimation and employment of these intellectual virtues and, second, the statesman who oversees the practice of the various arts and sciences must appreciate their role within a community. See *Posterior Analytics* i 33.89b7–9 for Aristotle's view of how the intellectual faculties are demarcated.

4. See *Posterior Analytics* i 1.71b9–12, *Physics* i 1.184a10–16, and *Metaphysics* i 4.983a24–26. Socratic crossexamination assumes that those who know something can give an account (*logos*) of it (see, e.g., Plato *Laches* 190c). For Plato, giving an account means (saying what X is in answer to a "What is X?" question) providing the cause or principle. The centrality of causes emerges for him particularly in *Phaedo* 95e–102a. For some contrast of ancient and modern understanding of the notion of cause, see Frede 1987, ch. 8 and Everson 1997, 45–55.

5. To the basic demarcation of the sciences as theoretical, practical, and productive, we may add the treatises known collectively as the *Organon* ("instrument"). These studies, now considered logic, were deemed by ancient interpreters as preceding and preparatory for the sciences.

6. Even mathematical entities have their principles in themselves and should not be viewed simply as our assumptions or "posits." Aristotle speaks of mathemati-

cal entities as having their being "by abstraction." Abstraction is the removal in thought of all the irrelevant aspects of those entities presented to our thought originally by sense perception. For example, perceptible bodies thought of apart from all particularity of feature and lack of uniformity leave us with mathematical units or figures. Mathematical principles thus are in the matters themselves and not in us.

7. His position contrasts with that of Descartes in 1637 when modern projects and their practical application began to fascinate research:

In place of the speculative philosophy taught in the Schools, one can find a practical one, by which, knowing the force and the actions of fire, water, air, stars, the heavens, and all the other bodies that surround us, just as we understand the various skills of our craftsmen, we could, in the same way, use these objects for all the purposes for which they are appropriate, and thus make ourselves, as it were, masters and possessors of nature. This is desirable not only for the invention of an infinity of devices that would enable us to enjoy without pain the fruits of the earth and all the goods one finds in it, but also principally for the maintenance of health, which unquestionably is the first good and the foundation of all other goods in this life; for even the mind depends so greatly upon the temperament and on the disposition of the organs of the body that, were it possible to find some means to make men generally more wise and competent than they have been up until now, I believe that one should look to medicine to find this means. It is true that the medicine currently practiced contains little of such usefulness; but without trying to ridicule it, I am sure that there is no one, not even among those in the medical profession who would not admit that everything we know is almost nothing in comparison to what remains to be known, and that we might rid ourselves of an infinity of maladies, both of body and mind, and even perhaps also the enfeeblement brought on by old age, were one to have a sufficient knowledge of their causes and of all the remedies that nature has provided us. (*Discourse on Method* part 6, p. 35 Cress trans.)

8. See Aristotle *Posterior Analytics* i 27 for his account of precision in science.

9. See, e.g., Aristotle *Politics* i 11.1259a9–18, Plato *Theaetetus* 172c–177c, and Xenophanes frag. 21B2 (Diels-Kranz).

10. On Aristotle's reliance upon *endoxa*, see Owen 1961, Nussbaum 1982, and Pritzl 1994. The classic Aristotelian discussion of the apprehension of principles is found in *Posterior Analytics* ii 19 and the importance of going through *endoxa* is made clear in *Topics* i 2.

11. Art is not restricted to fine arts; it includes any capacity for producing a product. In fact, Aristotle uses art (*techne*) more narrowly than did Plato. Plato sometimes extends the meaning of *techne* to cover any knowledge or science when he speaks of arithmetic, geometry, and so on as arts, along with arts that have a more specific product. See *Charmides* 165e–166a and Roochnik 1986.

12. See Aristotle *Nicomachean Ethics* i 1–2, and Plato *Republic* and *Statesman*. Today in developed countries, a combination of market forces and political oversight controls the practice of the arts.

13. The distinction between making and doing is related to Aristotle's distinction between motion (*kinesis*) and activity (*energeia*). Motion, for Aristotle, is a process taking time, heading for an end that terminates the process, and being complete only when the end is achieved. That end may be a change in place, in quality, or in quantity, i.e., locomotion, alteration, growth (or diminution). Activity is not motion at all but complete at each moment after its onset and continuable. An example is seeing: once we see, we have completed the activity of seeing and yet we may continue seeing what we see. Even a temporally extended object of an activity, as when we see the motion of an animal or are engaged in a long campaign in combat, need not interfere with the completeness of the activity; the seeing as such, or the choice of the brave deed, is complete at any moment. Because the ends of all activities lie within the activities themselves, activities pertain to soul. They include: activities of cognition (perceiving and thinking), affective activities (enjoying, desiring, having emotions), and actions (choosing, doing, and living happily). The rest of the activities are built upon cognition so that they have "intentional objects" rather than external ends (i.e., we must be aware of what we desire and choose). Further, because cognition for Aristotle occurs through reception of a sensible or intelligible form, which is a whole, any activity is somehow directed toward the whole. Hence Aristotle can insist that any activity is complete at every moment and continuable. For fuller treatment of these points regarding motion and activity, see Polansky 1983.

14. Analogous to the character of the individual governing the person's choices, the political community is viewed by some as having a character (its constitution or *politeia*) that shapes its collective action.

15. The emphasis of Plato and Aristotle on virtue and vice in relation to character and disposition concerns their understanding of securing good motives for action. They do not have a view of free will that seems to make each new choice independent of any that preceded but they suppose that our present choices are largely circumscribed by our previous choices. They are thus both more optimistic and more pessimistic than we tend to be. They believe that good persons will continue to do good things and can be relied upon to do such (their optimism), but they correspondingly believe that bad persons will continue to do bad things and can be expected to do such (their pessimism). Consequently, moral training—the early and continuing cultivation of character—seems so crucial. Most of Aristotelian ethics concentrates upon moral virtue and most of politics on the constitution, i.e., the arrangement of rulership. This is understandable because action is central for the life of the individual and community, and this action is shaped by the character of the individual or the form of the community.

16. Practical and political wisdom should order all the arts, but no higher science orders practical or political science. Yet since engagement in theoretical science may offer humans a divine sort of life and even greater happiness than practical activity, practical science is both for its own sake and for the sake of realizing the possibility of theoretical activity (see *Nicomachean Ethics* vi 13.1145a6–11). Aristotle suggests in the *Politics* that politics is always in danger of longing to be

like the arts and to accomplish some definite result. Instead of seeking virtuous action, conquest can easily become the aim of the community. To prevent this, only some aspiration for activity based on transcendent and universal principles, for the highest level of culture, seems likely to keep political life orderly and properly focused (see, e.g., *Politics* ii 7.1267a2–37 and vii 1–3, as well as Tress's discussion in this volume).

17. The greater precision of moral virtue than art is discussed more fully in Welton and Polansky 1995.

18. In post-Aristotelian thought, based partly upon Aristotle's suggestions (see *Topics* 105b19–29) and even earlier Platonic thought (see Long and Sedley 1987, i 160 on the role of Xenocrates), philosophy is often divided into logic, physics, and ethics in the effort to be fully systematic. This may be found among Stoics, Epicureans, Kant, as well as among some philosophers in our own age. Logic extends to what we call epistemology, and physics is construed expansively so that all the parts of philosophy are embraced. Such a division, rather than that of theoretical, practical, and productive realms, places more emphasis on the practical utility of all philosophy.

19. See the Hippocratic treatises *Law* 1 and *Decorum* 5.

20. Aristotle's comment is not unprecedented. Plato's *Timaeus*, after giving an account of the workings of the whole universe and the origins of humans, concludes with a view of human disease and health in light of the preceding account (82a–90de; cf. *Phaedrus* 270c,d). The Hippocratic corpus reflects frequently upon the degree to which medicine should be linked to natural speculation. See, e.g., *Ancient Medicine*; despite its seeming rejection of all speculation, ties its medical views to an understanding of the natural world. General claims have been made that Hippocratic medicine receives major inspiration from Presocratic philosophy. The emphasis upon regimen in disease and in health, rather than the earlier focus upon surgery and pharmacology (which could only be employed in limited cases), derives from the development of theories of health and disease by the philosophers of nature (see Frede 1987, ch. 12).

21. To the extent that architecture is envisioned as creating structures within a natural setting, and that poetry and painting are depicting natural things, the practitioners of these arts may also require considerable knowledge of natural science. See Vitruvius i ch. 1 on the demands upon the architect for broad knowledge.

22. Starting in the third century B.C. an empirical school of medicine rejected speculation and the rationalism of prior medicine, based on skepticism regarding knowledge generally. Since adherents of this school doubted any possibility of natural science, their medical practice accorded with their views about nature. Frede 1987, 239–240 explores how ancient physicians needing to persuade patients and to secure social acceptance as educated persons required medical theory, even if that theory was not closely linked to medical practice. Medical theory thus could play an important social role.

23. Greek art was less often the practical application of pure science than today's application of technology to the methods of modern science. For much of its existence ancient Greek medicine did not have the advantage of dissection, though much could be learned from observations of wounds, limited surgery, gynecological treatment, dissection of beasts, and so on.

24. Much ancient medicine spoke of health as a balance of the humors. There is much variety, however, about what the humors comprising the body are (see Phillips 1973, 48–52). The classic view of four humors—blood, phlegm, yellow bile, and black bile—appears in the Hippocratic corpus in *The Nature of Man* and in Galen. In some accounts, some of the humors appear only in disease.

25. Aristotle seems to have such passages in mind in *Nicomachean Ethics* i 13.1102a18–23 where he says, "clearly the student of politics must know somehow the facts about soul, as the man who is to heal the eyes or the body as a whole must know about the eyes or the body; and all the more since politics is more prized and better than medicine; but even among doctors the best educated spend much labour on acquiring knowledge of the body."

26. The Hippocratic corpus pays much attention to regimen both in health and in disease. See Frede 1987, 228–229. For discussion of medical aspects of the *Charmides*, see Coolidge 1993 and Annas, pp. 111–112 in this volume.

27. In *Nicomachean Ethics* iii 5 Aristotle argues that we are responsible for our habitual states of character, i.e., our virtues or vices. Though we do not choose to be virtuous or vicious, we do choose our various actions, which choices eventually mold our character. And though these choices begin when we are young and ignorant, yet we continue the pattern as we get older and so have responsibility for our character, though not perhaps the sort of responsibility that we have for the individual choices and actions. Similarly, we may have some responsibility for our physical condition, whether eating, drinking, and exercise, or our moral life generally affect it. Aristotle says:

But not only are the vices of the soul voluntary, but those of the body also for some men, whom we accordingly blame; while no one blames those who are ugly by nature, we blame those who are so owing to want of exercise and care. So it is, too, with respect to weakness and infirmity; no one would reproach a man blind from birth or by disease or from a blow, but rather pity him, while every one would blame a man who was blind from drunkenness or some other form of self-indulgence. Of vices of the body, then, those in our own power are blamed, those not in our power are not. (iii 5.1114a22–30)

28. The more we attribute disease to contagion and infection from external agents rather than to poor living, the less disease seems our responsibility. Perhaps, however, our vulnerability even to infectious disease (as well as injury) has something to do with how we live.

29. The body fundamentally individuates each of us: each of us has his or her own body. The body offers us our sexuality, our outlook on things, our mortality. The condition of our body, then, cannot be disentangled from the rest of our

life. Care for the body is therefore vital for the welfare of the soul. Plato aptly says in the *Timaeus*: "In determining health and disease or virtue and vice no proportion or lack of it is more important than that between soul and body" (87d) and one ought "not to exercise the soul without exercising the body, nor the body without the soul, so that each may be balanced by the other and so be sound" (88b).

30. Further, Gadamer 1996, 38 points out that modern science in contrast with ancient science seeks to dominate nature: "Our science is based not on the experience of life but on that of making and producing, not on the experience of equilibrium but on that of projective construction." Yet in spite of this remarkable change in the modern scientific viewpoint, "the art of healing remains ineliminably bound up with the presupposition that was still implied in the ancient concept of nature ... the science of medicine is the one which can never be understood entirely as a technology, precisely because it invariably experiences its own abilities and skills simply as a restoration of what belongs to nature" (Gadamer 1996, 39). Hence, some tension occurs between the modern scientific concept of nature as manipulable and the concept of nature operative in medicine as a healing art aimed at restoring natural equilibrium.

31. Aristotle's earlier discussion of the imprecision regarding good things and matters of conduct, and what sort of precision should be expected in accounts of these is in *Nicomachean Ethics* i 3.1094b11–27.

32. Medicine and navigation compare well with ethics and politics because they frequently operate in time-pressured and grave situations. The care for the condition of the body in medicine and the many options for care parallel the political concern for the soul. Navigation, like politics, directs the whole venture including the navigator himself. Compare Plato *Republic* iv and vi.

33. Bartz (pp. 15–17 in this volume) interestingly points out how the necessity of careful observation in ancient medicine for prognostics and healing requires trust and friendship not only of the doctor and patient but also of the doctor and the friends, servants, and relatives of the patient.

34. Phillips 1973, 120 comments about the emergence of ethical standards in ancient medicine:

These books dealing with medical ethics [i.e., parts of the Hippocratic corpus] show that, except in the important matter of enforceable discipline for members, something like a modern profession was gradually being created, with practitioners who were expected to be more than efficient craftsmen. The growing insistence on inner attitude after the Hippocratic age was an important advance in medicine. Such standards, which have been regarded as second nature for a good physician later in civilized ages, needed an effort to conceive and to attain, and much of the credit should go to the ethical thought of the philosophical schools ... Thus from the fourth century onwards philosophy in the form of ethics had an effect on medicine no less important than the earlier influence of another of its branches, that of speculation about nature.

Bartz p. 18 in this volume, however, suggests that the influence may have gone in the other direction, i.e., from medicine to philosophical ethics.

35. Ancient medical treatment was relatively inexpensive except possibly in time and human effort. Plato's discussion of medicine in book 3 of the *Republic* seems to emphasize the possibility of time lost from the performance of suitable social tasks by excessive medical treatment.

References

Barnes, Jonathan, ed. 1984. *The Complete Works of Aristotle*. Revised Oxford Translation. 2 vols. Princeton, N.J.: Princeton University Press.

Coolidge, Francis P. Jr. 1993. "The Relation of Philosophy to Σωφροσύνη: Zalmoxian Medicine in Plato's *Charmides*." *Ancient Philosophy* 13: 23–36.

Cooper, John M. ed. 1997. *Plato: Complete Works*. Indianapolis: Hackett.

Descartes, R. 1637. *Discourse on Method*. Donald Cress trans. 3d ed. 1993. Indianapolis: Hackett.

Diels, Herman, and Walther Kranz. 1954. *Die Fragmente der Vorsokratiker*. 3 vols. 7th ed. Berlin: Weidmannsche.

Everson, Stephen. 1997. *Aristotle on Perception*. Oxford: Clarendon Press.

Frede, M. 1987. *Essays in Ancient Philosophy*. Minneapolis: University of Minnesota Press.

Gadamer, Hans-Georg. 1996. *The Enigma of Health*. Translated by Jason Gaiger and Nicholas Walker. Stanford, Calif.: Stanford University Press.

Jones, W. H. S. ed. and trans. 1923. *Hippocrates*. 4 vols. Loeb Classical Library. Cambridge, Mass.: Harvard University Press.

Long, A. A., and D. N. Sedley. 1987. *The Hellentistic Philosophers*. Cambridge: Cambridge University Press.

Nussbaum, M. C. 1982. "Saving Aristotle's Appearances," 267–293 in *Language and Logos: Studies in ancient Greek philosophy presented to G. E. L. Owen*, ed. Malcolm Schofield and Martha Nussbaum. Cambridge: Cambridge University Press.

Owen, G. E. L. 1961. "*Tithenai ta phainomena*," 83–103 in S. Mansion ed. *Aristote et les problèmes de méthode*. Louvain: Publications Universitaires de Louvain [reprinted in G. E. L. Owen. 1986. *Logic, Science and Dialectic: Collected Papers in Greek Philosophy*. Ithaca: Cornell University Press].

Phillips, E. D. 1973. *Aspects of Greek Medicine*. New York: St. Martin's Press.

Polansky, R. M. 1983. "*Energeia* in Aristotle's *Metaphysics* IX." *Ancient Philosophy* 3: 160–170.

Porter, Roy. 1997. *The Greatest Benefit to Mankind: A Medical History of Humanity*. New York: W. W. Norton.

Pritzl, K. 1994. "Opinions as Appearances: *Endoxa* in Aristotle." *Ancient Philosophy* 14: 41–50.

Roochnik, D. 1986. "Socrates' Use of the Techne-Analogy." *Journal of the History of Philosophy* 24: 295–310.

Vitruvius. *The Ten Books on Architecture*. Trans. Morris Hickey Morgan, 1914. Cambridge, Mass.: Harvard University Press.

Welton, W. A., and R. Polansky. 1995. "The Viability of Virtue in the Mean," 79–102 in *Aristotle, Virtue and the Mean*, ed. R. Bosley, R. Shiner, J. Sisson. Special issue of *Apeiron* 25.

3

Phronesis and the Misdescription of Medicine: Against *The* Medical School Commencement Speech

Kathryn Montgomery

The contemporary understanding of medicine—within the profession and in society at large—is lodged in descriptions that are crude, incomplete, and unreflective. Medicine is conventionally labeled both a science and an art without much definition of either term. Those invited to address a medical school's graduating class often invoke the two in quick succession. You know the speech: "Medicine is a science," new physicians are reminded, "but it is also an art." Or the other way around: "Medicine is an art," the speaker tells them, adding only a little later, "above all, of course, it is a science." These descriptions are not so much wrong as ill defined and shallow. They are a reminder that medicine, the site of modern miracles, is poorly defined and poorly described by those who nevertheless practice it well.

The science-art split has an unintended effect. It creates distinct and difficult-to-reconcile parts—unequal ones at that—and suggests that these parts function as alternatives. Perhaps they are like the options in one of those rabbit-and-duck illusions: incommensurable, important in dissimilar situations. For how can it be literally true that a branch of knowledge is at once an art and a science? These speeches never include any suggestion of a continuum.[1] Are we then to understand the duality simply as a figure of speech? Literal or metaphorical, the science-art theme cries out for explication. Failing to receive that attention—sometimes elaborated but never examined—the trope survives, just barely viable, as hackneyed cliché. Medicine is left facilely described and (on the evidence) poorly understood. The split into science and art does not do justice to its character as a *practice*: the scientifically informed, experienced, well-reasoned care of sick people. The intellectual virtue of *phronesis*—the practical wisdom that is the pride of good clinicians—is overlooked in favor of an outmoded, rather Cartesian split between the good, hard, reliable stuff and the mushy but inescapable ineffabilities.

The tension between "art" and "science" as ritually used on graduation day points to an apparent paradox in medicine. Indeed, it is the paradox that commencement speakers are attempting to capture. Good medicine is a rational practice based on a scientific education and years of clinical experience. It is neither an art nor a science. Or, if it must be one of them, it must also be the other. The common understanding of "science" in medicine is Newtonian, a relic of nineteenth-century positivism: the replicable and invariant description of physical reality. There is a reason for this intellectual anachronism. Physicians have spent years studying human biology: anatomy, histology, physiology, microbiology and virology, pathology, pharmacology, and especially, cell and molecular biology. Yet, except for those few physicians who are engaged in bench research, "science," especially in medicine's limited definition of it, is not what physicians do. They diagnose and treat sick people, and that is not a science. Although with their white coats off they may know as much about the history and philosophy of science as any other college graduates, they claim the honorific label "science" for their professional activity because they need a warrant for their action. Clinical training is filled with strategies to minimize the inescapable uncertainty of their practice; one of these is to regard the best available information as real, dependable, and absolute (Bosk 1980; Montgomery Hunter 1997).

Yet medicine is not a science, not even today when it has become highly scientific and supremely technological. As patients, we know this. We do not look for a scientist when we are sick—not unless we are dying without recourse and we hear news of some long-shot, potential remedy fresh from the laboratory. People dying of cancer in the spring of 1998 were willing to take angiostatin straight from the bench scientist's vials, but this was not medicine. It would have been, at best, a clinical experiment, a kind of unofficial and unsupervised Phase I trial, one that establishes drug toxicity in human beings (the animal research having been completed) without promise of benefit to the experimental subject. That is scarcely what is meant by or hoped for from medicine. Physicians are expected to care for their patients and treat them more comprehensively: they must understand the human biology, investigate the patient's condition carefully, reach a diagnosis, understand the clinical research and its relevance to this particular individual, and then weigh the benefits and burdens of therapeutic choices. Such a practice is certainly rational, but it is not (by medicine's own Newtonian definition) science. It is that oxymoron, a science of individuals, that Aristotle in the *Metaphysics* declared an impossibility.[2] As such, it calls for a narrative rather than a purely hypothetico-deductive rationality that can take account of contextual features, accidental but nevertheless significant details, and alteration over time.[3]

Is medicine then an "art"? The definition of that term as it is used in medicine is fairly nonspecific. "The art of medicine" occasionally refers to behavioral attributes (such as a bedside manner or professional etiquette), to moral values, or to virtues manifested in physicians' demeanor or their habits of communication—all those aspects of physicianhood that may have seemed squishy and inessential during medical school. Sometimes the term "art" stands in for the "gut feeling" or hunch that experienced physicians have without knowing quite how (Dreyfus and Dreyfus 1987; Benner 1984). It is recognized as something more than knowledge of the science. It may be described as something intuitive (when that gender-tinged word is allowed) that is essential to good practice, a sort of know-how: an art!

Medicine is thus a learned practice that describes itself as a science[4] even though physicians have the good sense not to practice that way.[5] Commencement speakers are no doubt trying to capture this complexity when they invoke the science-art duality. On graduation day, after four years of inculcating the idea of medicine as a science, medicine's elders acknowledge publicly that "science" is not an adequate description for all they hope new physicians have learned. Still, the science-art duality persists, and the habit of splitting medicine into two parts, even though they are held in tension, shortchanges both medicine's complexity and the difficult practical education in which new graduates are still immersed.

What is medicine, after all? Richard Zaner, lamenting that an emphasis on abstract ethical principles preceded a thorough description of clinical practice, observes that "only a handful of serious efforts have been made

to understand the complicated discipline of medicine" (Zaner 1994, 211).[6]
Classical philosophy, Aristotle in particular, supplies a useful place to start.
In the *Nicomachean Ethics*, he likens moral knowing to knowing in med-
icine. Each is particular, circumstantial, and therefore uncertain:

> The type of accounts we demand should reflect the subject-matter, and questions
> about actions and expediency, like questions about health, have no fixed and
> invariable answers. And when our general account is so inexact, the account of
> particular cases is all the more inexact. For these fall under no craft or profession,
> and the agents themselves must consider in each case what the opportune action
> is. (Aristotle, Nicomachean Ethics ii 2.1104a3–9)

It is not that certainty or fixed and invariable knowledge is undesirable,
but that *episteme* or scientific reason is not "appropriate to the occasion"
in fields like medicine or morals, law or meteorology, that are themselves
uncertain. *Episteme* is proper to stable physical phenomena that can be
known through necessary and invariant laws. *Phronesis*, or practical reason, by contrast, is the virtue of working out how best to act in particular
circumstances that are not (and cannot be) expressed in generally applicable rules. Scientific reason has as its goals precision and replicability; practical reason enables the reasoner to distinguish the better from the worse
choice in a given situation. The first is lawlike and generalizable, the second inescapably particular and narratable.

Clearly, medicine draws at need on both sorts of reason. Scientists in
their labs with the vials of angiostatin as well as clinical investigators conducting approved Phase I trials are concerned with replicability, generalizability; of necessity, the individual case cannot concern them. Medical
practice is different. While not a science per se, clinical medicine is undoubtedly scientific: based on science, it relies in its practice on what
scientists know and learn. To be a good clinician, the physician will need
to be familiar with the results investigators obtain and add it to the store
of well-established knowledge of the human body, sick and well, from the
fields of human biology. Much remains to be discovered, but such knowledge is to some degree "fixed." Even so, its use in the care of patients is
not simply "application." Science is abstract and its rules are timeless,
while patients are astonishingly variable—as are diseases and the results of
therapy. Clinical judgment involves the tactful deployment of the knowledge and experience relevant to determining what is wrong with one par-

ticular patient and deciding what action is best to take on the patient's behalf. Far less certain than even the slippery facts of human biology, the clinical realities of diagnosis and therapy require a flexible, situated, and reinterpretable means of knowing (Montgomery Hunter 1996).

The organization of medical education embodies this complex relation of science to medicine. It begins with two years of intensive study of human biology, but it only begins there. The next two years are devoted to the inculcation of *phronesis*, the clinical judgment that enables physicians to act wisely and for the good of their patients. Students spend their days in the hospital learning to read not from science or clinical generalization to patients' symptoms but the other (and at first confusing) way around: from symptoms to diagnosis and the science, then back again to therapy. Residents spend at least three years more accumulating experience in this interpretive activity, slowly assuming responsibility for the diagnosis and treatment of patients. They are exercising *phronesis*, acquiring not "facts" but good judgment about what is to be done. As Eric Cassell observes:

Knowledge ... whether of medical science or the art of medicine, does not take care of sick persons or relieve their suffering; clinicians do in whom these kinds of knowledge are integrated.... [M]edicine needs a systematic and disciplined approach to the knowledge that arises from the clinician's experience rather than artificial divisions of medical knowledge into science and art. (Cassell 1991, xi)

I propose that *phronesis* be recognized as the culminating virtue toward which medical education and the profession itself aim. It is this virtue, clinical judgment, not medicine's vague "art" and inexact "science," that students should be reminded of on the day they become physicians. Physicians would be scientists, able to deploy knowledge of fixed matters, if they could. The trouble is that medicine is radically uncertain. A century of clinical research and the recently renewed emphasis on application of that research to patient care in evidence-based medicine have not altered this. We very much wish it were otherwise, especially when those we love or we ourselves are ill, but despite its miracles—and they are legion—medical knowing is not a knowledge of fixities. Nor is it likely ever to be. If the day comes when the last molecular function is understood, the genome explicated, and cancer curable, the diagnosis and treatment of sick people will still not be simply the application of science.

Patients will continue to present with demographically improbable symptoms of diseases that entail toxic therapy, and treatment will be delayed; tests will still be balanced between their sensitivity to marginal cases and the specificity with which they can identify them; therapies of choice will be second choice for some patients and may not cure quite everyone.

Diagnosis and treatment will continue to call for *phronesis*: a hermeneutic, narrative, practical reason—a means of knowing that is flexible, situated, and reinterpretable. The physician's goal in the clinical encounter remains the discovery of what is going on with this particular patient. Events of body, mind, family history, and environment are reconstructed as the physician constructs the case. Scientific knowledge is necessary; logic is essential; but they take their place in an activity that is narrative and interpretive. The clinician must grasp and make sense of events occurring over time even as he or she recognizes the inherent uncertainty of this quasi-causal, retrospective, but unavoidable strategy. Piecing together the evidence from the patient's symptoms and the physical signs to create a recognizable pattern or plot is imprecise and subject to all the failings of historical reconstruction, but it is the best—the logical, rational best—they can do. This is not science, and if it is an art, it is a very particular kind. Those who know Aristotle's distinction recognize it as *phronesis*.

Why has the science-art theme persisted? Despite stereotypes, many physicians have had a good liberal education, including the classics. Yet recent graduates who were immersed in cultural studies are no more likely to resist the science claim (with or without the art hedge) than those who majored in biomechanical engineering or business administration. I believe there are two reasons for this, one deeper than the other. The first is that medicine's status depends in large part on the scientific character of its knowledge. To claim to be a scientist in our culture is to stake out authority and power. Physicians have begun to suffer the ill effects of this hubris: as patients and as public we expect them to be far more certain than either their practice or the science on which it is based can warrant.[7] Nor do they seem to be aware of the late twentieth-century debate about the status of scientific knowledge or its representation of reality. The history and philosophy of science has not altered the prevailing presumption in the profession that medicine is a science—the old-fashioned, positivist sort that delineates a transparently knowable, quantifiable, concrete reality. It is as if, having embarked on a perilously uncertain practice characterized by ungeneralizable rules and exceptions that erupt like hydraheads, physicians cling for justification—indeed for their social and interpersonal power—to the shards of a historical but by now metaphoric and inapplicable certainty.

The other reason for the claim to "science" is pedagogical. Science is the "gold standard" of clinical medicine precisely because it promises reliability, replicability, objectivity—in short, the certainty that is available in an uncertain field. For physicians, science models the cool impersonality, the thoroughness, even the nonjudgmental, democratic openness that are among the goals of medicine. To claim medicine as a science is pedagogically useful. How could the medical faculty teach overtly—even if it occurred to them—-that clinical medicine is irreducibly uncertain and ultimately a matter of judgment and still inculcate the near-obsessive attention to detail, the drive to know all that can be known, the dedication to the best possible care for each patient that mark the good clinician? It is a problem. Do we want physicians who lead off with the declaration that their knowledge is incomplete, its application to our case imprecise, and its usefulness uncertain? Not unless our complaint is very minor (Bursztajn et al. 1981). We want to think of them as powerful, dedicated, perfect figures. We do not even want to call into question their dedication to the care of patients by instituting work shifts or limiting hours for residents. And even when we know the assertion is necessarily suspect, we want to go on hearing them say, "We've done everything possible."

Nevertheless, for medicine as a science, the image of the gold standard—so widely used in the profession as an expression of supreme value—is ironically apt. Gold has not been the monetary standard for decades. Indeed, gold no longer backs any major world currency. It has gone the way of positivistic science: although it is still available for the invocation of value, money was long ago relativized, conditioned, understood as the product of its social use.

How, then, are physicians to be educated? Clinical education, in fact, is wonderfully sophisticated, finely calibrated to instill and reward the development of clinical judgment in the face of uncertainty.[8] The claim to be a science is a part of professionalization just as scientific knowledge is

essential to the vocabulary that marks out that terrain. But what is important is the discretion, the tact,[9] the educated common sense that sometimes
rises to intuitive insight or even genius when exercised in the diagnosis and
treatment of a person who is ill. This is neither science nor is it art; it is a
virtue carefully cultivated through the long clinical apprenticeship. It is
phronesis.

Is it possible to educate good physicians while recognizing science as a
tool rather than the soul of medicine? I believe it is, especially if that education is framed formally (as it now is tacitly) as a moral education: a long
and scrupulous preparation for choosing the better action in an uncertain
field of knowledge (Bosk 1979). A first step might be scrapping the
science-art dichotomy, which ignores all that medicine shares with moral
reasoning and reinforces a contemporary tendency to split ethics from
medicine. Moral choice is the essence of clinical practice, inextricably
bound up with the care of the patient. In medicine, morality and clinical
practice are a seamless whole; both require *phronesis*, the practical reason
that characterizes the good physician and the reliable moral agent.[10]

The ideal commencement speech should point out that medical education already is a moral education that has as its aim the cultivation of
phronesis. The acquisition of clinical judgment in the treatment of people
who are ill requires a knowledge of human biology, a store of clinical
experience, good diagnostic and therapeutic habits, and a familiarity with
the vagaries of the human condition. In such a practice, moral knowledge
is an aspect of clinical knowledge. Neither is a science; neither is an art.
They are distinctive practical endeavors whose "phronesiology" deserves
understanding and recognition, especially in the oratory that marks the
physician's entry into the world of practice.

Notes

1. The "binary economy" of art and science is a trope of Western culture. See
Jones and Galison 1998, 2ff. and Burnett 1999.

2. Aristotle discusses this in several places. See especially *Metaphysics* III
6.1003a12–17 and XIII 10.1086b32–37.

3. Jerome Bruner (1986) explicates William James's distinction between narrative
and hypothetico-deductive reasoning; see especially chapter 2, Two Modes of
Thought, 11–43.

4. Or at least the "youngest science"; see Thomas 1983. In fact, there are other, chronologically newer sciences—computer science for one—and were when Thomas wrote.

5. This point has been made by Michael Alan Schwartz and Osborne Wiggins with regard to the biomedical model that George Engel famously found wanting (Schwartz and Wiggins 1985, 334ff.).

6. Although medical ethics tends to ignore medical sociology, Zaner's observation still has merit.

7. Charles Taylor points out that the misunderstanding of practical reasoning generally has had ill effects for the concept of reason: if the "model of practical reasoning ... [is] based on an illegitimate extrapolation from reasoning in natural science," little can meet its criteria, and skepticism about reason itself is the consequence (Taylor 1989, 74–75).

8. In addition to Bosk and Montgomery Hunter cited in note 2, see Renée Fox 1957.

9. Hans-Georg Gadamer, maintaining that practical wisdom is not (as Giambattisto Vico implied) a matter of probabilistic reasoning, cites Helmholtz's description of this mode of knowing as "a kind of tact" that is as judicious in its omissions as in its selection of experiential information (Gadamer 1984, 16–17).

10. See also the essays by Alex London and Ronald Polansky in this volume for further clarification of this point.

References

Benner, P. 1984. *From Novice to Expert: Excellence and Power in Clinical Nursing Practice*. Reading, Mass.: Addison-Wesley.

Bosk, C. 1979. *Forgive and Remember: Managing Medical Failure*. Chicago: University of Chicago Press.

Bosk, C. 1980. "Occupational Rituals in Patient Management." *New England Journal of Medicine* 303: 71–76.

Bruner, J. 1986. *Actual Minds, Possible Worlds*. Cambridge, Mass.: Harvard University Press.

Burnett, D. G. 1999. "A View from the Bridge: The Two Cultures Debate, Its Legacy, and the History of Science." *Daedalus* 128: 193–218.

Bursztajn, H., R. I. Feinbloom, R. M. Hamm, and A. Brodsky. 1981. *Medical Choices, Medical Chances*. New York: Delacorte Press.

Cassell, E. 1991. *The Nature of Suffering and the Goals of Medicine*. New York: Oxford University Press.

Dreyfus, H. L., and S. E. Dreyfus. 1987. "From Socrates to Expert Systems: The Limits of Calculative Rationality," 327–350 in *Interpretive Social Sciences: A Second Look*, ed. P. Rabinow and W. M. Sullivan. Berkeley: University of California Press.

Fox, R. 1957. "Training for Uncertainty," 207–241 in *The Student-Physician*, ed. R. Merton, G. G. Reader, and P. L. Kendall. Cambridge, Mass.: Harvard University Press.

Gadamer, H.-G. 1984. *Truth and Method*. 2d ed. New York: Crossroad.

Irwin, T. 1985. *Nichomachean Ethics* and *Metaphysics*. Indianapolis: Hackett.

Jones, C. A., and P. Galison. 1998. *Picturing Science, Producing Art*. New York: Routledge.

Montgomery Hunter, K. 1996. "Narrative, Literature, and the Clinical Exercise of Practical Reason." *Journal of Medicine and Philosophy* 21: 303–320.

Montgomery Hunter, K. 1997. "Aphorisms, Maxims, and Old Saws: The Paradoxical Inculcation of Clinical Judgment," 215–231 in *Stories and Their Limits: Narrative Approaches to Bioethics*, ed. H. L. Nelson. New York: Routledge.

Schwartz, M. A., and O. Wiggins. 1985. "Science, Humanism, and the Nature of Medical Practice: A Phenomenological View." *Perspectives in Biology and Medicine* 28: 331–366.

Taylor, C. 1989. *Sources of the Self*. Cambridge: Harvard University Press.

Thomas, L. 1983. *The Youngest Science: Notes of a Medicine-Watcher*. New York: Viking.

Zaner, R. M. 1994. "Experience and Moral Life: A Phenomenological Approach to Bioethics," 211–239 in *A Matter of Principles? Ferment in US Bioethics*, ed. E. R. DuBose, R. P. Hamel, and L. J. O'Connell. Valley Forge, Pa.: Trinity Press International.

4

Aristotle, *Phronesis*, and Postmodern Bioethics

David Thomasma

The clever men at Oxford
Know all that there is to be knowed.
But they none of them know not half as much
As intelligent Mr. Toad!
—Kenneth Grahame (1909)

Phronesis in bioethics has been getting a lot of press lately.[1] This is a good thing, as the methods and structure of clinical ethics have long been recognized to parallel closely those of clinical judgment in medicine. For many years I have claimed that although medical ethics and bioethics may be seen as forms of applied ethics—that is, ethics applied to issues in medicine—clinical ethics by contrast is actually a branch of medicine itself. What is more, postmodern bioethics has blocked the establishment of any new system of ethics for medicine; in its stead are many competing voices for authenticity about the nature of medicine in society today, as well as conflicting theories of bioethics. This rupture in the ancient fabric of medicine, the Hippocratic ideals of beneficence and nonmaleficence, has created what the late Cardinal Bernardin of Chicago, in an address to the AMA, called a "crisis in medicine" (1988), and Pellegrino has called a moral vacuum in contemporary health care (unpublished manuscript).

Thus we have two, among many, important movements converging at a propitious time. On the one hand, the clutter of apodictic systems and arrogant thinking in ethics in medicine is being cleared out. On the other hand, renewed interest is mounting in the nature of the practice of medicine itself (MacIntyre 1990) and in virtue ethics as possibly providing some norms for bioethics today (Thomasma 1980). At one juncture of the two aspects of that renewed interest lies Aristotle's notion of prudence or *phronesis*. Before turning to what it is and how it can be helpful in a post-modern era, I will first set the context for this discussion, clarify some key concepts about postmodernism and antifoundationalism, and then make some initial claims.

Context of Crisis

The postmodernist movement creates a sense of crisis in bioethics and in ethics generally because of its questioning of any foundations for ethics. For some neoAristotelians, *phronesis* represents a possible way out of the problem.

Jonsen and Toulmin (1988) alerted bioethicists to the thin support for principled ethics and held out a promise that casuistry and practical reason could provide a great deal of the consensus sought by public policy-makers. The two ethicists based their argument for securing moral agreement among policymakers on the central role of *phronesis* and *phronesis* alone. This argument stemmed from the experience of developing principles for and positions about bioethical issues on the National Commission for the Protection of Human Subjects of Biomedical and Behavioral Research that began meeting in 1974 and issued the *Belmont Report*. Both Jonsen and Toulmin served on this Commission.

Before this joint work, Toulmin argued in his pathbreaking essay on how medicine saved the life of ethics (1982) that he was struck by the remarkable way the commissioners were able to agree regarding complex and delicate ethical issues, not by appealing to ethical principles but through close attention to the texture of specific types of cases. In other words, persons of disparate backgrounds and conviction were able to weigh and balance the important values in cases despite their different reasons for doing so. As Toulmin notes, "Only when the individual members of the commission went on to explain their own particular reasons for supporting the general consensus did they begin to go seriously different ways."

This primacy of practical reasoning over moral theory is central to my thesis as well. However, Beresford (1996) points out that in order for *phronesis* to secure the agreements promised by Jonsen and Toulmin, and needed in health-care ethics, it must pay attention not only to details of cases—the concreteness stressed throughout this essay—but also must focus on the central substantive goods in the case. The latter, he argues, continue to be elusive.

Separately, Jonsen (1991), Toulmin (1981), and MacIntyre (1981, 1988, 117) have sought to develop a *phronesis*-based ethics centered on exercising "judgments in particular cases." The very intransigence of the particular means that one cannot explain *phronesis* in procedural terms. Aristotle is quite explicit that the complexities of particular cases make them impossible to capture in any of the best-available rules. Thus, the very requirement to exercise judgment arises in the absence of objective certitude that even the mathematical sciences have difficulty providing. Aristotle reminds us that we should not seek a degree of exactitude that a given area or discipline might not be able to provide (*NE* 1094b20–27).

My argument enters at this point. A search for foundations for clinical ethics must turn to the experience of patients and physicians in medical practices and in terms of their developing and evolving existential and experiential a prioris. Thus, to answer Beresford, substantive goods can be discoverable through practical experience and wisdom. Before exploring the possible source of such goods, I now turn to clarifying key ideas of postmodernism, antifoundationalism, and the problem of competing ethical theories in bioethics.

Postmodernism

As many understandings of the movement we loosely call "postmod-ernism" are available as are proponents for it and opponents of it (Connor 1989; Hoy and McCarthy 1994). In general, postmodernism is a reaction to systems of thought that brought about the modern era—the industrial and now postindustrial age. After World War II, and especially after Russian and Eastern bloc communism collapsed, this reaction turned into a political alarm about any systems that led to supposed certitude about the truth and the oppression of those who somehow did not understand or comprehend that particular "truth." Postmodernism is, therefore, both a moral and a political reaction to authority, the authority of systems and those who act in their name, as well as the authority of rationality, standards, and norms. As a combination of politics and morality, it returns to more ancient conceptions of moral wisdom that connected individual conduct with society and the commonweal. But it is a connection with a difference.

Although this movement may be characterized in many ways, the principal convictions of postmodernism are that all philosophical systems are suspect: moral and cultural pluralism must be recognized, and even appreciated, such that no overarching standards of conduct or "objective morality" are possible; and no foundational proposals for the theory of any human activity, much less a public policy can be allowed (Critchley 1992). All of these convictions, in turn, rest on a belief that the industrial ethic and the appeal to reason and natural law found in the Enlightenment project of finding an objective basis of morality is dead (Beiser 1997).

Also behind much of postmodern thought is either a nostalgia for a presumed, somewhat romanticized past[2] or a delight in skepticism that ignores its obvious violation of the principle of contradiction. Nostalgia possesses, in the words of Tamara Plakins Thornton, "bittersweet memories of a past when moral certainty still seemed possible" (Thornton 1996; Mallon 1997). The skeptic revelers, by contrast, seek a clean sweep of outdated moral certitudes as a way of life and thought for coping with a pluralistic world. If it is a contradiction to speak apodictically by saying that nothing can be spoken about with certainty, then so be it.

A third group of persons who might accept the moniker "postmodern" are neither nostalgic Romantics nor intensely skeptical theorists. They are simply cautious naturalists or pragmatists (Nielsen 1997). They are aware of the limitations of their own knowledge and beliefs, and their thinking remains open to new possibilities and discoveries (Horgan and Tienson 1996).

This is not the place to explore the postmodernist challenge in detail. Note, however, that awareness of multicultural competition for standards and norms is not new. Indeed, Roman and natural law were founded on the notion of international standards in the face of the many cultures ruled or absorbed by the Roman Empire. The clash of great cultures and civilizations often has been explored as a key to world history. Right now Western concepts of the rule of law, separation of church and state, respect for individual freedom, honoring pluralism by the virtue of tolerance and civility, and the other characteristics of Western democracy that are over one thousand years old are in a struggle with traditionally religious cultures such as the Orthodox East, Islam, and the communitarian cultures of China and Japan (Huntington 1996).

Thus, postmodernism arises not just in the recognition of multiculturalism but in the egalitarianism of that recognition. In the United States, for example, until the 1920s, the majority considered its own white and Nordic culture to be superior to minority cultures. Around the third decade of the twentieth century, a shift occurred such that various cultures were considered of equal value. One's preferences were held to arise, without apology, from feeling comfortable about one's own roots rather than from a judgment of superiority about one's cultural values over another (Michaels 1995). The problem engendered by this shift is that one must accept relativism as a necessary adjunct to a multicultural sensibility, i.e., there can be no dominant or "primarily" valid viewpoint. One is then left without crosscultural standards or any valid moral principles. Individual roots provide the only moral norms for a person's behavior (Thomasma 1997a; de Wachter 1997).

One characteristic underlying all of postmodernism is an intense suspicion of any rational effort to ground ethics in crosscultural or transhistorical realities (Norris 1993)—a suspicion played out in the field of bioethics in many ways. A good example right now is the effort to establish standards for bioethics consultations. What is the ethics consultant doing? If he or she brings to bear a set of moral and objective standards to bear on a tragic circumstance of human suffering in order to make a recommendation, then that is seen as "imposing" moral values on others, which is *de rigeur* out of touch with postmodern sensibilities. Yet if he or she does not bring some viewpoint to the negotiations, or has no aim in facilitating a good outcome, then why invite such a person to consult at all?[3] Is not bioethics supposed to help make our moral judgments internally coherent as well as rationally justifiable and to provide a guide for sound public policy?

The focus on an awareness of moral and cultural pluralism also leads to profound questioning of fundamental assumptions of medicine itself (see Thomasma 1997b). Some of these assumptions have been held for centuries—for example, the sanctity of human life, the goal of the preservation of life, and professional commitments to altruism. The postmodern critique requires more than a critical reflection on competing theories (Veatch 1989). If we take the postmodern challenge seriously, reiterating rational grounds for bioethics and the moral theory of medicine is insufficient. Something else is needed, and that something seems to reside within individuals not theories. I will return to this point later.

Antifoundationalism

Postmodernism is closely allied to antifoundationalism that also characterizes our age. Indeed as a moral response to the challenge of pluralism and relativity, postmodernism can be seen as one form of antifoundationalism. A closer but brief look at the "foundations" against which antifoundationalism deconstructs the rationalist Enlightenment Project and philosophy in general shows that at least four kinds exist. All of them are relevant with respect to a more Aristotelian view of all disciplines and ethics itself.

Cartesian Rationalism

The most obvious example of foundationalism is Cartesian rationalism: the explicit assumption that permanent, absolute, and comprehensive systems of knowledge with overarching principles exist. This assumption led to an identification of what is good or true with what is perceived as universal, absolutely certain, and permanent (Toulmin 1982), and explicitly left behind the particularities of context and culture. Cartesianism is also essentially rationalistic to the extent that what is good and true is that which is clear and distinct, uncluttered with the "dirty linen" of everyday reality. With regard to specific practices like medicine, through its history or in its dealing with caregivers and patients, the level of abstraction in Cartesian rationalism is judged to be too great.

Part of Kant's original effort to develop a foundation (*Grundlage*) for ethics was to preserve it from the encroachments of science. Because science was becoming so successful in the age of Enlightenment, it appeared that ethics would be judged as irrelevant. It seemed to follow that ethics should be more scientific and ground its validity in conformity to principle, to universalizability. Again, what counts as the Good in this rationalist system is an appeal to an abstract, scientific conception: Reaction against such superrationalism is a good thing.

Scientism and Logical Positivism

A second foundational "system" occurred in reaction to historicism when the nineteenth-century fascination with history led to a desire by thinkers like Russell, Moore, and Quine to try to find unchanging structures underlying the flux of time. Their initial efforts focused on logic and mathematics and later, on language itself.[4] We now call this scientism, or in some instances, logical positivism. Oddly, the search for these structures was also perceived as a reaction to Cartesian rationalism since the source of meaning lay not with unchanging substantive structures but with the content of propositions and their necessary connections.

About both of these first two examples of foundationalism Toulmin writes, "most philosophers chose to disregard *utterances* of particular writers/speakers to particular readers/audiences on particular occasions" (Toulmin 1982, 737). For Toulmin, this is anathema, as he approvingly quotes Aristotle arguing for the necessity of reading everyday utterances and statements *pros ton kairon*—"with an eye to the occasion" (Toulmin 1982, 739). In other words, for Toulmin, the meaning of a moral dilemma must be gleaned not from principles, theories, and other abstractions but from the context in which the concerns arise. This attempt has been largely missing in principled bioethics, not necessarily in clinical ethics, which must deal with the context and complexities of a case. Toulmin's turn toward *praxis* as that context is an important further step away from the isolated individualism of the Cartesian. For the moment, though, recall that Aristotle also developed an entire discipline of ethics around higher levels of abstraction than just the context—upon, for example, the virtues, the nature of the person, the objective reality of human ends.

Radical Anti-antifoundationalism

Although the debate between foundationalism and antifoundationalism is at least as old as the first philosophers who disputed issues of permanence versus flux, the "lightening rod" (Rockmore 1992, 3) of the debate today is the idea of Richard Rorty that philosophy is no longer a viable discipline (Rorty 1989). Antifoundationalism itself would not be a viable philosophical option for Rorty either, but rather, the resulting failure of what was once a correct approach to foundationalism. His work could be characterized as fully deconstructed, post-postmodernism. If there is any characterization of this movement, it would be a naturalist pragmatism, not a complete skepticism.

For Rorty, however, the whole question of the grounding of moral thought is a nonissue, the type of thing, he might aver, that philosophers do when they get together to discuss things, but hardly one that makes for a living reflective thought. To attribute antifoundationalism to Rorty is a mistake as he finds neither it or its opposite, foundationalism, of interest for a live philosophy.

Elimination of Morality

A fourth form of antifoundationalism is more specifically aimed at ethics. For some time now, ethicists have been arguing that behind ethics, at its foundation, is simply assertion and counterassertion. A good example of this claim is that made more than twenty years ago by Alasdair MacIntyre (1979). At the time his claim arose from a consideration of pluralism. MacIntyre's more recent thinking has led him to consider spheres of moral enquiry in which certain values hold sway, but outside of which and across which they do not (MacIntyre 1990).

An even more radical rejection of morality comes from ethicists today who hold that bioethics is futile and misguided. Anne Maclean, for example, in her scathing attack on those who claim that ethical problems are in principle resolvable, argues against medical ethics as practiced by utilitarians. The purpose of utilitarian, indeed of all medical ethics is seen as resolving problems raised by medical practice. Maclean says:

The objection I wish to make to the bioethical enterprise is a fundamental one. It is that philosophy as such delivers no verdict upon moral issues; there is no unique set of moral principles which philosophy as such underwrites and no question, therefore, of using that set to uncover the answers which philosophy gives to moral questions. When bioethicists deliver a verdict upon the moral issues raised by medical practice, it is their own verdict they deliver and not the verdict of philosophy itself; it is their voice we hear and not the voice of reason or rationality. (Maclean 1993, 5)

Here we stare directly in the face of postmodernist thinking. If this is to be considered a form of antifoundationalism, Maclean would argue—as she does, in an old-fashioned Pyrrhonist way, that at the foundation there is no truth of the matter in ethics. At best what we have are attitudes, not reasons, for why we do or should do certain things (Maclean 1993, 35). This view has much in common with that of the philosopher Bruce N. Waller. He holds a version of "noncognitivism" claiming that "when ethical disagreements are run to ground in the search for resolution, ultimately there will remain only basic value preferences that cannot be rationally justified, and alternatives to which that can be favored without violating reason" (Waller 1994, 59–60). "Basic value preferences" perhaps may not be able to be rationally justified, but they do stem from experience in a practice and, as such, emerge from a store of practical wisdom or *phronesis* of many individuals.

Phronesis in Aristotle

Aristotle's *Nicomachean Ethics* is grounded in his notion of *phronesis.* Indeed, this notion suffuses his psychology, political philosophy, and his notions of friendship and the common life. At the heart of *phronesis* is the notion of a role-model teacher, a person who possesses the wisdom required and can teach younger persons by doing rather than by words alone.

Today's bioethicists tend to recognize the importance of the idea, especially since it grounds ethics within a particular context, family network, social and cultural support system, yet parallels W. D. Ross's notion of "moral instinct" (1930) either as a rational judgment or rational faculty. Nonetheless, a corresponding postmodern tendency is present to dismiss *phronesis* as elitist, since Aristotle argued that only the person with a complete moral life of virtue could exercise this virtue as well. Remaining after such a dismissal of the *virtue* of prudence is the rational facility of practical reason alone.

The elitist dismissal is puzzling. Are not some positions better than others, some persons held in more esteem than others for their probity or courage or dedication? They are indeed "better" than others in some respect. Aristotle's concept rightly implies that some moral judgments and some moral acts are better than others. In this sense, then, ethics itself implies an "elitism" of moral character. Nonetheless, in a properly functioning community, whether pre- or postmodern, many gifts and many persons are admirable—this one for humility, that one for probity, another for courage, still another for wisdom—and this is not undemocratic. Indeed, respect for individuals and their talents, their very individuality, moral and otherwise, is at the heart of a democratic community.

Response to Supposed Elitism in the Notion of *Phronesis*

Throughout all cultures and according to the mores of each time and place, the most important virtue for human beings has been moral wisdom. For the most part, this was based on a shared conception of the Good, such that communities could train, support, promote, and honor their citizens without a great deal of self-critical analysis about whether the contents of the Good were justifiable (Charvet 1995). Even in the advanced civilizations of Greece and Rome, with their explicit debates about the Good, unanimity existed that there was, indeed, such a reality, and that morality was achievable in pursuit of it.

Postmodernism directly challenges both convictions: first, that such an objective, publicly accessible Good exists; and, second, that morality consists in pursuing such a Good. In its stead, the moral life is said to consist in devising one's own plan for a morally good life. In the absence of a generally accepted notion of the Good, pursuit of one's own plan is incredibly difficult to achieve. Confronting the obstacles, à la Ayn Rand, requires a strongly motivated, autonomous person with great gifts, among them the thorough exercise of practical wisdom (Kekes 1997). So, by turning away from a publicly shared good to a private moral imagination and public courage, the notion of *phronesis* is hermeneutically reinterpreted to stand for individual moral probity, no matter what the goal, rather than a unique networking judgment, a habit of conjoining the abstract and socially shared conception of the Good with the everyday and practical exercise of it. As St. Thomas Aquinas argued, practical reason is *quasi conclusio syllogismi practici*—"like a conclusion of a practical syllogism."

Despite taking the high moral ground, the egoist position actually succumbs on at least two counts. First, in the absence of a shared good the construction and pursuit of one's own plan is intensely solipsistic, such that all forms of reprehensible social behavior, up to and including the Holocaust, could be justified as just such an "authentic" pursuit of a plan.

After all, as Erich Loewy has argued against "care ethics," the Nazis truly cared about their pogroms (Loewy 1995). Second, the requirements of moral imagination, courage, and dedication to one's private life plans and goals may produce saints, but it will also produce sinners—those who singlemindedly pursue ethnic cleansing or kill for a Chicago White Sox jacket worn by a rival gang member or an innocent teen. Even this elemental observation betrays the need for objective standards. As I understand postmodernism, however, it is not the fact that we do have standards that puzzle its adherents so much as the lack of rational justification for such standards and rules when subjected to the lens of honest multicultural appraisal.

Realizing this, most postmodern ethicists require that decisions must be checked through peaceable dialogue and only those decisions reached by consensus might be judged to be appropriate (Engelhardt 1996). At this point, however, one is quite rudely thrown back out onto the community, at least the community of interlocutors, and one's thinking is subjected to at least minimally communitarian checkpoints. The moral is necessarily linked to the political, as Aristotle held. Further assumptions about the Good reappear in such accounts as "side constraints," or conditions of possibility for moral dialogue, respect for pluralism, respect for persons, authentically listening even in disagreement, respect-for-liberty interests, and not violating the autonomy of another person unless he or she consents. These requirements for dialogue and/or a peaceful social existence—in a word, civility—are actually experientially constructed "goods" arising from activities in public life. I will return to this point later. We can now examine the element of practice in *phronesis*.

Practice

Praxis is an essential feature of *phronesis*. What is important about the virtuous or excellent individual is how that person functions day to day, gradually through experience developing the practical wisdom that others around him or her may lack to some degree. A virtuous person is not one filled with abstract knowledge about ethical theories but one skilled at making prudent judgments for the good of others, oneself, and the community. As St. Thomas Aquinas says in this regard, "Prudence, which is right reason about things to be done, requires that a man be rightly disposed with regard to ends; and this depends on rightness of appetite" (Aquinas II, Iiae, q. 57, a. 4).

How do "disposition" and "rightness of appetite" come about? These prerequisites for prudence develop through at least three means (a fourth means is proposed by religious faiths—namely, Divine inspiration or assistance in the form of grace and the supernatural virtues; with their development in respect to medicine, see Pellegrino and Thomasma 1996). For Aristotle, the first is the innate psychological structure of persons such that they have appetites or emotions that impel them toward particular goods or rewards. These appetites in our nature will control us without a more powerful direction from our higher intellect and will. The second means to acquire the virtue of prudence is through precept and example in the community. A third way to achieve prudence is through reflection on one's choices in life and resolutions to improve these choices next time through repeated practice.

All three pathways work together in complex ways. Practical knowledge is experiential, progressive, and developmental. These characteristics, it seems to me, are lacking in the denuded form of *phronesis* that is seen not as a virtue but only as a reasoning facility. *Phronesis* comes about from doing right things and wrong things in life, and learning from them. Moral beliefs, too, arise from this source of practical knowledge, as do theories, principles, and rules (Wallace 1996). From this collected experience we are able to raise and train our children and provide for social stability. In medical ethics, inductive methods of analyzing particular conundrums lead to wisdom in clinical ethics and medical judgment (Graber and Thomasma 1989).

The main point is that particular practices themselves, like medicine, acquire a collection of norms and standards. The justification of these norms and standards does not lie, as postmodernists rightly argue, in systems or theories of ethics but, rather, in the practical realm of "doing" medicine, the doctoring and patienting activities that bring about healing. I will come back to this practical realm in the final section

Acquired Skill

Phronesis is an acquired skill. Like all human endeavors that need practice, one needs a mentor or guide who is himself or herself a model of practical reasoning and experience. Glenn McGee explores this point by examining the problem of learning clinical ethics. In asking himself how one learns clinical ethics, he notes that moral learning takes place in any field through mentorship and practice. Indeed, as already noted, Aristotle's conception of *phronesis* requires this mentorship. The excellence of any person is tied to the long-term behavior of that person functioning in the community and society. When one acknowledges the moral excellence of any person, especially physicians, one attributes to them the wisdom of experience and practical judgments made every day about mundane as well as the occasional dramatic matters (McGee 1996).

Relation to Medicine

In my introduction, I noted that clinical ethics can be seen as a branch of medicine itself. Why is this so? Dan Davis argues that while clinical reasoning and clinical medicine are sometimes referred to as a *techne* (or art) or as an *episteme* (or science), the best way to construe clinical medicine and reasoning is as *phronesis*. Although portions of the discipline of medicine can be described as an art or a science, the best paradigm is that of practical reasoning, since this notion fits better with the ways of knowing and doing carried out by the physician in a relationship with the patient (Davis 1997). Davis's argument is anchored in the philosophy of medicine as a healing relationship conducted for a right and good decision for the patient, i.e., grounded in a beneficent professional healing encounter with the patient (Pellegrino and Thomasma 1981, 1988).

Phronesis **as Response to Postmodernism**

Most efforts at correcting antifoundationalism compound the problem by not accepting the view that all foundations are relative; instead, these efforts focus on rearticulating and redefending epistemological or metaphysical foundationalism (Chisholm 1982; Habermas 1988). Yet important arguments are to be considered in ethical foundationalism as well (Tollefsen 1995).

First, the postmodernist critique of a Cartesian certitude in philosophy, ethics, or indeed in any form of human knowledge, should be taken as valid. It is helpful to face honestly the slippery foundation of all truth-or-fact claims. This is especially true in ethics. Even Kant, the most rigorous of all moralists, recognized this by holding that we do not really know "*Das Ding an Sich*," and that in ethics, the fundamental principle, the categorical imperative, requires us to "act as if."

The reason that there can be no Cartesian-like principles and norms in ethics is not that there can be no principles, norms, and standards at all but, rather, because all reality, and our concepts of that reality, is other-referent. By that I mean that it is relational, having built into itself referents to other realities from which it came, to which it currently attends, and for which it will dissolve. In our conceptualization of these realities we cannot imagine even abstract truths that do not relate to one another. In metaphysics, the good, the true, and the beautiful are all transcendentals, i.e., they cannot be defined without reference to one another. In Einsteinian geometry and in relativity theory, the curvature of space means that no item can be defined without a referent to another. In mathematics, as Gödel's theorem attests, no purely deductive mathematics is possible, since for every "x" there must be a "y" interpreting the meaning of "x" (Wang 1996).

Turning to ethics, then, we could not imagine any choice that does not involve a balancing of goods or cherished values. There is no "one good" in which all other goods are reconciled unless we turn to theology and belief. As Sir Isaiah Berlin said:

> The notion of the perfect whole, the ultimate solution, in which all good things coexist, seems to me to be not merely unattainable—that is a truism—but conceptually incoherent; I do not know what is meant by a harmony of this kind. Some of the Great Goods cannot live together. That is a conceptual truth. We are doomed to choose, and every choice may entail an irreparable loss. (Berlin 1991, 2)

Hence, the rich concept of practical reason lies at the heart of ethical decision making. This entails not only the reasoning so essential to balancing the Goods in this particular situation, but also the emotional maturity and integrity required to appreciate the gains and to grieve for the losses during one's acceptance of the choice as it proceeds to affect the rest of one's life. That is why the meaning of *phronesis* is essentially that of a virtue: it requires practice, and it signifies an habituation toward and development of one's standards and norms. Further, the choices made are incorporated into one's life as well as into other judgments by which values are measured, weighed, and acted upon. Further still, the balancing of values occurs within the social context such that others are affected as well. The best postmodern ethics must therefore be one of connectedness, not just *difference* (Bauman 1993).

Second, as a social judgment, practical reason is nothing less than the same virtue in lawmakers who have the power to enforce a judgment for the common good. As Aquinas argued, law itself is defined as a kind of public *phronesis*, a power of practical reasoning lodged in public authorities and/or legislators who can enforce standards on the community (*Summa Theologiae* II, II, Q. 91). Aquinas shared with Aristotle this vision of law being a rational application of a universal rule to particular circumstances. Aristotle says: "Each [type of] just and lawful [action] is related as a universal to the particulars [that embody it]; for the [particular] actions that are done are many, but each [type] is one, since it is universal" (*NE* 1135a5–7). Traditionally, the structure of social order has been seen to reflect some order in nature itself. Thus, the development of a natural law theory for social and personal order seems to rest on a psychological need in individuals to find some order in the social and natural chaos that surrounds them (Smith and Weisstub 1979). The ultimate interpretation of Aristotle's notion of rationality in law and ethics is seen in Aquinas's view of a purposive universe in which all creatures are providentially governed. This is precisely what is denied in postmodernism. Yet appeal to rationality still grounds most of our legal theory. In international bioethics, for example, the International Bioethics Committee of UNESCO bases its arguments about the right not to be discriminated against on the basis of genetics on universal principles like "the intellectual and moral solidarity of mankind," and "the common welfare of mankind" because these, in turn, are "indispensable to the dignity of men and constitute a sacred duty which all the nations must fulfill" (UNESCO 1997). Rationality is essential for the inductive process itself because of the fit between innate psychological capacities and the causal structure of the world (Kornblith 1993).

A third point is relevant. The observation of postmodernists that the Enlightenment project is dead is an important one. This means not only that there will be no chance to develop a completely rationally coherent basis for ethics and law in society but also that such efforts produce deadly results. Ironically, the eighteenth-century Enlightenment was itself a reaction against absolutism, most particularly politically absolutist claims made by Kings in the mid-1600s. Grounding authority in individuals, their rights, and their inherently rational nature was a radical break with the notion of external authority in society (Academy of Humanism 1996). But the Enlightenment only transferred authority; it did not eliminate it entirely. Individuals appealed to the natural order, to "Nature and Nature's God." The deadly results are formed by the systems of thought in which reason dominated all other versions of reality, eliminating the emotional, irrational, impulsive, and incoherent features of human beings and nature itself.

An example would be the habit arising from the Western manner of solving problems by objectification—breaking them into smaller, more manageable parts, and then manipulating and commodifying them (James 1996). This general description fits, for example, our search for the genetic basis of disease, transplant technology, or the approach of a clinician toward treating an appendicitis attack (without the commodification step, of course). While this approach has positive results in many cases, the habit itself has led to horrible consequences more specific to bioethics—for example, with respect to prolonging a dying patient's life or pursuing reproductive technologies that treat living matter as an object of study (Crewdson 1997).

Behind this objectification is a more general danger: accepting any one vision means accepting what passes for objective verity in its pursuit of the Good. The postmodern warning is that this truth and that good are only based on subjective preferences or unexamined cultural assumptions (in the final analysis). Not to recognize this contingency at the root of all systems is to suspend doubt and to rush down the road of progress provided by the Enlightenment pursuit of objective reality. What practical reason supplies to this broadly painted dialectic is a discovery of truth and goods within the concourse of human relationships and experience. Neither totally objective nor totally subjective, the ethics that arises from *phronesis* develops its wisdom over the course of a life for individuals, and over the course of a society and civilization for a community.

But what experience is present that might transcend individual preferences with regard to bioethics? In medicine, and thereby in medical ethics, it is the existential principle of human finitude. We all share in this finitude and its effects—illness, decay, health itself (which is always a temporary condition), disability, vulnerability, and death. These existential conditions are not alien to the postmodern speaker and listener; they constitute the conditions of physical existence that define our lives. While we can debate the proper responses of a community to these conditions, they are undeniable facts of life that medicine addresses. The responses to these conditions create the standards to which we must and should appeal as fellow humans in any ethical discussions about medical theory and practice. These standards arise from experience with making practical judgments about values in that medical context.

These are, then, the irreducible medical realities with which every bioethical theory must deal. They are common to the human experiences and predicaments that have given rise to the need for medicine in every time and culture. These realities are the phenomena of medicine, making it a special kind of human activity, with special and distinctive moral characteristics (Pellegrino and Thomasma 1981). These standards are more than just role-specific duties taken on through public profession and promise keeping (Thomasma 1996). They are rooted in vast and universal human experience.

Given these reflections about one path out of the postmodernist challenge to truth in clinical ethics, a path directed by Aristotle's *phronesis*, what contributions can it make to preserving some standards in ethics? Instead of looking either to defend or reject the "correspondence theory" of truth in ethics, one can reinterpret that theory such that truth in ethics corresponds to learning and to developing in accordance with one's being and relationships. A search in this direction is not an abandonment of the search for truth but, rather, its proper path. Further, as Bernard Williams argues, some concepts become "thicker" than others to the degree to which others converge with it as it moves toward objectivity (Williams 1985). The thicker the concept, the more validity it has for general application in the sense that it has been tested and converges with other experiences. These experiences remain time and culture bound, but as they pass from century to century they acquire a validity that approaches "objective" truth. In my view, this is the greatest and only form of "objectivity" that ethics can approach: "generally for the most part true" (Aristotle, *NE* 1094b21).

Built into this level of abstraction is hard-fought contingency flagged for us by postmodern thinkers. No principle in ethics should be posited without its individual and cultural referent. An example might be the rule against killing. The rule is shorthand for a statement that should read, if spelled out, "Generally, for the most part, it is evil to kill." This rule arises from our personal and cultural experience that killing destroys both the sacredness of the life of the victim and the boundaries that each individual should place on his or her own being in consort with others in the community. I call this the "experiential a priori" that should be present on the table of all negotiation and discourse about values.

This inductive process leads to a practical truth, then, a truth of standards inductively drawn that are for a single individual "generally for the most part true," based on her life experience and her relations among family, friends, acquaintances, business, social, and cultural worlds. The broader her experiences and the more complex her choices, the "wiser" she becomes compared to others with less practice. Similarly, a society can grow (and decline) in practical wisdom for many of the same reasons. Some societies possess practical wisdom, a rule by law, that is better than others where chaos prevails. Compare today's Netherlands, Denmark, and Germany, for example, with Bosnia, Albania, and Chad.

Turning these points to bioethics and postmodernism, several problems persist with the noncognitive views of bioethics I outlined earlier in the discussion of postmodern challenges. The first is Maclean's identification of bioethics with utilitarianism (1993). Only a few bioethicists may be said to follow this approach—John Harris, James Rachels, Peter Singer, and R. M. Hare, for example. One could object to Maclean's arguments on their behalf, as did John Harris (1995), who holds that her view is fundamentally flawed. One might expect this critique from him, as he is one of the principal thinkers against whom Maclean argues.

Without becoming embroiled in the arguments, this debate is interesting for my purpose because it sheds light on an almost mechanistic process of cataloguing and resolving ethical questions in medicine. In their efforts to appeal to reason, utilitarians are vulnerable to the critique that the appeal to reason is really an appeal to schema they have designed that precisely take away the moral struggle. Consider, for example, Hare's proposal of a canon of moral rules people must follow to think rationally about ethics. He claims that everyone who follows this method correctly, Maclean argues, "will come to the same moral conclusions" (Maclean 1993, 114). One can readily see why Maclean objects to this kind of rote reasoning. As Cornford put it in his spoof of academe, "Plainly, the more rules you can invent, the less need there will be to waste time over fruitless puzzling about right and wrong" (Cornford 1953, 10). Of course we would like standards gleaned from past experience, as conscience provides for individuals, but these standards should not be grounded so much in the more abstract rules of reasoning well about ethics as in practical experience. This is the realm of prudence.

Second, Maclean concludes, in the words of another reviewer, Elizabeth Telfer, that "Moral philosophy's proper role in medicine is only one of clarification" (Telfer 1995). That is to say, philosophers should analyze problems in everyday language, and then propose to moral agents, such as patients or policymakers, the many possible answers. The moral agents would then make up their own minds.

This view is close to that of clinical ethics theory, the purpose of which is to propose to patients and physicians a number of courses of action that are supportable. A recommendation is made by the ethics consult service members or, more rarely, by an ethics committee. Nonetheless, our experience indicates that some courses of action are judged to be better than others and that clinical ethicists, too, are moral agents and not just moral bystanders. At the very least, they are officials of the health-care system that offer a recommendation to the patient and physician. They, too, have a stake in the enterprise as a whole, not to mention their membership in the moral community itself, a concept that cannot appeal to antifoundationalists at all.

The clinical ethicist participates in medical responsibilities. Physicians carry with them a clinical responsibility arising both from public dedication and from the existential a priori of human finitude to, in the words of Schultz and Carnevale, "sincerely strive to help their patients in a way that fits the circumstances of the situation at hand" (1996, 193). This involves more than the desire to help the patient, a kind of altruism and beneficence to be sure. Rather, it requires a commitment to working through the patient's medical narrative, entering the patient's life story and value system. This entering of another's physical and social life is guided by what Schultz and Carnevale call practical health-care wisdom, or "clinical *phronesis*." What makes *phronesis* stand out from normal forms of rationality is "its creative use of difference rather than simply neutralizing it." This creativity includes the use of moral imagination and various ways of perceiving, including, but not limited to, "expert clinical observation" (Schultz and Carnevale 1996, 193–194).

Third, the "value preferences" that Maclean finds at the foundation of bioethics, or that noncognitivists ethicists accept as forming the root of moral debates, are not simple personal and subjective assertions if they are grounded in the values of patients and doctors about healing illness and disease—the existential *a priori* of human finitude I continue to emphasize. Such "preferences" are cognitive and experiential a prioris for a moral philosophy of medicine. They stem from centuries of medical practice, centuries of physicians and patients caring for illnesses common to all persons, across time and across cultures.

Further, the utilitarians are correct in positing the existence of rules of right thinking. If there are no foundations, for example, some irrefutable principles that are necessary or necessarily true—such as Aristotle's principle of contradiction or the law of the excluded middle term—then reasoning itself becomes chaotic. A necessary set of principles must be present that ground all claims to know or to ascribe meaning. Regarding knowledge and reasoning, antifoundationalism contends that no set of principles is inherent in knowing: all such have been derived from the human act of achieving knowledge itself. This point is valid, as I have argued, since these principles have evolved from the habits of thinking and reasoning over time and have been tested as valid by human experience. In this regard, antifoundationalism is important for a moral philosophy of medicine because it rests on rejection of the one-dimensionality and reductionism to universally abstract principles of thought and action.

Conclusion

The problem of postmodernism arises when the rejection of rationalistic reductionism itself goes too far by asserting that there is no such thing as medicine in general, or ethics in general, or physics in general, or any discipline in general. This strikes me as absurd. Crosscultural and transhistorical disciplines do exist. They can be studied and learned and applied in many contexts. While their value assumptions are too often ignored, or accepted without question, the disciplines themselves are distinct from each other and from other forms of human activity.

Practical ethical reasoning can produce valid principles that can be rationally defended. Their application to human life has meaning, and one is ethical according to the degree to which one acts on such principles. The desire for a clear and distinct, abstract, and universal knowledge, and a corresponding absolute certitude in ethics about right and wrong, is misplaced. It transcends too far beyond the human condition into the realm of ideals and Idealism, and cannot bear the weight of its own justification. All knowledge, disciplines, principles, norms, and axioms are historically developing artifacts. In ethics, the maximum level of certitude possible is, as Aquinas taught, *ut in pluribus,* generally for the most part true (Aquinas I, I. Q. 23, art. 7, obj. 3).

In contrast, the level of generalizability is much higher for all disciplines, including bioethics, than the current antifoundationalists permit. Part of postmodernism harbors the fiction that a radical and disjunctive change in human culture from the past has occurred and that the history of thought and culture can have little or no bearing on the present. Rejecting this view does not mean we should remain blissfully unaware of dramatic changes in practice and thought. Nonetheless, our cultural and personal history at the very least can contribute negative principles, or principles of limits, arising from our past history and experience. I have called these precepts existential and experiential a prioris and have explored how they arise inductively from the reasoning and habit of *phronesis*—in individuals, in practices like medicine, and in society and culture itself.

Notes

1. This virtue is examined in Pellegrino and Thomasma 1994 as well as the essays in this volume by Ronald Polansky and Kathryn Montgomery.

2. Consult, for example, the first endnote in Engelhardt 1991, in which he bemoans the losses of certainty and ritual in the Roman Catholic tradition. Reading his work leaves a distinct feeling that Engelhardt wishes secular pluralism were not the case but is ruthlessly honest that it is. His thinking takes the loss of the Enlightenment project seriously (see also Engelhardt 1997).

3. See the articles on ethics consultations in *Journal of Clinical Ethics* 1996, 7(2), especially Fletcher and Siegler 1996; see also Society for Health and Human Values/Society for Bioethics Consultation 1998 and Aulisio et al. 1998.

4. This was also the path taken by Husserl (1934–1937), especially in his concerns about the future of sciences and the humanities; see Husserl 1991.

References

Academy of Humanism. 1996. *Challenges to the Enlightenment: In Defense of Reason and Science*. Amherst, N.Y.: Prometheus Books.

Aquinas, T. 1952. *Summa Theologiae*, vols. I and II, trans. Fathers of the English Dominican Province; rev. D. J. Sullivan. Chicago: Encyclopaedia Britannica.

Aulisio, M. P., R. M. Arnold, and S. J. Youngner. 1998. "Can There Be Educational and Training Standards for Those Conducting Health Care Ethics Consultation?" in *Health Care Ethics: Critical Issues for the 21st Century*, ed. J. F. Monagle and D. C. Thomasma. Gaithersburg, Md.: Aspen.

Bambach, C. R. 1996. Review of *The Genesis of Heidegger's* Being and Time by Theodore Kisiel. *American Catholic Philosophical Quarterly* 70(3): 442–447.

Bauman, Z. 1993. *Postmodern Ethics*. Oxford/Cambridge, Mass.: Blackwell.

Beiser, F. C. 1997. *The Sovereignty of Reason: The Defense of Rationality in the Early English Enlightenment*. Princeton, N.J.: Princeton University Press.

Beresford, E. B. 1996. "Can *Phronesis* Save the Life of Medical Ethics?" *Theoretical Medicine* 17(3): 209–224.

Berlin, I. 1991. "The Pursuit of the Ideal," 1–19, in I. Berlin. *The Crooked Timber of Humanity: Chapters in the History of Ideas*. New York: Knopf.

Bernardin, J. 1988. *The Consistent Ethic of Life*. St. Louis, Mo.: Catholic Health Assn.

Charvet, J. 1995. *The Idea of an Ethical Community*. Ithaca, N.Y.: Cornell University Press.

Chisholm, R. M. 1982. *The Foundations of Knowing*. Minneapolis: University of Minnesota Press.

Cornford, F. M. 1953. *Microcosmographia Academia: Being a Guide for the Young Academic Politician*. 5th ed. Cambridge: Bowes & Bowes.

Crewdson, J. 1997. "U.S. Fires Research Over Use of Embryonic DNA." *Chicago Tribune*, Sec. 1:4, Jan. 9.

Critchley, S. 1992. *The Ethics of Deconstruction: Derrida & Levinas*. Oxford/Cambridge, Mass.: Blackwell.

Connor, S. 1997. *Postmodernist Culture: An Introduction to Theories of the Contemporary*. 2d ed. Oxford/Cambridge, Mass.: Blackwell.

Davis, F. D. 1997. "*Phronesis*, Clinical Reasoning, and Pellegrino's Philosophy of Medicine." *Theoretical Medicine* 18(1/2): 173–195.

de Wachter, M. A. M. 1997. "The European Convention on Bioethics." *Hastings Center Report* 27(1): 13–28.

Engelhardt, H. T. 1991. *Bioethics and Secular Humanism.* Philadelphia: Trinity Press International.

Engelhardt, H. T. 1996. *The Foundations of Bioethics.* 2d ed. New York: Oxford University Press.

Engelhardt, H. T. 1997. "The Crisis of Virtue: Arming for the Cultural Wars and Pellegrino at the Lines." *Theoretical Medicine* 18(1/2): 165–172.

Fletcher, J. C., and M. Siegler. 1996. "What Are the Goals of Ethics Consultation? A Consensus Statement." *Journal of Clinical Ethics* 7(2): 122–126.

Graber, G. C., and D. C. Thomasma. 1989. *Theory and Practice in Medical Ethics.* New York: Crossroads.

Grahame, K. 1909. *Wind in the Willows.* London: Methuen.

Habermas, J. 1988. *Nachmetaphysisches Denken: Philosophische Aufsätze.* Frankfurt a/M: Suhrkamp.

Harris, J. 1995. "The Elimination of Morality." *Journal of Medical Ethics* 21: 200–224.

Horgan, T., and J. Tienson. 1996. *Connectionism and the Philosophy of Psychology.* Cambridge, Mass.: MIT Press.

Hoy, D. C., and T. McCarthy. 1994. *Critical Theory.* Oxford/Cambridge, Mass.: Blackwell.

Huntington, S. P. 1996. *The Clash of Civilizations and the Remaking of World Order.* New York: Simon & Schuster.

Husserl, E. 1991. *Die Krisis der Europäischen Wissenschaften und die Transzendentale Phänomenologie Ergänzungsband: Texte aus dem Nachlass 1934–1937.* Dordrecht, Holland/Boston: Kluwer.

Irwin, T. 1985. Trans. Aristotle, *Nichomachean Ethics.* Indianapolis, Ind.: Hackett.

James, C. 1996. Sex and Reason: Bertrand Russell, Passionate about Both. *New Yorker* 72(38): 104–117.

Jonsen, A. R. 1991. "Casuistry as a Methodology in Clinical Ethics." *Theoretical Medicine* 12(4): 295–307.

Jonsen, A. R., and S. Toulmin. 1988. *The Abuse of Casuistry: A History of Moral Reasoning.* Berkeley: University of California Press.

Kekes, J. 1997. *Moral Wisdom and Good Lives.* Ithaca, N.Y.: Cornell University Press.

Kornblith, H. 1993. *Inductive Inference and Its Natural Ground: An Essay in Naturalistic Epistemology.* Cambridge, Mass.: MIT Press.

MacIntyre, A. 1979. "Why Is the Search for the Foundations of Ethics So Frustrating?" *Hastings Center Report* 9(4): 16–22.

MacIntyre, A. 1981. *After Virtue: A Study in Moral Theory.* Notre Dame, Ind.: University of Notre Dame Press.

MacIntyre, A. 1988. *Whose Justice, Which Rationality?* Notre Dame, Ind.: University of Notre Dame Press.

MacIntyre, A. 1990. *Three Rival Versions of Moral Enquiry.* Notre Dame, Ind.: University of Notre Dame Press.

Maclean, Anne. 1993. *The Elimination of Morality: Reflections on Utilitarianism and Bioethics.* New York: Routledge.

Mallon, T. 1997. "Minding your 'P's and 'Q's." *The New Yorker* 72(45): 80.

McGee, G. 1996. "*Phronesis* in Clinical Ethics." *Theoretical Medicine* 17(4): 317–28.

Michaels, W. B. 1995. *Our American Nativism, Modernism, and Pluralism.* Durham, N.C.: Duke University Press.

Nielsen, K. 1997. *Naturalism without Foundations.* Amherst, N.Y.: Prometheus Books.

Norris, C. 1993. *The Truth About Postmodernism.* Oxford/Cambridge, Mass.: Blackwell.

Pellegrino, E. D. Unpublished Manuscript. "Bad Ethics Makes for Bad Law: A Critique of the Moral Arguments of the Second Opinion of the Ninth Circuit Court," in *Compassion in Dying in State of Washington.*

Pellegrino, E. D., and T. McIlhenny, eds. 1982. *Teaching Ethics, the Humanities, and Human Values in Medical Schools: A Ten-Year Overview.* Washington, D.C.: Institute of Human Values in Medicine/Society for Health and Human Values.

Pellegrino, E. D., and D. C. Thomasma. 1981. *A Philosophical Basis of Medical Practice.* New York: Oxford University Press.

Pellegrino, E. D., and D. C. Thomasma. 1988. *For the Patient's Good: The Restoration of Beneficence in Health Care.* New York: Oxford University Press.

Pellegrino, E. D., and D. C. Thomasma. 1994. *The Virtues in Medical Practice.* New York: Oxford University Press.

Pellegrino, E. D., and D. C. Thomasma. 1996. *The Christian Virtues in Medical Practice.* Washington, D.C.: Georgetown University Press.

Rockmore, T. 1992. *Antifoundationalism Old and New.* Philadelphia: Temple University Press.

Rorty, R. 1989. *Contingency, Irony and Solidarity.* New York: Cambridge University Press.

Ross, W. D. 1930. *The Right and the Good.* Oxford: Oxford University Press.

Schultz, D. S., and F. A. Carnevale. 1996. "Engagement and Suffering in Responsible Caregiving: On Overcoming Maleficence in Health Care." *Theoretical Medicine* 17(3): 189–207.

Smith, J. C., and D. N. Weisstub. 1979. "The Evolution of Western Legal Consciousness." *International Journal of Law and Psychiatry* 2: 215–234.

Society for Health and Human Values/Society for Bioethics Consultation. 1998. *Core Competencies for Health Care Ethics Consultation: The Report of the American Society for Bioethics and Humanities*. Glenview, Ill.: American Society for Bioethics and Humanities.

Telfer, E. 1995. "The Elimination of Morality." *Philosophical Books* 36(3): 204–206.

Thomasma, D. C. 1972. *Pre-Conceptual Knowledge and Hermeneutics*. Ann Arbor: University of Michigan Microfilms.

Thomasma, D. C. 1980. "The Possibility of a Normative Medical Ethics." *Journal of Medicine and Philosophy* 5(3): 249–260.

Thomasma, D. C. 1996. "Promise-Keeping: An Institutional Ethos for Healthcare Today." *Frontiers of Health Services Management* 13(2): 5–34.

Thomasma, D. C. 1997a. "Bioethics and International Human Rights." *Journal of Law, Medicine and Ethics* 25(4): 295–306.

Thomasma, D. C. 1997b. "Antifoundationalism and the Possibility of a Moral Philosophy of Medicine." *Theoretical Medicine* 18(1–2): 127–143.

Thomasma, D. C. Forthcoming. "Medical Ethical Theories." In *Textbook of Military Medicine*, ed. Washington, D.C.: Office of the Surgeon General.

Thornton, T. P. 1996. *Handwriting in America: A Cultural History*. New Haven Conn.: Yale University Press.

Tollefsen, C. 1995. *Foundationalism Defended: Essays on Epistemology, Ethics and Aesthetics*. Bethesda, Md.: Cambridge University Press.

Toulmin, S. 1981. "The Tyranny of Principles." *Hastings Center Report* 11(6): 31–39.

Toulmin, S. 1982. "How Medicine Saved the Life of Ethics." *Perspectives in Biology and Medicine* 25: 736–750.

UNESCO. 1998. "Universal Declaration on the Human Genome and Human Rights." *Journal of Medicine and Philosophy* 23(3): 334–341.

Veatch, R. M. 1989. "Hospital Pharmacy: What is Ethics?" *American Journal of Hospital Pharmacy Quarterly* 46(1): 109–115.

Wallace, J. D. 1996. *Ethical Norms, Particular Cases*. Ithaca, N.Y.: Cornell University Press.

Waller, B. N. 1994. "Noncognitive Moral Realism." *Philosophia* 24(1–2), 57–75.

Williams, B. 1985. *Ethics and the Limits of Philosophy*. Cambridge, Mass.: Harvard University Press.

Wang, H. 1996. *A Logical Journey from Gödel to Philosophy*. Cambridge, Mass.: MIT Press.

5

Confessions of an Unrepentant Sophist

Tod Chambers

In the basement of a church, following a potluck lunch, I was one of three panelists to address the issue of physician-assisted suicide. The first to speak was a physician, who was a member of the congregation; she explained that as part of the medical profession, she felt that physician-assisted suicide was morally objectionable. The second speaker was a lawyer who worked for the ACLU; he claimed that people had a right to die with dignity and therefore people had the right to commit suicide if they wished. When it was my turn, I briefly explained that I thought this community's first duty was to care for the dying and to do so in a manner that reflects the teachings of Christ. The issue of physician-assisted suicide, I argued, directs us away from the Christian responsibilities of caring for those most vulnerable and of addressing the pain and suffering of the dying. Following my comments, a large number of the audience applauded. The ACLU representative seemed flabbergasted. He rejoined that everyone was not Christian in this society and that the issue was about allowing each of us individually to decide. (The audience, of course, was not persuaded by his appeals.)

I do not, however, regard myself a Christian. My Jewish mother and Christian father resolved their religious differences by not raising my brothers and me in either of the faiths. Although I am not in favor of legalizing physician-assisted suicide, my opinion against it is not in any manner informed by Christian theology. My belief, I suspect, is more likely the result of my upbringing in the midst of New England conservatism, which generally distrusts radical change. I have obviously drawn upon the symbols and theology of Christianity simply to persuade these people, who do not share my own worldview—a move that might be characterized by some as an act of "pure sophistry." I know well from looking in my dictionaries that if I were to accept such a characterization, I should be deeply ashamed, for by admitting to being a sophist, I am admitting to advancing specious arguments. But I am not. In this essay I wish to counter the negative associations we have with the sophistic position and argue that the discipline of bioethics has much to learn from the original sophists.

A parallel exists between sophistry and casuistry in terms of how these approaches historically have acquired negative connotation. Both of the approaches have received negative connotations (ones that can be found in most dictionaries) because of attacks by prominent philosophers. In the case of casuistry, the attack was from Pascal. Tom Beauchamp and James Childress (1994) note how surprising it is that casuistry was capable of being resurrected in medical ethics. To illustrate this, they quote a 1945 entry on casuistry in *An Encyclopedia of Religion* by Edgar Sheffield Brightman: "1) The application of ethical principles to specific cases. 2) Quibbling, rationalization, sophistry or an attempt to justify what does not merit justification." Beauchamp and Childress go on to say how the casuists consider their position to be the reverse of Brightman's perspective—"a system of justification that tries to surmount the sophistry of 'applying' principles" (1994, 93). Similarly, Mark Kuczewski, commenting on the relation between rhetorical methods and casuistry, notes that "casuistry must constantly face the challenge that it may degenerate into mere sophistry" (1997, 68). While the term *casuistry* in recent years has been reevaluated, sophistry seems still to be a categorical insult. The most renowned critic of the sophists was Socrates, and in many of Plato's dialogues, the sophists are the targets of Socrates's arguments. These perhaps unwilling participants in Plato's philosophical dramas included some of the most prominent sophists of the day, such as Gorgias and Protagoras. Of late, an attempt has been made in rhetorical studies not only to defend the sophists but to use their ideas in response to contemporary problems (Enos 1976; Poulakos 1984; Crowley 1989; Foss 1989; Jarratt 1991). In a similar manner, I wish to admit that what I do *is* mere sophistry and why we in bioethics should be doing a lot more of it.

From Autonomy to Auto Nomos

Contemporary medical ethics in North America has been fixated on preserving individual rights, which are justified upon purely secular grounds. Although this moral liberal tradition arose in some ways in response to a plurality of moral values in American society, it has its roots in a concept of the person as a singular being radically separate from others. Individuals are held to have the freedom to pursue any goal they wish as long as it does not interfere with the goals of others. In medical ethics this has come to be summarized as the concept of "autonomy." Beauchamp and Childress discriminate "being autonomous" from "being respected as an autonomous agent," explaining that "To respect an autonomous agent is . . . to acknowledge that person's right to hold views, to make choices, and to take actions based on personal values and beliefs" (1994, 125). This idea of respecting a person's right to make decisions about health care based upon his or her value system has been the linchpin of contemporary bioethics, and for many health-care professionals in the United States the concept of respect for autonomy has come to be the principle that trumps all other principles. So firmly has this moral liberalism become a part of how Americans conceive of medical ethics that it has dominated the manner in which problems have been framed. Consider, for example, how the idea of individual rights is used in our language: "a right to health care," "a right to die," "a right to be informed," "a right to life," and "a right to choose."

The development of this liberal moral vision for medical ethics is epitomized by such philosophers as H. Tristram Engelhardt. His *The Foundations of Bioethics* stands as a clear example of an attempt to construct morality that does not depend on individuals sharing a common moral background. Engelhardt distinguishes "community" from "society." In a community, persons share a common moral perspective, and although they may not always agree on particulars, they do agree upon the general idea of what is good and also share methods for arriving at the answers to questions of morality. Society is an association of persons who do not share a single moral vision. Engelhardt's interest is in attempting to discern a morality for society, but his general conclusion is that the best we can do is a procedural morality based on respect for autonomy.

In recent years this liberal tradition has come under attack from a variety of perspectives. One of the dominant critiques has been from a group of thinkers who fall under the umbrella term "communitarians." Communitarians have been critical of the emptiness of the concept of autonomy as the point of departure for moral inquiry. Their stance has even included a radical attack from this perspective on such elementary concepts as rights and individualism. The communitarians ground moral reasoning within the context of communities. Acknowledging the Aristotelian idea of human beings as essentially political animals, the communitarians see the liberal concepts of autonomy and personal choice as illusions. They argue that, ironically, the quest for the resolving moral issues is a sign of the root cause of our current problems. We must repudiate the liberal moral perspective, which perpetuates interminable moral debates, and return to a concept of common goods and communal responsibility that acknowledges our fundamental social nature. Daniel Callahan reflects this perspective in proclaiming that "there is no such thing as a 'common good' under a reign of autonomy; there is only the aggregate of individual goods" (1984, 42). Ezekiel Emanuel in *The Ends of Human Life* argues that such conceptions of a neutral, procedural morality, as Engelhardt promotes, must be replaced with an "alternative political philosophy," which is defined through a common concept of the Good. Emanuel's final vision for health care is a liberal communitarian one in which there are "thousands of community health programs (CHPs), each made up of a few thousand to a few tens of thousands of citizen-members" (1991, 178). Emanuel's vision of a solution to health-care allocation—and one suspects probably for most of our moral dilemmas—consists of moving toward clearly defined communal activity that would consist of interacting with those that share our vision of the good life. This move, however, is not that far from Engelhardt's perspective.

In the second edition of his book, Engelhardt renames the principle of "autonomy" the "principle of permission" in order to make sure that readers do not see him as promoting radical individualism. As a result, his vision of the moral world is not different from that of the communitarians. Although he sees his own task as attempting to create a safe world where "moral strangers meet as individuals" (1996, xi), Engelhardt also seems to promote a movement toward entering into a community-based way of life. He states: "If one wants more than secular reason can disclose—and one should want more—then one should join a religion and be careful to choose the right one. Canonical moral content will not be found outside of a particular moral narrative, a view from somewhere" (1996, xi). Engelhardt then provides the reader with a glimpse of his own moral perspective in terms of the Orthodox Catholic tradition. For Engelhardt, if the reader also wishes to live a life that has a content-full moral life rather than only a procedural one, then one must stop spending one's time only with strangers (which consists merely of getting permission) and, instead, develop friendships.

Thus, in an odd manner, although the intellectual descendants of Kant and those of Aristotle seem to end up in the same place, ultimately I think one finds their worldview in some manner wanting. The result of their moral vision is a nation of insulated communities that do not seem to share much contact with one another. I am sure that neither the communitarians such as Emanuel or MacIntyre or the Kantians such as Engelhardt would wish to suggest that people not speak with their neighbors, but a form of exhaustion results from finding nothing outside relativism, the limits of rationality, and unending moral disagreement.

Speaking with One's Neighbors

In the conclusion to *The Foundations of Bioethics*, Engelhardt leaves the reader with a telling image, one that shows the limits of his concept of moral dialogue. After noting the "virtue of being a member of an actual and concrete moral community," Engelhardt states that:

If one's only contact with secular pluralist morality occurs when one walks to the property line of one's peaceably established moral exclave . . . , one can be seen as acknowledging secular moral constraints insofar as one does not carry the imposition of one's viewpoint beyond that line and insofar as one expects reciprocal tolerance of one's own way of life. (Engelhardt 1996, 422)

This image reveals that Engelhardt conceives of the social life of humanity as a habitat where people have clearly defined fences and one does not engage one's neighbors in any form of discussion, beyond perhaps "good morning" and "how nice it is we have such high fences." This seems, in one way, a peculiar vision of social life and in another an unrealistic one, as if one only lived in a single community. Engelhardt's description seems unable to provide us with an understanding of how a gay, right-wing, Cuban-born Catholic man lives within his world, a world where he can in a single day move from one community to another and from one subcommunity to another. Our social boundaries are just not so neatly defined. Engelhardt's description is also not a helpful vision of the social world, for discussions with one's neighbors do not merely entail where the property lines are but also what kind of things will go on in the public park. Engelhardt's vision is limited to the kind of world that results from the theories of liberalism and communitarianism.

A world of various independent communities is close to the world in which the sophists lived—an environment of independent *poleis*, or city states (ironically, the root for our word autonomy). The sophists were highly aware of the diversity that existed from one community to the next, and one can speculate that much of the sophistic perspective was a response to the diversity they found in their travels. One of the common jobs of the sophists was teaching the Greek youth so that they could participate in this new democratic political world. In this political environment, the capacity to persuade became far more important than one's family or class (Poulakos 1993, 57). The sophists provided the tools that this new class of politicians needed in order to gain power in a world that gave it to those who could reason together. Eric Havelock argues that although the sophists taught rhetoric, their central concern was far closer to a form of pragmatic politics.

> If there is one quality which identifies them, and yet which is wholly incompatible with their traditional reputation, it is a sense of social and political responsibility. Beginning with the sociology attributed to Protagoras with its rationality, its humanity, its historical depth, continuing with the pragmatism which seeks to understand the common man's virtues and failings and to guide his decisions by a flexible calculus of what is good and useful, and ending with a theory of group discourse as a negotiation of opinion leading to agreed decision, we are steadily invited to keep our eye not upon the authoritarian leader, but upon the average man as citizen of this society and voter in his parliament. (Havelock 1964, 230)

For Havelock the sophistic worldview was not "unscrupulous persuasion" but, rather, the political techniques necessary to the creating of consensus. A useful contrast is with Plato's political perspective, which had its power grounded in the elite. Susan Jarratt observes that the sophists' proficiency in teaching the art of rhetoric "derived in part from their experiences of different cultures; they believed and taught that notions of 'truth' had to be adjusted to fit the ways of a particular audience in a certain time and with a certain set of beliefs and laws" (1991, xv).

The accusation that the sophists were relativists was generally true, but one could counter that it was similar to the methodological relativism that cultural anthropologists developed in the 1920s and 1930s. This methodological relativism, which argued against the innate superiority of particular cultural moral patterns, led to anthropology's capacity to demonstrate accurately the cultural diversity in the world's societies (Marcus and Fischer 1986, 19–20). In an analogous fashion, the sophists on their travels found diversity not as something to promote but simply a description of the way things are, a fact that should be recognized in order to operate effectively in the world. Mario Untersteiner summarizes this intellectual discovery: "There is gradually emphasized the contradiction between the traditions, usages and customs of different peoples, which by mutual comparison lose their universality in the contingent nature of chance or occasion" (1954, 21). Ethical relativism, which continues to be one of the most feared concepts in medical ethics, describes the way the world is, and one feels that many in bioethics are akin to those who simply want to wish away this basic truth. Protagoras's famous statement that "man is the measure of all things" typifies the belief of many of the sophists that truth could not be established on objective grounds. Instead, truth, they held, is relative to each person. Aristotle interpreted Protagoras's statement "meaning simply and solely that what appears to each man assuredly also *is*" (quoted in Guthrie 1971, 171).

An intriguing parallel may be seen between Protagoras's belief in the relativity of goodness in each individual and the Hippocratic perspective on medicine. Laszlo Versenyi observes that both emphasize "that their arts are necessary because of the difference between one man and another … and that there is a resulting relativity of what is good for each. Both hold that 'our present way of life' (laws, customs, regimen) is not by nature but 'has been discovered and elaborated during a long period of time'" (quoted in Guthrie 1971, 167–168). Consequently, Versenyi notes, they both aim to "find what is useful, appropriate, fitting, or due to the nature … so as to promote healthy, harmonious and undisturbed life" (quoted in

Guthrie 1971, 168). When a sick person approaches a physician with the problem that food tastes unpleasant, according to Protagoras, the food *does* taste bad. The physician, with the consent of the patient, attempts to change the patient's experience of food. This does not mean that the food is objectively "good," but that the patient's life can be changed by changing his or her experience of the food.

Two analogous insights demonstrate the usefulness of this sophistic view for bioethics. First, rational discussion will not change the patient's perspective; one cannot talk the patient out of the bad taste. Second, in order to persuade patients to undergo medical treatment, one must be able to, well, persuade them. This does not mean coercing individuals or using physical force against them. Neither does this lead one to a complete relativity of goods, since the concept of rhetoric and persuasion as morally appropriate means also indicates that one is against the use of force as a way of achieving change within a society. A parallel case exists in the question of forcible treatment of children. One could make a case, which has often been made, that one should take possession of children whenever the parents are not making decisions that are in keeping with "standard" medical treatment. The danger of such a position is that the parents may never show up if they fear the child will be taken from them.

Protagoras believed in the capacity to use persuasion in communal life and that such persuasion was one of the central tenets of human social existence. In Plato's dialogue, Protagoras tells of a myth in which human beings lived in a chaotic world; lacking protection from the other beasts, human beings receive special gifts from Zeus that make them capable of practicing the art of politics, and subsequently they can live in harmony.

The sophistic perspective thus contains two insights for medical ethics. First, the sophists recognized the pluralism in the social world and, furthermore, could teach a way to persuade within that pluralism. Second, the capacity to persuade is essential in the working of a democracy that functions through a duty to respect individual autonomy.

Kairos, Nomos, and Moral Persuasion

One of the primary difficulties in surmising what the sophists believed is that we have only fragments of the ideas of their most prominent thinkers.

The other main source of information has been the writings of Plato. The degree to which Plato accurately presents the sophist perspective is debatable; he does not, however, allow them to win arguments against Socrates. John Poulakos (1993) addresses the issue of the literal fragmentation of sophistry and proposes analyzing key terms. Drawing on the work of Richard Weaver (1953), he suggests that the study of key terms can "help us make some sense out of the sophists' textual remains" (Poulakos 1993, 55). The key terms I would like to apply to the issues in bioethics are *kairos* and *nomos*.

Time and place are important concepts to keep in mind in acts of persuasion. The concept of *kairos* as elaborated by Plato in *Gorgias* means shaping one's speech to fit within the particular historical moment within a community. Untersteiner claims that Gorgias's concept of *kairos* can be summed up as "'that which is fitting in time, place and circumstance,' which means the adaptation of the speech to the manifold variety of life, to the psychology of speaker and hearer" (1954, 197). Acknowledging *kairos* in the act of moral persuasion means recognizing that "speech exists in time and is uttered both as a spontaneous formulation of and a barely constituted response to a new situation unfolding in the immediate present" (Poulakos 1993, 63). One need only think of how different a reference to "socialism" would have been for much of the American public during the 1930s compared to the 1950s and to the 1990s. Today the concept retains rhetorical power: one need only recall the use of the concept of socialism as what Kenneth Burke referred to as a "devil term" during the attempt at health-care reform in the United States in the early 1990s. As significant as knowing the particular time is knowing the rhetoric of location. Here once again the concept of socialism has different meanings in the United States, China, and the Netherlands.

Nomos can be translated in a variety of ways. For my discussion, I draw upon its meaning as the norms, customs, and laws of a community. In their various travels, the sophists became aware of how understanding the *nomos* of the community they were within was essential to being able to persuade. *Nomos* by its definition makes one cognizant that "making sense" is contingent upon following the rules established by the community. As Susan Jarratt observes:

The sophists translated the natural scientists' observations about the temporality of human existence into a body of commentary on the use of discourse in the function of social order: i.e., they concentrated on the power of language in shaping human group behavior explicitly within the limits of time and space. Sophistic rhetoric, then, as an instrument of social action in the *polis* was bound to the flux. (Jarratt 1991, 11)

The sophistic belief in attending to the historical norms and customs of community placed them in direct contrast to the beliefs of Socrates and Plato, who taught of an unchanging ideal reality that one should be able to appeal to regardless of time and place. If one believes in an unchanging reality, then the arguments of the sophists appear to be a form of deception, attempting to persuade people without regard to Truth. If one doubts the existence of this Truth, then persuading (without the use of force) through attention to *kairos* and *nomos* are "truly" the only thing one can do to live in harmony with others.

Some might respond that I have merely demonstrated in my argument to the Methodist congregation the practices that have given sophistry a bad name in philosophy; that is, I seem willing to say anything as long as it is possible to get my way in a debate. Furthermore, because I am unwilling to accept the presence of Truth (or at the least our capacity to demonstrate the presence of the Truth), the only precepts that will guide my decisions are social harmony and situational morality. The problem with this concern is that it seems to confuse relativism as descriptive with relativism as normative. Just because we accept the sophist perspective that a multitude of communities with differing worldviews exist and that one cannot simply appeal to reason as a way of resolving all problems does not, on a personal level, affect my day-to-day life. This position, I believe, is close to what Clifford Geertz refers to as "anti antirelativism." According to Geertz, one can be against a position "without thereby committing oneself to what it rejects" (1989, 13). The sophists were not *pro*relativism; they were, in Geertz's sense, anti-antirelativism—against those who were against it. But can one even be a prorelativist? The literary critic Stanley Fish, who refers to himself as a "modern-day sophist," argues that while relativism is

a position one can entertain, it is not a position one can occupy. No one can *be* a relativist, because no one can achieve the distance from his [or her] beliefs and assumptions which would result in their being no more authoritative *for him [or her]* than the beliefs and assumptions held by others ... there is never a moment when one believes nothing, when consciousness is innocent of any and all categories of thought, and whatever categories of thought are operative at a given moment will serve as an undoubted ground. (Fish 1980, 319–320)

As much as I might wish to convince myself that my way of seeing the world is contingent on social and historical categories, I cannot enter a mode of being that doubts the existence of modes of being. Fish states that his response to those who fear relativism is "not challenging, but consoling—not to worry" (1980, 321). Once one accepts, first, that people hold different values and, second, that there is nothing to worry about in recognizing this, the next issue is how one can not merely live next to others who hold different concepts of the Good but live with others.

The answer, I believe, lies in the sophistic concept of *nomos* and, in turn, the ability to translate one's own concept of the Good into the *nomos* of others. If one accepts that one cannot be a relativist, then one can believe that translating one's idea of the Good into the *nomos* of another does not lead one to accept that alien worldview. Instead, one cannot change worldviews as one can change clothes: the values held are so tied into the way one exists in the world that a transformation in worldview represents an extraordinary life-transforming event. One can hold in abeyance one's worldview to understand how another sees existence, but to live one's life in accordance with that other worldview is simply not something human beings can do. To return to my opening example, the *nomos* of the group I was talking to was different from my own (which lacks the mythic meaning of the Christian vision of God's relation to the world), but because this worldview is known to me, I could translate my own concerns about physician-assisted suicide into their concerns. Lacking this knowledge, I would have to resort to an argument that moves purely from rights, one that does not hold as much meaning to this group as an appeal to the concept of caring for the suffering of others.

We in medical ethics must become self-conscious as well of the *nomos* of Western medicine and of bioethics. Here the work of a variety of social scientists has been particularly helpful. Charles Bosk (1979) examines the way physicians "manage" their failures. Robert Zussman (1992) looks at the way moral decisions are made in intensive care. Renée Fox and Judith Swazey (1978) examine the culture around organ transplants. Ethnographers such as Fox, Swazey, Arthur Kleinman, Patricia Marshall, and Barbara Koenig point out the distinctly American character of bioethics and how it affects the way we "do" bioethics. One feature of the bioethics field not often noted is that we have tended to move it forward through a battle of paradigms: principlism against contextualism, care perspective versus the justice perspective, casuistry versus communitarianism. Bioethicists do not tend to see one paradigm adding to another; instead, we tend to see approaches in diametric opposition to others. There is a sense within bioethics that we could solve all our moral problems if only we could uncover the master paradigm. Part of the *nomos* of American bioethics includes a fixation on constructing paradigms.

Of Witches, Unicorns, and Rights

I would like to return briefly to the issue of rights in moral discussions. What could be called a backlash has arisen against the concept of rights in moral philosophy. Mary Ann Glendon (1991) argues that Americans are obsessed with "rights talk" and this, in turn, has seriously impoverished our moral language. Warren Reich finds rights language lacking because of (1) the difficulty in identifying the duty-bearers, (2) a tendency for rights to be adversarial, and (3) the abstractness of the framework (1987, 282–283). Fox and Swazey observe that in American bioethics:

The concept and language of "rights" prevail over those of "responsibility" and "obligation" in bioethical discourse, and the term "duty" does not appear often in the bioethical vocabulary.... The strongest appeals to responsibility are concentrated on requirements for the protection and promotion of individual rights (Fox and Swazey 1984, 354).

MacIntyre in *After Virtue* challenges the notion that "human rights" exist even: "there are no such rights, and belief in them is one with belief in witches and in unicorns" (1981, 69).

Concerning the narrative with which I began this essay, it would seem that appealing to rights does not persuade audiences such as the Methodist congregation described. I find the antirights arguments compelling, especially since so many of those making this argument wish simply to supplement our moral languages. In discussing end-of-life issues with different generations of Thai Buddhists in the Chicago area, I was struck by the lack of rights language among foreign-born Thai-Americans and the tendency of the generation born in the United States to speak almost exclusively in this way. In this single temple community, two separate *nomoi* existed, different in generation and thus experience. The foreign-born Thai-Americans often argued with each other through general concepts of the family and their shared belief in a Buddhist worldview; the American-born group tried to persuade each other through an appeal to conflicting rights. I am not sure if MacIntyre would put the rights talk and the metaphysical talk on the same level as the unicorns and witches, but in some cultures those entities certainly have a reality to the people who believe in them. In a similar way, I believe that for most Americans, people have rights in the same manner they have a spouse, have a pain, have concerns, have faith. Simply stating that rights are an illusion does not seem a more productive way of countering the American-born Thai-Americans than it would be to argue against the reality of Buddha's teachings to the foreign-born group.

To abandon rights language may seem a good way to provide a more complex view of moral problems in the academic *nomos*, but in order to apply one's moral concepts (as I believe has been the objective of bioethics) in the public arena, one must use rights language. I do not think that if the *kairos* was different—that is, if I had been addressing the issue of physician-assisted suicide to a group of Christians, Buddhists, and Muslims—my reference to the Christian *nomos* would have been helpful. Instead, the right to practice religion, I suspect, would be a far better way of making this argument. One wonders how far MacIntyre would get if he was addressing a group of contemporary New Age witches on the issue of communitarianism. One would suspect that the dialogue would be odd in that they would agree on the existence of his abstract concepts but he would seem unable to acknowledge their existence.

Conclusion: Persuasion and Bioethics

In this discussion, I have argued that the sophistic perspective on persuasion and moral discourse provides important insights for bioethics. The sophists assisted the youth of Greece to work within the new democracy of the time. Youth's ability to function within the new power base was rooted in their ability to persuade others of the correctness of their positions. Power was gained not through force, money, or birthright but through gaining the support of the majority. I mention the tie between the sophists and democracy because it seems that although bioethicists claim that they do their philosophical thinking "in the trenches," the field has become insulated from average conversations on moral matters outside of the clinical setting. We have spent little time talking with the public who may employ rights language or perhaps are persuaded by a different *nomos*. The sophists came to their opinions through their travels throughout the various city-states, and it seems that bioethicists should also begin to travel and encounter those whose worldview forces the discipline to construct new ways of talking to one's neighbors. I hope that this essay has been able to defend my actions with the Christian community and to persuade others of the importance of persuading others.

References

Beauchamp, T. L., and J. F. Childress. 1994. *Principles of Biomedical Ethics*. New York: Oxford University Press.

Bosk, C. L. 1979. *Forgive and Remember: Managing Medical Failure*. Chicago: University of Chicago Press.

Callahan, D. 1984. "Autonomy: A Moral Good, Not a Moral Obsession." *Hastings Center Report* 14(5): 40–42.

Crowley, S. 1989. "A Plea for the Revival of Sophistry." *Rhetoric Review* 7: 318–334.

Emanuel, E. J. 1991. *The Ends of Human Life*. Cambridge, Mass.: Harvard University Press.

Engelhardt, H. T. 1996. *The Foundations of Bioethics*. 2d ed. New York: Oxford University Press.

Enos, R. L. 1976. "The Epistemology of Gorgias' Rhetoric: A Re-examination." *Southern Speech Communications Journal* 42: 35–51.

Fish, S. 1980. *Is There a Text in This Class? The Authority of Interpretive Communities*. Cambridge, Mass.: Harvard University Press.

Foss, S. K. 1989. *Rhetorical Criticism: Exploration & Practice*. Prospect Heights, Ill.: Waveland Press.

Fox, R. C., and J. P. Swazey. 1978. *The Courage to Fail*. Chicago: University of Chicago Press.

Fox, R. C., and J. P. Swazey. 1984. "Medical Morality Is Not Bioethics: Medical Ethics in China and the United States." *Perpsectives in Biology and Medicine* 27: 336–360.

Geertz, C. 1989. "Anti Anti-relativism," 12–34 in *Relativism: Interpretation and Confrontation*, ed. M. Krausz. Notre Dame, Ind.: University of Notre Dame Press.

Glendon, M. A. 1991. *Rights Talk*. New York: Free Press.

Guthrie, W. K. C. 1971. *The Sophists*. Cambridge: Cambridge University Press.

Havelock, E. A. 1964. *The Liberal Temper in Greek Politics*. New Haven: Yale University Press.

Jarratt, S. C. 1991. *Rereading the Sophists: Classical Rhetoric Refigured*. Carbondale: Southern Illinois University Press.

Kuczewski, M. G. 1997. *Fragmentation and Consensus: Communitarian and Casuist Bioethics*. Washington, D.C.: Georgetown University Press.

MacIntye, A. 1981. *After Virtue: A Study in Moral Theory*. Notre Dame, Ind.: University of Notre Dame Press.

Marcus, G. E., and M. M. J. Fischer. 1986. *Anthropology as Cultural Critique*. Chicago: University of Chicago Press.

Poulakos, J. 1984. "Rhetoric, the Sophists, and the Possible." *Communication Monographs* 51: 215–225.

Poulakos, J. 1993. "Terms for Sophistical Rhetoric." 53–74 in *Rethinking the History of Rhetoric*, ed. T. Poulakos. Boulder, Colo.: Westview Press.

Reich, W. T. 1987. "Caring for Life in the First of It: Moral Paradigms for Perinatal and Neonatal Ethics." *Seminars in Perinatology* 11(3): 279–287.

Untersteiner, M. 1954. *The Sophists*. Oxford: Basil Blackwell.

Weaver, R. M. 1953. *The Ethics of Rhetoric*. Chicago: Henry Regnery.

Zussman, R. 1992. *Intensive Care: Medical Ethics and the Medical Profession*. Chicago: University of Chicago Press.

6
Philosophical Therapy, Ancient and Modern

Julia E. Annas

In the ancient Greek and Roman world, a widespread model for philosophy, especially in the Hellenistic period, after Aristotle, is that of *therapy*, with the philosopher standardly compared to a doctor. The roots of this idea are older, but in later Greek philosophy the idea is taken for granted. Here is a statement of it by Chrysippus, the second founder of Stoicism after Zeno.

It is not true that whereas there is an art, called medicine, concerned with the diseased body, there is no art concerned with the diseased soul, or that the latter (art) should be inferior to the former in the theory and treatment of individual cases. Therefore just as the physician of the body must be "inside," as they say, the affections that befall the body and the proper cure for each, so it is incumbent on the physician of the soul to be "inside" both of these (things) in the best possible way. And a person might understand that this is so, since the analogy with them was set up at the start. For the correlative affinity with them will also make evident to us, as I think, the similarity of the cures and in addition, the analogy that the two kinds of healing have with each other. (Chrysippus, quoted by Galen)[1]

This passage makes the point, by the way, that ancient academic prose can be just as awful as modern academic prose; Chrysippus was a famously bad writer. We can see here that he takes it for granted that the philosopher can be compared to the doctor; the philosopher cures the soul of what troubles it just as the doctor cures the body. A point of comparison which he takes to be important is that both of them must be "inside," as he puts it, what has gone wrong; they must understand what is troubling the patient, from the patient's point of view, if they are to be able to cure it.

Nowadays, of course, philosophers do not set themselves up as doctors of the soul. Most philosophers would regard the idea as strange, probably pretentious and even harmful. We claim, as philosophers, to do various things—clarify ideas, solve puzzles, get students to think about problems. To present ourselves as able to "cure" problems not only seems to lay claim to an expertise that most of us would hesitate to say we possessed, but it seems also to presuppose that those who come to us already have something wrong with them—an idea that would probably offend most of our students.

What, then, do we make of the ancient idea that the philosopher is, in important ways, like the doctor? This idea is probably familiar to many through Martha Nussbaum's well-known book *The Therapy of Desire* (1994), in which she discusses the therapeutic aspects of the best-known philosophies of the Hellenistic period—Stoics, Skeptics, and Epicureans. Some of us may have the thought, voiced by Bernard Williams,[2] that philosophy as therapy—as something that can actually help people overcome problems and live their daily lives—is not an idea that we can take seriously and, to the extent that ancient philosophies adopted this model as part of their self-conception, we are bound to find them alien and have difficulty taking them seriously.

Whether we find this a reasonable reaction will, of course, partly depend on what we think philosophy is. Someone whose model of philosophy is the rigorously analytical dissection of logical problems will probably disdain the idea that this could help or cure anybody. But we would have to have an extremely narrow and unsympathetic conception of philosophy to think that doing philosophy is utterly irrelevant to the way we live our lives. If we try to get our students to think for themselves rather than handing over what we think are correct answers, it is because we think that the former, rather than the latter, is a better lesson for them to learn and apply in the way they approach problems that they will face in their lives. Even if we shrink from thinking that we can "cure" our students, we surely think that their philosophy courses are not just intellectually interesting for them but also of some use in their lives. This is true, at any rate, for most teachers of ethics courses.

The major problem in our taking seriously the therapy model for philosophy, I think, is less our conception of philosophy, which in many ways is surprisingly continuous with ancient philosophy, as with our conception of therapy and what the doctor does. Obviously, whatever it is that philosophy does for you cannot be compared with going to the doctor with an infection and being prescribed an antibiotic. Unsurprisingly, it is aspects of ancient medical practice which are being appealed to in the idea that the philosopher is like a doctor, and many of these are unfamiliar or alien to us, though I suggest by the end of this discussion that they may have more appeal for us than we might be inclined at first to suppose.

Ancient medicine has a long tradition, from the fifth century B.C. beginnings of the Hippocratic corpus to the late Roman Empire; moreover, many different schools of medical thought flourished. During the heyday of the therapy analogy for philosophy, the main schools of medical theory—Rationalist, Empiricist, and Methodist—existed in competition, fighting for both theoretical prominence and for patients. So there is no one tradition of medical theory or practice that can be appealed to.

Moreover, as soon as we raise the issue of the analogy of philosophy and medicine, we confront a frustrating fact about method. The analogy is one that philosophers welcome and find obvious, but it is not one that interests the doctors, who do not point out that what they do is like what philosophers do with their arguments.[3] Perhaps on some points at least philosophers idealize medical practice in taking it to be analogous to their own practice. It is unlikely, however, that they would invent wholesale about what doctors do in order to present themselves as a kind of doctor; an analogy that everyone can see to be false is one that will fail. The therapy model offered by philosophy, however, continued robustly for centuries. On this point, therefore, the philosophers are, in a broad sense, right about the relevance for them of medical practice.[4]

I will begin with one point on method that is very important for philosophers who make the analogy; it emerges in Plato's dialogue *Charmides*. Socrates has been told that the boy Charmides is suffering from headaches and says that he knows a cure, a particular herb; but it will not work unless you also recite a spell. He then begins to expand on what the spell is.

You see, Charmides, it's the sort of spell which cannot cure the head alone. Perhaps you too have heard what good doctors say when a patient comes to them with sore eyes. They say, I think, that they cannot attempt to heal his eyes alone, but that they must treat his head too at the same time, if his sight is to recover. They say too that to think that one could ever treat the head by itself without the whole body is quite foolish. On that principle, then, they apply their regimens to the entire body and attempt to treat and heal the part in conjunction with the whole. You do realize that this is what they say and that this is in fact the case, don't you? (Plato, *Charmides* 156b3–c6)

Socrates expands further on what a spell would have to be like to work. He claims to have got this one, when in the army, from a Thracian doctor, who claimed that Greek doctors were on the right track but did not go far enough:

… just as one shouldn't try to heal the eyes without the head, or the head without the body, so one shouldn't try to heal the body without the soul either; and that this is the reason why many diseases baffle doctors in Greece—because they ignore the whole, which they ought to take care of, since if the whole is not well, it is impossible for part of it to be so.[5] (Plato, *Charmides* 156e1–6)

Here Socrates is clearly expanding imaginatively on the common practice of accompanying a cure with a magic spell, and he goes on to suggest that the real spell that cures the whole person is nothing less than philosophical discussion. I am interested here not in this nice but fanciful idea but in the ascription to good doctors of a holistic method—that they cure a particular ailment not in isolation but in the context of the study of the whole body. Socrates's expansion on this to include the soul as well takes the familiar Greek form of ascribing wisdom to the foreigner. Presumably, however, some Greek doctors were willing to talk about the soul as well as the body, or Socrates's reference would lack sense. After all, the ordinary Greek conception of the soul is simply of that which makes a living thing be alive. For the general use of holistic procedure, Socrates appeals to "good doctors," but we can find no exact reference.[6]

The Stoics took over this idea of holistic method—of examining the entire body when seeking a cure for a particular diseased part—not just into the idea of what philosophy does generally but into a specific part of their ethics, their theory of the emotions. Stoics view an emotion as involving a false belief because they think that emotions always involve a false estimation of the objects of our emotions. They compare emotions to diseases, explaining our tendency to emotion by the overall unsatisfactory state of our psychological health. It is because of overall psychological weakness that we give in to emotion on particular occasions. The standard example of this is Menelaus, who was determined to punish Helen but crumbled in the face of her beauty because of his overall weak and irresolute character.[7]

The idea that a particular diseased part of the body can be cured only in the context of an examination of the entire body goes naturally with another very basic assumption of ancient medicine, namely, that health is conceived of as a matter of overall balance and harmony of all the elements of the body. This idea is first found in the words of doctor and preSocratic philosopher Alcmaeon of Croton. In a famous fragment, we find his belief that

> ... health is conserved by egalitarianism (*isonomia*) among the powers—wet and dry, cold and hot, bitter and sweet and the rest—and that autocracy (*monarchia*) among them produces illness; for the autocracy of either partner is destructive. And illness comes about *by* an excess of heat or cold, *from* a surfeit or deficiency of nourishment, and *in* the blood or the marrow or the brain. It sometimes occurs in them from external causes too—water of a particular kind, or locale, or fatigue, or constraint or something else of that sort. Health is the proportionate blending of the qualities. (Alcmaeon, frag 4)[8]

Here we find that although external factors are relevant, health or the loss of it depends on the correct balance of the body's own powers. Later this idea developed into the view that health depends on the correct balance of the four "humours," which was its most influential and lasting version.[9]

This idea is, of course, familiar (perhaps overfamiliar) to us through Plato's extensive use of the idea in the *Republic*, where he uses health of the body as an analogy for virtue as the harmony and health of the soul. We might suspect that in the *Republic* this view of bodily health is already somewhat influenced by the desired parallel with the soul. However, we can find the idea readily enough elsewhere—in a passage in the *Sophist*, for example, where bodily sickness and ugliness are said to be kinds of ways in which the body is afflicted by disproportion. (Slightly later, gymnastics is said to be a remedy for ugliness, so Plato must be thinking of people who are out of shape rather than facially unattractive.) "Presumably," says the Eleatic Visitor, the main speaker, "you regard sickness and discord (*stasis*) as the same thing, don't you?... Do you think that discord is just dissension among things that are naturally of the same kind, and arises out of some kind of corruption (*diaphthora*)?... And ugliness is precisely a consistently unattractive sort of disproportion?" (Plato *Sophist*)[10]

This is a powerful, intuitive picture of health and disease and, as R. J. Hankinson (1995) points out, its success in some measure explains why ancient doctors never developed the idea that disease is transmitted by infection. Although the ancient world certainly had a transmission model to hand, in the idea of pollution, doctors were never moved to postulate the idea that disease could be transmitted from one person to another. This occurred partly because they lacked a convincing mechanism (as did all doctors until the discovery of germs) but also because of the intuitive appeal of the idea of health as a balance and harmony of elements. Disease, consequently, was viewed as upsetting this balance. Hankinson (1995) writes:

Health, then, is a balance of key bodily forces; disease occurs when that balance has been upset, usually by facts to do with the patients' regimen.... Almost all of ancient medicine is allopathic in conception.... And while there were many variations on this basic theme, and one or two departures from it ... all ancient doctors who busied themselves in any degree with theoretical issues ... thought of disease as some form of mechanical interference with the body's proper functioning. Either some humour gets out of hand, or some blockage prevents normal operation.... Galen, whose exemplification of this style of explanation (and of the corresponding therapy) dominated medicine until the Renaissance (and in some respects much later) even defines disease as the impairment of some natural function.

This model of health and disease is manifestly very different from ours. It is tempting to think that, given our knowledge of germs and infection (not to mention the vastly better understanding we have of the biological and chemical basis of bodily conditions), the ancient model is simply useless, and can cast no light on any notion of philosophy useful for us. But this would, be premature. Clearly, the idea of health as harmony and balance of bodily elements is of no use if you have to go to the doctor with a broken leg. Now we find it of no use when we go to the doctor with pneumonia or jaundice. But it does not follow that the model has no resonance for us at all; although it does not serve as a model of health and disease in general, we shall see that in some cases we, as well as the ancients, can see the point of what ancient philosophers were appealing to in making their analogy.

The ancient model of health and disease has two important implications for the relation of patient and doctor. The first springs from the point that disease is not regarded as an invasion of the body from outside but as some kind of internal blockage or failure. Because of this, it cannot be understood without understanding the entire system within which there has been such a failure or blockage (as with the Stoic account of the emotions). Nor can it be properly explained, without dealing with the entire system. Plato emphasizes this in another passage in the *Sophist* (230c5–d4): Doctors who work on the body think it can't benefit from any food that's offered to it until what's interfering with it from inside is removed. The Visitor infers from this the analogous case of the soul: you will gain no benefit from learning new knowledge unless your soul has previously been purified and cleansed by having someone refute and remove your false beliefs.

This point about treatment of the whole system emerges in the stress, among the medical writers on "regimen" as part of a cure. As well as treatments such as bleeding and purging, which themselves are aimed at improving overall state rather than specific problem, doctors pay great attention to diet and overall regimen of the patient's life.[11] These treatments seem strange to us because we are more used to the very different model of illness as an invasion of the body from without, by viruses or microbes, and hence of cure as a localized response, by means of antibiotics or the like, to this localized disturbance. In the modern view, overall health is a background to both invasive disease and counteracting cure. Within the ancient model, disease, even if local, already is a loss of overall health.[12]

How do we understand disease and cure using this model? Suppose you go to the doctor complaining of fatigue and shortness of breath. The doctor examines you and tells you that your heart is under stress. This is not an isolated fact about you, she points out: you are grossly overweight, eat and drink too much, take no exercise, and smoke heavily. It is quite clear here that and how your overall state is contributing to your problem. Moreover, the doctor cannot cure the problem in isolation from the overall state. Whatever she prescribes will not get rid of your problem unless you also make a complete overhaul of your regimen and living habits. You need, for a start, to eat and drink less, to eat low-cholesterol and low-salt food, stop smoking, and regular exercise. If you are not willing to do all this, then the doctor cannot successfully deal with your problem. The model of health as an overall condition, in other words, brings with it the idea that you are partly responsible for at least some of the things that go wrong if you have brought your overall condition into a bad state. It is up to you to eat reasonably, exercise, and so on; if you do not, you cannot be very surprised if you experience a failure of health. Obese smokers can hardly be surprised when they get heart problems. Just as you are partly or largely responsible for bringing about a failure of your overall health, so you are partly or largely responsible for regaining your health by undertaking an overall revision of your habits and way of life; nothing short of this will do. If you do not cooperate with the doctor by changing your habits, the doctor cannot help you.

This point is recognized relatively early by Democritus: "Men pray to the gods for health, but do not realize that they have within themselves the power to have it. By doing the opposite in weakness of will, they become traitors to their health, in the interests of their desires."[13] This is especially interesting in that Democritus also holds that philosophy is analogous to medicine: "Medicine cures the body of diseases, and wisdom clears passions from the soul." (Democritus, frag. B 31 Diels-Kranz fr B 31).

Secondly, even though you need the doctor when you are ill and cannot manage on your own, you do not just hand the problem over to the doctor to deal with while you carry on as before. The doctor is not, according to this model, a professional who comes in and fixes what has gone wrong with part of the system without worrying about the rest. For this model, the doctor cannot understand the local problem without achieving understanding of the global condition. Nor can the doctor just fix the problem locally; she needs the patient's cooperation in reorganizing the whole of her regimen: the local problem comes from global imbalance.

Much of modern medicine, of course, does not fit this model—being prescribed an antibiotic, getting a vaccination, and so on—because we understand the nature of many diseases a great deal better and can reasonably see them as local invasions of health that can be locally cured. But there remain, as my example indicated, some failures in health that the model of overall balance fits well. Moreover, some modern doctors are becoming more sympathetic to one idea behind the overall-balance model—namely, that local invasions of the body, whether by infections or by antibiotics, do have global impact on our health, and global considerations may be more relevant than has sometimes been thought.

One corollary of this is that, just as the doctor cannot cure you without your overall cooperation, so he cannot just lay down the law as to what you should do locally to become healthy and then go away (or get you to go away). He must get you to understand what the nature of the overall problem is and how it can be tackled, or you will not understand his instructions and will not recover your health. An effective doctor will not order you about since merely following instructions to the letter will not provide the understanding you need to recover your overall health by paying the right attention to your regimen. It is scarcely enough, for example, to be told, "Lose weight" or "Stop smoking" without any attempt to tell you why you need to do this, how to put it into practice, and how it relates to other aspects of your overall condition, such as the need to exercise.

Plato is the source of many famous passages about doctors in which the implication is that these stand to the body as philosophers stand to the soul. Unfortunately, the most famous passages are rather misleading from the present perspective. In the *Republic*, we find the idea that the doctor is the expert, and that you should do what the expert says if you are not an expert, whether you understand it or not. The doctor in these passages appears, along with the navigator, as the person whose expertise entitles him to others' obedience (*Republic* vi 489a–c). This idea is repeated and reinforced in the *Statesman*, where the Eleatic Visitor says that a doctor who fails to persuade his patient and forces him to accept a new course of treatment is justified by his expertise.[14] But Plato is interested here not so much in realistic views about doctors as in a position that the expert is entitled to rule.

In the *Laws*, where Plato does not have this concern, there are two remarkable passages where he contrasts the actual practice of doctors with that of their assistants. The doctor investigates the patient's problem from the start, discussing it with the patient and his family, both learning from the patients and instructing them. He gives no instructions without obtaining the patient's consent, which ensures that the patient is persuaded to submit to the treatment before continuing it. Those who are used to more rough-and-ready methods find this ludicrous; they contend that the doctor is educating the patient as much as curing him, as though he wanted to turn him into a doctor, too.[15] Here Plato discusses methods of doctoring in a way that does not serve as a model for authoritarian expectation on the part of a ruler. (Indeed, the political moral we are to draw is quite different: rulers must *persuade* their subjects.) We can see that doctoring could serve Plato as an example of a cooperative relation between expert and nonexpert, one in which the expert must take time both to understand the whole of the nonexpert's difficulty and to ensure that the nonexpert understands his response to it.

Thus the model of health as overall balance of bodily elements has quite extensive and interesting implications for the relationship of doctor and patient. The patient needs to take responsibility for his overall condition as part of the process of curing the problem and producing a satisfactory condition of health, and the doctor needs to make the patient aware of the global problem and to get his consent and continuing cooperation in the process of therapy and his own role in it. The patient *ex hypothesi* needs the doctor; but the doctor will not be able to produce a cure without the understanding and cooperation of the patient. There is thus a real sense in which the patient has to bring about his own cure.

To return to the analogy of medicine with philosophy, we can find this illustrated in a very interesting passage comparing the philosopher with a doctor that comes from some time in the first century B.C. It is from Philo of Larissa, the last head of Plato's Academy, which until its end was, in ancient terms, skeptical—that is, its members held that philosophical activity proper consisted of arguing against the positions of others, rather than in putting forward positions of one's own. This is important for our understanding of the passage. Since Philo is an Academic, he does not hold philosophical positions of his own, and thus his lengthy comparison of a philosopher with a doctor is not just something *he* believes; it provides a framework that both he and his opponents would accept: that is, the comparison is good evidence not only that philosophers were thought of widely as having a therapeutic role, but also that it was widely thought of as taking something like this form:[16]

[P]hilo says that the philosopher is like a doctor. Just as the doctor's job (*ergon*) is first to persuade the sick person to accept the therapy and secondly to undermine the arguments of those whose advice is in conflict with this, so it is with the philosopher. Each of these tasks, then, belongs to what is called the argument of conversion (*protreptikos*), since the conversion argument encourages people towards virtue. Of this part indicates the enormous benefit of virtue, while the rest refutes those who criticize or blame or in some other way behave badly towards philosophy.

Second is what comes next in the analogy with medicine. After persuading the person to accept therapy, the doctor must apply it. Part of therapeutics[17] is removing the causes that are producing illness, and part in installing what is productive of health. It is similar with this branch of knowledge; after the conversion part, [the philosopher] attempts to apply what is therapeutic, and to this end applies considerations which motivate the person, in two parts. He applies argument to eliminate the false beliefs which have come about, due to which the soul's judging faculties have become ill, and then argument to install beliefs which are sound. Second, therefore, is the topic of good and bad things; conversion is about this and comes about by means of it.

The third part of philosophy is again analogous to the third part of medicine. [M]edicine's whole effort is directed at its end, that is health, and philosophy's whole effort at happiness. Following the argument about ends is the argument about lives. With medicine it is not enough to introduce health; there is also a need to provide instructions (*parangelmata*) about health; people who pay attention to these will keep the good condition of their bodies. Similarly with one's life there is a need for some principles (*theoremata*), through which one will be able to keep to one's end.[18]

The doctor's first step is to persuade the patient that something is wrong with him, that the doctor is right about what it is, and that other doctors are wrong. Then she must persuade the patient to undergo therapy of a particular kind to remove the source of the problem and introduce what will enable a cure to be accomplished. This is followed up by advice, which will of course differ from case to case, as to how successfully to carry out the policies designed to produce health and to keep healthy once the therapy is successful. If we are to apply the point, we must ignore the many cases in which the Greeks would not have succeeded in producing a cure this way, and think of a kind of case where it would. The obese heavy smoker with chest pains has first to become convinced—really convinced—that he has a problem, that his way of life is not just one alternative among others, but one that is working badly and will predictably lead to severe illness or death. Then, he must be convinced to do what is necessary to remove the bad condition: diet, give up smoking, exercise. Thirdly, he must solidify this result by acquiring and living by various rules that sustain this condition: he must adopt a new way of life, with different ways of exercising, eating, and so forth, and stick to this.

The Philo passage provides an attractive picture of the doctor-patient relationship. Nowadays, even obese smokers tend to find doctors telling or ordering them what to do, presenting themselves as entitled by professional expertise to lay down the law as to the rules the patient must follow. The ancient picture (which of course may be idealized—and, as stressed, we are taking our lead from the philosophers rather than actual doctors) is more cooperative: the doctor is aware at every point that if the patient ceases to follow the advice, the therapy will not be successful, and thus the patient must be convinced all along the line. Philo, as head of Plato's Academy, may have approved of Plato's passage in the *Laws* about doctors educating their patients, however pointless this might seem to more ruthlessly practical-minded people.[19]

Philo takes the philosophy/medicine analogy to be relevant to moral philosophy and has nothing to say about logic or metaphysics. How well does it even fit moral philosophy? In ancient terms, it fits it well (presumably a reason for the widespread acceptance of the analogy implicit in Philo's use of it). The ancients thought of moral philosophy as beginning with what I have called in the opening of *The Morality of Happiness* (Annas 1993) "the entry point for ethical reflection." The assumption is that at some point, each of us will begin to reflect on our life—how it is going and whether we think that our priorities are the right ones, or whether we should live differently. Puzzling about ethics is not assumed to begin from nothing or to have no developed views to contend with; it is what someone does who is already adult, or at any rate adolescent, and thus already equipped with a set of ethical beliefs and habits. The philosopher's task is to show the person who has begun to reflect in this way that yes, she does indeed have a problem and that philosophical reflection and theory are needed for a satisfactory solution to her reflections. Here we might feel that an initial worry returns. Is this not arrogant? Why are not ordinary ethical beliefs all right the way they are? It is now clear, however, that there is not much distance between ancient and modern philosophy on this issue: I cannot think of any major ethical theory which holds that the ethical beliefs held by ordinary people are all fine as they stand, that nobody should worry that her ethical beliefs might be problematic, and that moral philosophy should not alter them in any way.

Ethical reflection is supposed to have practical results; thinking philosophically is supposed to change your life. The result of engaging in ethical reflection is taken to be like a cure in that your overall intellectual state is now satisfactory rather than unsatisfactory, and you now see your way to an answer for problems that troubled you. You have thought about your views overall, and have at least begun to discard beliefs that you now find to be false, as well as attitudes based on them. If you do not change yourself in response to ethical reflection, then it was pointless to embark on it. This is a point common to ancient theories that see themselves as therapeutic; Epicureans, Stoics, and Skeptics all have differing views as to what beliefs will cause distress to ordinary people, and what the theory requires that will render them free from that distress. But it is not alien to many modern conceptions of moral philosophy, which may not use the language of cure but which certainly assume that the ethical beliefs of ordinary people are faulty, which will emerge in inadequate responses to ethical problems, and that learning the correct theory will lead to living differently and in a way that the person will characterize as an improvement.

Philo is open about the point that the philosopher, in persuading people that they need to think about ethics and ethical theory, will employ exhortation and criticism of others. We might think that exhortation has no place in philosophy, and it is true that analytical philosophy avoids open appeals to rhetoric; but even the most austerely analytical approach to ethics will employ something analogous. Commonly, introductions to ethics get the student or reader to focus on problem cases in order to convince her that she needs to think about such problems and think about them philosophically. Moreover, books on ethics, whether introductory or advanced, criticize some theories and present others as rationally preferable, and will present grounds for accepting some theories rather than others. Moral philosophy takes it for granted that ethics is a disputed area and that no theory can be presumed to get general acceptance. Not only do thoughtful people have to be persuaded that they should think philosophically about ethical problems, but they have to be faced with the fact that there is a number of competing theories and that puzzlement is succeeded not by authoritative reassurance but by the need to think rationally about the advantages and disadvantages of a number of options.

The second and third stages in Philo follow up what happens when the student realizes that his own ethical reflection has been inadequate and that he needs to learn about ethics in order to improve his own values. The philosopher uses arguments to show what is wrong with some theories and also to support others—in particular, the one that he believes to be the best theory. And finally, there is followup. The philosopher does not assume that one philosophy course, say, will turn an earnest but confused student into someone who thinks clearly about ethics and has a well-reasoned set of values to live by. So as well as arguments to convince the student as to the correctness of the theory, more detailed work is required on the theory and on the ways in which it is applied in everyday life. We need to go on learning and deepening our understanding of our ethical theory and the numerous ways in which holding it affects, and changes, our lives.

Nowadays we are likely to be suspicious of the implication in the philosophy/medicine analogy that the philosopher has the correct answer, just as the doctor has the right cure. But it is not so clear that we should be frightened of this point. There are different schools of thought envisaged in the doctor case. Rationalists, Empiricists, and Methodists compete for patients, with very different approaches. The doctor believes that his theory of the disease and its treatment is the best, but so do others with competing views. The patient must consider competing arguments and show judgement in choosing one kind of treatment rather than another, and he then needs to keep up informed discussion of competing approaches. Similarly, in philosophy there are always controversies, particularly in moral philosophy. Few philosophers have no commitment to the superiority of their own theory, but they are aware that there is little agreement and that they will always be trying to convince people against the background of conflict. Moreover, because the conflict continues, it is not enough to make an informed decision at the start and stick to it; new arguments and considerations are always being brought forward, and you need to keep abreast of these to feel that you are holding your ethical views rationally rather than merely relying mindlessly on past convictions.

I also think that some interesting points emerge from the Philo passage, and, in general, from the appeal of the ancients to therapy as a model for ethical philosophy at least. The model takes seriously two points that can be neglected in modern moral philosophy and some ways it is taught. One is that we do not come to ethics a blank sheet of paper; by the time we get to doing ethical philosophy we are grown up and already have ethical habits and views. What starts us reflecting seriously about ethics is often a combination of dissatisfaction with the inadequacy of our own views and an awareness of competing ethical theories that claim to explain and remove that dissatisfaction. This is not the only way we come to do moral philosophy but it is common enough and, presumably, is generally felt to be a good way into the subject, given that introductions to moral philosophy often try to produce this dissatisfaction in students who do not already feel it by presenting them with difficult moral problems.

However, resolving the dissatisfaction we feel is not a simple matter. To think seriously about moral philosophy requires not just a local puzzling-out of a few problems but thinking radically about one's values and how they hang together (or fail to). The person who takes ethics seriously has to be prepared to think profoundly about their whole system of values and the way they live their life. This is something the ancients realized and took seriously; it informs their whole view of ethical philosophy. In an obvious way, it fits their use of the therapy model. A person who comes to ethics hoping to clear up intellectual problems about abortion, say, but has not the faintest intention of letting the results affect her life is like the obese smoker who hopes to have her heart fixed without changing any of her habits. To sum up, the ancient therapy model, by stressing the importance of the whole system of our beliefs, emphasizes three critical elements: (1) the profundity and importance of philosophy—at least of ethics; (2) the way in which a commitment to it involves examining one's beliefs and values seriously; and (3) taking seriously the idea that accepting certain conclusions might imply making and sustaining deep changes in oneself.

Finally, the ancient model provides an attractive and realistic role for the philosopher. He is not a professional fixer who can come along and solve your puzzles for you, or remove from you the burden of thinking about your problems and how to solve them. Nor is he a guru figure who requires complete obedience to his demands. He is someone who can help you but who in the end helps you by enabling you to help yourself. You need him or her (or their books) to get the process going, given that it is unlikely that most people wil be able to reflect for themselves in the way required to get them to see that their own lives, and their understanding of them, are unsatisfactory. But philosophy is not a source of pat answers or local cures, and people who think it is are misunderstanding its nature. In fact, philosophy requires you to do the hard work for yourself. The ancient therapeutic model presents philosophy as the answer you need for intellectual problems and dissatisfactions but it is not presented as convenient or comforting. The aid it provides is austere.

We can, in the end, still find the ancient therapy model useless on the grounds that it covers so little of what we think of as central cases of disease, weakening the force of the analogy. But even if we think of the model as having limited scope, it still offers interest in two ways. It perhaps gets us to reflect on the far more technological and expertise-oriented view of doctors and therapy that we have; and the way in which a picture of disease as a local invasion of the body, to be dealt with locally, has directed attention away from some valuable aspects of the more global model of health. The idea that a philosopher is a doctor of the soul may lead us to rethink some of our views about health.

It may also perhaps make us think again about philosophy, particularly the claim that we cannot take seriously the idea of philosophy as therapy nor the ancient philosophies that conceived of themselves in this way. Once we see what picture of therapy the ancient philosophies espoused, we can see that it does not turn philosophy into a quick fix for our problems—something that would indeed be implausible. Rather, it gives us a picture of philosophy as something important and central to us and to our well being, and as the only finally satisfactory way of answering problems that trouble us. The answers are difficult and disputed, and while we need philosophers and their theories, they do not remove the need to think about central questions for ourselves. Just as we need the doctor, but must take his advice over into the whole way we live our lives if we are to get better, so we may have to be stirred to philosophical thought by problems and to learn from others, but we must, in the end, do the most important part of the work ourselves if we are to get any benefit and to live lives that are improved.

Notes

1. Chrysippus, quoted by Galen in *On the Doctrines of Hippocrates and Plato* (*PHP*), v, 2, 21–25, translated by Phillip de Lacy.

2. See his exchange with Richard Sorabji on Stoic philosophy as psychotherapy in Sorabji 1996.

3. Galen is an exception here, being both a doctor and someone with philosophical interests (though as a philosopher he is less than impressive). His short treatise, *The Best Doctor Must Be a Philosopher*, values philosophy for the methodological understanding of medicine that it provides. Longrigg 1993 discusses various ways in which philosophy influenced ancient medicine. Ludwig Edelstein discusses the therapeutic analogy to be found in both disciplines toward the end of "Ancient Philosophy and Medicine" (1967), emphasizing that philosophy may come to unwelcome conclusions, just as a medical cure may hurt. He takes the analogy, moreover, to have more authoritarian implications for the role of the doctor than I do.

4. For actual medical attitudes, the Hippocratic corpus is a valuable source.

5. I have used the translation of *Charmides* by Donald Watt in the Saunders edition, substituting "spell" for Watt's "charm."

6. Similarly, in *Phaedrus* (270c), Hippocrates tells us that we cannot understand the body (never mind the soul) without understanding the nature of the whole. Opinions differ as to whether "the whole" is the whole body or the whole universe; see Phillips 1973, 30–32.

7. Stoics differed as to whether the overall state of the person who succumbs to emotion should be described as being like that of a person whose constitution is sickly and already to some extent undermined by disease, or like that of a person whose body is healthy but prone to disease of various kinds, particularly of intermittent kinds. See Galen, *PHP* v 2, for the differing views of the early Stoic Chrysippus and the later Stoic Posidonius on this point.

8. Alcmaeon, frag 4 (Diels-Kranz 24), translated by Jonathan Barnes (1987, 90). The fragment comes from Aetius (Diels-Kranz 442).

9. The humoural theory is found in the Hippocratic treatise *The Nature of Humans*, possibly influence by Empedocles; see Longrigg 1993, ch. 4.

10. *Sophist* (227d13–228a11), translated by Nicholas White.

11. Cf. Longrigg 1993, 53: "[A]s a result of the 'balance' theory, dietetics, in its widest sense, was accorded a role of primary importance within Greek medicine. The doctor, to restore health and redress the imbalance, would prescribe for the patient not only a specific diet (in the modern sense) but also a comprehensive regimen of life." Many of the treatises in the Hippocratic corpus reflect this concern.

12. Cf. Phillips 1973, 75, where he distinguishes three epochs in therapy:

... the first, when disease was ascribed to invading demons, the second, when it was thought to arise from a lack of balance among the humours, and the third, when new invaders of the body were discovered in the form of microbes and viruses.... Incantations or other forms of magic were used against the demons; bleeding, purging, emetics and diet were intended to remedy the imbalance among the humours; and now antiseptics and antibiotics are employed against the hostile parasites that are seen to penetrate the body. On the assumptions of its age, each one of these methods has its justification."

13. Democritus (Diels-Kranz 68), B 234. Cf. "A Regimen for Health" in *Hippocratic Writings*, ed. Lloyd 1978, 276, 12–15. "A wise man ought to realize that health is his most valuable possession and learn how to treat his illness by his own judgement."

14. Similarly, a statesman who fails to persuade recalcitrant citizens of a salutary course of action and compels them to accept it is justified by his expertise (*Statesman* 296a–297c). Along with the doctor, the ship's captain is introduced as an example of expertise, as in the *Republic*. In the *Statesman*, the expertise of the individual ruler is defended against the rule of law as being sensitive to the particular case, and therefore more accurate and correct, whereas law, being general, often applies inadequately to particular cases.

15. *Laws* IV.720c–e, IX.857c–d. This method is contrasted with that of the assistants, who are slaves and are doctors to slaves. Since slaves do not have control over how they spend their lives, but have to minister to those of their employers, there is no point in the assistants giving them anything but instructions; they do not have time for anything more elaborate.

16. Philo may have had a less detached and *ad hominem* attitude to the philosophical positions he discusses than earlier Academics such as Carneades. His own position raises a number of interpretative problems that I cannot go into here. However, this does not affect the point that it would be pointless for Philo to discuss at length a philosophical framework that was not both widely accepted and the framework for philosophical discussion.

17. Translating [*tou men therapeutikou*] omitted by Heeren and Wachsmuth, restored by White.

18. Philo, as reported in Arius Didymus, in Stobaeus, *Eclogae* ii 39.24–41.7. The passage continues with the interesting point that this would suffice if everyone could be a wise person, but there are many ordinary people who lack the requisite time and leisure, so that there is also a role for potted advice in handbooks to give them continuing instruction. I have translated part of this passage in *The Morality of Happiness* and am grateful to Stephen White for letting me see his forthcoming translation of it.

19. He would be aware of the passages from the *Republic* and *Statesman*, but unlike many modern readers of Plato, would not privilege them at the expense of other dialogues such as the *Laws*.

References

Annas, J. 1993. *The Morality of Happiness*. New York: Oxford University Press.

Barnes, J. 1987. *Early Greek Philosophy*. London: Penguin.

Edelstein, L. 1967. "Ancient Philosophy and Medicine," 349–366 in L. Edelstein. *Ancient Medicine*. Baltimore: Johns Hopkins University Press.

de Lacy, P. trans. 1981. Galen, *On the Doctrines of Hippocrates and Plato*, Akademie-Verlag, Berlin, *Corpus Medicorum Graecorum* V, 4, 1, 2.

Hankinson, R. J. 1995. "Pollution and Infection: an Hypothesis Still-Born." *Apeiron* 28: 25–65.

Lloyd, G. E. R., ed. 1978. *A Regimen for Health in Hippocratic Writings*. London: Penguin.

Longrigg, J. 1993. *Greek Rational Medicine: Philosophy and Medicine from Alcmaeon to the Alexandrians*. London: Routledge.

Nussbaum, M. C. 1994. *The Therapy of Desire*. Princeton: Princeton University Press.

Phillips, E. D. 1973. *Greek Medicine*. London: Thames and Hudson.

Saunders, T., ed. 1987. *Early Socratic Dialogues*, trans. D. Watt. London: Penguin.

Sorabji, R., ed. 1996. *Aristotle and After. Bulletin of the Institute of Classical Studies*, Supplementary volume.

White, Nicholas P. trans. 1993. Plato, *Sophist*. Indianapolis, Ind.: Hackett.

II

The Heuristic Value of Classical Approaches

7

Thrasymachus and Managed Care: How Not to Think about the Craft of Medicine

Alex John London

Surely, then, no doctor, insofar as he is a doctor, seeks or orders what is advantageous to himself, but what is advantageous to his patient? We agreed that a doctor in the precise sense is a ruler of bodies, not a money-maker. Wasn't that agreed?
—Socrates in Plato's *Republic* 342d[1]

At the present time the United States is witnessing something of a crisis in the field of health care. The trust that was once a central feature of the doctor-patient relationship and a hallmark of the medical profession has been seriously eroded in recent years.[2] One particularly potent element driving this sense of distrust is a growing awareness that business and economic concerns are playing an increasingly important role in the practice of medicine and in medical decision making. On the one hand, the leaders of business and industry, along with a number of public policymakers, have spearheaded a campaign to reform what they see as traditional medicine's lavish use of resources that are becoming increasingly scarce. The increased effectiveness of our medical technology has come with an equally increased price tag, and with the ability to accomplish new medical wonders has come the realization that we may no longer be able to dispense health care on the basis of individual need without breaking the bank. On the other hand, the cost-cutting measures that many managed care organizations (MCOs) have implemented in response to these concerns have been decried for pitting the interests of doctors against the interests of patients. Those who defend the sanctity of the doctor's role as caregiver against the invidious influence of business and economic concerns argue that asking physicians to ration health care at the bedside is asking them to forsake their role as caregiver and patient advocate.

Doctors, we are told, cannot serve two masters (Levinsky 1984). As it stands, doctors, patients, politicians, businesspersons, and ethicists alike are struggling to understand the physician-patient relationship in a way that will allow them to balance the interests of the individual patient against the myriad interests with which they are now competing.

In the discussion that follows, I argue that the ancient conception of medicine as a craft (τέχνη), and of the physician as a craftsman, when properly understood, provide a way of conceptualizing the doctor's role as caregiver that will allow physicians to practice medicine within an environment of fiscal scarcity while at the same time preserving and illuminating the physician's role as caregiver and patient advocate. I also argue that this view provides a conceptual framework within which potential conflicts of interests can be exposed and, hopefully, resolved.

The idea that medicine is a craft and the physician a craftsman is as old as medicine itself. However, I will not be drawing on the Hippocratic corpus for my conception of the medical craft.[3] Instead, I begin by looking at part of Socrates's argument with Thrasymachus in Book I of Plato's *Republic*. There Socrates argues that each craft brings with it its own particular sort of benefit and that any benefit that all craftsmen receive in common must come from their practicing a common craft. For example, insofar as doctors practice the craft of medicine, they look after what is advantageous for the patient; and insofar as they look after their own benefit and earn money they practice the art of wage earning (346c–d). On its face, this argument might seem to support the view that doctors are either exclusively concerned with their patients' best interests, or they are looking after their own interests or the interests of some third party. I argue that this is not the case and that a proper understanding of the relationship among the science of medicine, political science, and what Plato calls the art of wage earning provides us with the conceptual tools necessary to tackle some of the very difficult questions surrounding the role of economics in medicine.

Crafts and the Art of Politics

Although the science and technology of medicine have changed considerably since the time of Plato, medicine still aspires to improve itself as a form of craft knowledge. For Plato, a craft is a body of knowledge (ἐπιστήμη) that ranges over a specific domain. As such, the craftsman possesses specialized knowledge about the nature of the craft's subject matter and about the relevant causal mechanisms concerning that subject matter. So, the physician possesses specialized knowledge about the functioning of the body, the proper order and condition of its parts, the ways in which those parts can be injured or afflicted, and the way in which those injuries and afflictions can be ameliorated. Second, each craft represents a power or an ability (δύναμις) to bring about a specific result within that domain (see 346a2–3). The knowledge of a craft includes the knowledge of how to use an array of specialized tools and materials in order to accomplish this goal. In the case of carpentry, various woodworking tools and various types of wood and metal are used in order to produce a house. In the case of medicine, various diagnostic devices are used in order to detect illness or injury and then therapies of different kinds are brought to bear in an effort to restore the patient's health. Third, the craftsman can give an account or explanation of these things. In the case of medicine, this means that the physician can give an account of the nature of an illness or injury, its causal origins, and can explain the mechanisms by which he or she will attempt to ameliorate the problem. Fourth, this specialized knowledge is something that is more or less uniquely possessed by practitioners of the craft. The knowledge of the best way to make excellent shoes is unique to the craft of cobbling just as the knowledge of the best ways to restore a body to its state of proper functioning is unique to the craft of medicine.

In what follows, however, I will need to make use of two additional and important features of crafts such as medicine. The first is that all other crafts are subordinated to the art of politics.[4] The second is the claim that all crafts look after the good of that over which they are set. Let me say a few words about this first feature before exploring the second.

Both Plato and Aristotle emphasize the fact that crafts are complex, interlocking social practices and that, as such, no craft operates in a social vacuum. Many crafts are subordinated to other crafts because they rely on those superordinate crafts to supply the specifications for the good they produce, to direct them as to when and where and how many such goods are to be produced, and to provide the resources with which the subordinate craft will have to work.[5] So, for example, imagine we must construct a new public building. The local blacksmith receives instructions from the carpenter as to how many of the various tools and supplies the builders will need. The carpenter, however, must first receive instructions from the architect as to what kind of structure is to be erected, in which place, at which time, and at what cost. In like manner, the architect receives this information along with the specifications for the kind of structure to be designed and built from the political body, which has decided that a need exists for the new building, that a certain sum of money should be allocated to finance its construction, and that this should be accomplished within a certain time frame.

This example highlights the hierarchical nature of the relationship between certain crafts and illustrates the way in which the quality of the work that the subordinate crafts can accomplish is often determined in part by the resources that the superordinate crafts make available to them. In our example of a public project, it falls to the most architectonic craft, the political craft, to determine the amount of resources to be allocated to the project, and each subordinate craft must fulfill its function within the constraints of the resources they are allocated.

Because crafts do not exist in a vacuum, and because the quality of the craft's work will be affected to some degree by the resource constraints under which it works, the excellence of the craftsman will be judged not by how closely her work approximates the ideal per se but by the quality of the work she is able to accomplish with the tools and supplies available.[6] As Aristotle puts it, "it is not the function of medicine to make a man healthy, but to put him as far as may be on the road to health. For it is possible to give excellent treatment even to those who will never enjoy sound health" (*Rhetoric* 1355b12–14). The reason he gives for this is that in every craft the function is not simply to produce a product but rather it is "to discover the means of coming as near such success as the circumstances of each particular case allow" (1355b10–12). Just as the most skillful cobbler is the one who makes the best shoes with the materials at hand—not the one who makes the best shoes per se—so, too, the best physician is the one who can provide the best care with the available resources.

For our purposes, the two most important features of this hierarchical relationship are (1) that often the resources available to the subordinate craft are limited or determined by the superordinate craft and (2) that the function of the craftsmen is to make the most excellent use of the available resources. In a moment I will argue that the fact that medicine is subordinated to the political art in this way is of considerable importance. First, however, I want to distinguish the relationship of medicine and politics from the relationship between medicine and the craft of wage earning. To do this we need to turn to Socrates's dispute with Thrasymachus in Book I of Plato's *Republic*.

Socrates and Thrasymachus on the Structure of a Craft

In the *Republic*, Socrates's view that justice benefits the just person as well as others is contested by Thrasymachus, a sophist who claims that justice is really the benefit of another and that only through injustice does one benefit oneself. The details of this argument are important for my purposes because I contend that at the heart of Socrates's debate with Thrasymachus is an argument about the relationship between crafts and craftsmen that will enable us to construct two competing views of the physician's relationship to third-party payers and to the patient—a Thrasymachean and a Socratic conception of medicine.

To begin with, we need to understand the level at which Socrates and Thrasymachus carry out their dispute. When Thrasymachus gives his account of justice he says first, that justice is the advantage of the stronger (338c) and second, that justice is the advantage of the established rule (339a). Socrates is quick to point out that rulers can make mistakes and that when they do, they legislate laws that are not in fact to their own advantage. By making the populace obey such laws the people are made to work against the ruler's true interests (339e). As Cleitophon suggests, Thrasymachus could reformulate his position so as to claim that the advantage of the stronger is what the stronger believes to be his advantage (340a–b). But Thrasymachus rejects this option. Instead, he offers what he calls a "strict account" of what it means to be craftsman. In the strict account, a craftsman never errs. Whenever a doctor or a politician makes a mistake it is not as a doctor or a politician that he or she makes that mistake. A ruler is a kind of craftsman, and it is just to obey the laws the ruler legislates only insofar as that person is exercising the craft of ruling (340d–341b).

In rejecting Cleitophon's proposal and opting for his own alternative view, Thrasymachus is effectively situating the discussion of the nature of justice within a larger discussion of the nature and function of a craft. If we are to understand whose advantage justice looks after, then we must understand who benefits from the exercise of the political craft. Furthermore, Thrasymachus is making a conceptual point about the nature of a craft. He recognizes that people who are physicians and rulers commonly make mistakes. For instance, after he says that no craftsman ever errs, he says: "It is when his knowledge fails him that he makes an error, and in regard to that error he is no craftsman" (340e). His claim is not that if someone makes a mistake she is not a doctor or a ruler. Doctors and rulers make mistakes all the time. His point is that when this happens it is because they have failed at their craft. Here is why.

A craft is a body of knowledge (ἐπιστήμη) that represents a power or ability (δύναμις) to bring about a specific end (346a2–3). Each craft (τέχνη) is set over (ἐπί) or concerned with some subject matter, and the function (ἔργον) of the craft is to produce or improve that over which it is set. Conceptually, then, each craft is defined in terms of its specific function (345e–346b). Bungled treatments, misdiagnoses, and even bad scientific information are not parts of the craft of medicine since the function of medicine as such is to bring about health (346a). Because a craft is defined functionally in terms of the end to be realized, the imperfections of actual practice are extrinsic to the concept of the craft. Similarly, a craftsman is someone who performs the function of realizing the end of a craft by internalizing the norms and techniques internal to that craft. The excellence of the craftsman is being able to perform the function of the craft as well as possible. Actual craftsmen can fail to realize the ends of their crafts on occasion, but this is a fact about actual people and not about the function or purpose of a craftsman qua craftsman. Therefore, Thrasymachus is not flouting common beliefs about the various craftspeople.[7] Rather, he is making a conceptual point about the relationship between a craft, a craftsperson, and the actual people who instantiate those roles. I am proposing that Thrasymachus rejects Cleitophon's suggestion because it locates the focus of the argument with the people who realize these roles and what they actually do. The suggestion is rejected because Thrasymachus's thinking is motivated in large part by a certain conception of the function of a craft and what it means to be a craftsman.

Now that we see that Socrates and Thrasymachus are arguing about the nature of a craft on a conceptual level, we can turn to the substance of their disagreement. Thrasymachus argues that those in power will make laws that benefit themselves. Democracies make laws that benefit the majority; tyrants make laws that benefit tyrants, and so on (338e). If the politician is the one who benefits from ruling, and the politician is a craftsman, then Thrasymachus seems to be committed to the thesis that it is the craftsman who benefits from the exercise of her craft. Socrates then asks: "Is a doctor in the precise sense, whom you mentioned before, a money-maker or someone who treats the sick? Tell me about the one who is really a doctor" (341c). Thrasymachus admits that the doctor is someone who treats the sick and looks after bodies. Our bodies are not self-sufficient; they have a certain virtue or excellence (ἀρετή), namely, health, and the function of medicine is to restore this virtue to bodies. For example, the virtue of the eye is sight, and the doctor's function is to restore sight to the eyes (341e–342b). Unlike those things on which crafts work, the individual crafts themselves are self-sufficient. They do not need some further craft to look after their own excellence. So Thrasymachus agrees that crafts rule over and are stronger than the things with which they are concerned (342c).

Now, we are told that he assents to this very reluctantly or with great difficulty (μάλα μόγις). His difficulty, however, is not with the truth of the premise itself but with the fact that he knows that his own position will be weakened if he accepts it. In fact, I want to suggest that this is a premise that Thrasymachus has accepted all along either explicitly or implicitly. After all, Thrasymachus claims that justice is both the advantage of the stronger and the advantage of the established rule. As Annas (1981, 40–41) points out, this seems to presume that in all cases the established rulers will be the stronger party. The premise that a craft is stronger than that over which it rules helps to explain why Thrasymachus might be led to identify the advantage of the stronger with the advantage of the rulers. Let me explain briefly.

Thrasymachus is concerned with justice on the political level as primarily predicated of laws and social institutions.[8] If part of the function of a ruler is to make laws and set up institutions that govern the organization of the rest of society, then the craft of ruling involves establishing the laws and institutions that effectively determine what is just and unjust. Because

Thrasymachus also believes that rulers rule in their own interests, he thinks that they will erect institutions and make laws that are to their own benefit. Every craft is stronger than that over which it is set in that a craft is a body of knowledge (ἐπιστήμη) representing a power or an ability (δύναμις) to bring about a specific end within a given domain (see 346a2–3). Because of their craft, craftsmen can use the implements and materials at their disposal to bring about a certain result with respect to their subject matter. Since every craft is stronger than that over which it is set, insofar as a ruler is practicing the craft of ruling, justice will turn out to be the advantage of the stronger. This, then, is not so much an empirical point about the ability of any given ruler to wield the most power in his society as it is a conceptual point about the relationship of justice to the art of politics. Justice is a property of the political institutions that are the subject matter of the craft of politics and because Thrasymachus thinks that politicians qua politicians should always legislate in their own interests, justice is the advantage of the established rulers.[9] Therefore, even if Thrasymachus did not explicitly believe that crafts rule over and are stronger than that over which they are set, this is nevertheless a belief that is latent in his own thinking about politics. He is reluctant to accept it as a premise only because he does not want to accept the conclusion of Socrates's argument. This is why, just a few lines later, we are told that "he tried to fight *this conclusion*, but he conceded in the end" (342c, emphasis added).

The conclusion he is reluctant to accept is that because each craft looks after the good of what it concerns, and because each craft rules over and is stronger than its subject matter, justice is not the advantage of the stronger. To illustrate the point, Socrates says: "Surely, then, no doctor, insofar as he is a doctor, seeks or orders what is advantageous to himself, but what is advantageous to his patient? We agreed that a doctor in the precise sense is a ruler of bodies, not a money-maker. Wasn't that agreed?" (342d). By this point the structure of the argument is clear. Thrasymachus thinks that justice is the advantage of the stronger because he believes that justice is produced by the craft of politics and that politicians legislate in their own interests. In arguing against him, Socrates has been mining Thrasymachus's own knowledge of the conceptual relationships that hold between crafts, their products, and craftspeople—namely, crafts look after the advantage of that over which they are set by making sure that those things attain the completion that is their proper virtue or excellence. And the function of the craftsman is to fulfill the function of her craft. Moreover, he is trying to show how Thrasymachus's way of thinking about politics misconstrues these relationships.

This is illustrated in the way he deals with Thrasymachus's rejoinder to his general argument. Seeing that his argument has been turned into its opposite, Thrasymachus rather rudely scolds Socrates for having missed the sense in which he takes politicians to be concerned with the welfare of their people. Politicians, he tells us, care about their citizens in the way that shepherds care about their sheep. The shepherd cares for and fattens his sheep so that either he or his employer can sell or eat them. In the end, the shepherd and the politician look after what is best for those under their care only to the extent that it serves their own overall good. As Socrates summarizes the view, "You think that, insofar as he is a shepherd, he fattens sheep, not looking to what is best for the sheep but to a banquet, like a guest about to be entertained at a feast, or to a future sale, like a money-maker rather than a shepherd" (345c). Socrates has already argued that it is the purpose of a craft to look after the good of the things that it concerns. Thrasymachus is claiming that the good of one's people, one's sheep, or one's patients is secondary or subservient to the good of the politician, shepherd, or physician, respectively. On Thrasymachus's view, although craftsmen seek to practice their craft well and must thereby look after the good of whatever it is that their craft concerns, nevertheless, their primary interest in practicing a craft is their own good.

Socrates's response is to claim that although Thrasymachus went through all the trouble of giving a strict account of what it means to be a doctor, he has not bothered to stick to this strict account when it comes to shepherds (345b–c). In other words, Socrates thinks that Thrasymachus is confounding a point about the people who actually instantiate the role of craftsman with a conceptual point about what it means to be a craftsman. If each craft has its own specific function and brings about its own particular sort of benefit by fulfilling that function, then any benefit that all craftsmen receive in common must be secured by means of some other craft (346a–d). At first, this may strike us as counterintuitive. However, the point is again a conceptual one. A craft, as such, is defined by the end that it functions to bring about. Socrates's point is that, although actual craftsmen earn money by practicing their crafts, earning money is not itself a part of their craft as such. Each actual craftsman may have to set the price of the products she produces, or set a wage for the use of her time and her skill, but this is an activity not governed by the craft itself. No amount of expertise in cobbling, as such, will make one a shrewd marketer because developing a head for business is a matter of learning a different set of skills and norms.[10] This is why the best cobbler may not make the most money; she has not mastered the art of making money as some less talented artisans may have.[11]

Both Socrates and Thrasymachus agree that politicians are craftsmen and that by exercising their craft they can produce justice in their society. However, they differ on the question of whose good the politician looks after (among other things). Because the politician is a craftsman, and all craftsman are concerned with the good of those things that their craft concerns, Socrates argues that the politician is concerned with the good of those ruled. This argument is his way of making perspicuous the distinction between practicing a craft and benefiting from the practice of that craft. It is also part of a larger attempt to show that Thrasymachus's beliefs about the role of the politician are inconsistent with his own understanding of the nature and function of crafts in general. Before trying to show how this discussion is relevant to the present state of the doctor-patient relationship, a few words follow concerning how Thrasymachus's beliefs about the role of the politician came to be inconsistent with what he himself knows about the role of a craftsman.

As Socrates points out, Thrasymachus's thinking about the role of the politician has been corrupted because he has confused the behavior or motives of some who are actual politicians with the role of the politician qua craftsman. A major motivating force behind this confusion is Thrasymachus's belief that people "desire to outdo others and get more and more" (πλεονεξίαν) and that "this is what anyone's nature actually pursues as good" (359c).[12] In this view, we are all primarily self-interested beings in competition for resources, riches, and power. This view of human nature puts pressure on the concept of a craftsman as someone who, as craftsman, is concerned with the good of those things over which his craft is set: it requires those who enact these roles to act in ways that seem contrary to their nature and that seem to be in conflict with their natural conception of the good. Thrasymachus wants to hold both that the politician, as politician, acts in accordance with his human nature and that the politician is a craftsman. This leads him to claim that the function of the politician, qua craftsman, is to look after his own advantage.[13]

Thrasymachean Tendencies in Modern Medicine

In the portion of the first book of the *Republic* we have been considering, Socrates is at great pains to disentangle the craftsman's end qua craftsman from the end of making money. Insofar as she is a doctor, a doctor is a healer of the sick and injured; insofar as she is a businessperson, a doctor seeks to support herself and earn a living. Socrates is particularly careful to show that these are conceptually distinct roles or functions and that we must not lose sight of this fact. But we have to be very careful in the way we understand this point. Socrates is not saying that physicians, as actual individuals, must be wholly altruistic. Nor is he saying that physicians cannot be concerned about their own financial well being. Remember, he says that every doctor practices two crafts, medicine and wage earning. His point is that these are two *conceptually* distinct enterprises, and although we may practice them both at the same time, we must be careful not to confound them conceptually. Socrates is not saying that we cannot practice medicine in a market economy and he is not saying that it is wrong for physicians to make money at their craft. What he is saying is that the actual physician must not lose sight of the fact that she is first and foremost a doctor. The physician's relationship with a patient must be organized around the goal of providing that patient with the most excellent medical care available. This is not a point about the resources available to a given patient; discussion of that point will follow. For now, the point is simply that the benefit a physician or her employers receives from the use of available medical resources must come either as a result of successfully administering excellent patient care or at least must not conflict with this end. When the physician's primary interest in utilizing available medical resources is her own profit or the profit of a third party, then the physician has, in effect, ceased to practice medicine and has begun to practice the craft of wage earning instead. Let me elaborate.

Some argue that a fee-for-service system provides systematic incentives for physicians to profit by overtreating their patients. As I have explained Socrates's argument so far, we could describe this as the temptation of physicians to let the practice of the craft of wage earning dictate how they practice the craft of medicine. In other words, in a fee-for-service system a systematic temptation lurks to make some individual medical decisions based not on the effect of that decision on the patient's health but on the effect of that decision on the physician's profit margin. Recognizing this potential, managed care organizations have implemented various policies meant to counterbalance these incentives and provide alternate incentives for physicians to better manage their resources. I want to suggest, however, that some of these policies make the same error in the opposite direction.

Take, for example, the practice of capitation. Under this system, an MCO allots a fixed amount of money per patient per year to its various participating health-care institutions. When physicians spend less than the capitation rate on a patient in a given year they can keep the remainder. If they spend more, the excess money must come from their own budget. The policy is intended to provide physicians with an incentive to manage their resources more efficiently and it has proved to be an effective cost-cutting tool. However, in many instances this policy has fostered a Thrasy-machean view of the craft of medicine. That is, in some cases this policy has succeeded in regulating the way doctors dispense care by focusing their attention directly on their own financial advantage when making individual treatment decisions rather than on the interests of the patient. For example, an HMO in San Antonio is reported to have paid $600 to obstetricians whose patients remained in the hospital for three days after delivery whereas physicians whose patients left the hospital within 24 hours received $1025 (Hirshorn 1986). This vast disparity between reimbursements provides a systematic pressure to discharge individual patients even when those patients may have complications. This is a Thrasymachean view of medicine because it goes beyond merely trying to motivate physicians to practice fiscally conscious medicine. Rather, it has the effect of pressuring physicians to make individual treatment decisions based not on the effect a specific decision will have on the patient's health but on the effect that decision may have on the physician's pocketbook. In this way, the conception of the patient as a vulnerable individual in need of caring medical treatment is circumscribed by the view of the patient as a budget expense and cost-containment problem.

This should not be understood as an argument holding that the practice of using incentives is inherently wrong. The point is that the use of such incentives carries an inherent risk of fostering a Thrasymachean view of medicine. If we are going to use incentives, they must not be used in such a way that they encourage the craft of wage earning to dictate the outcome of individual treatment decisions.[14] We can structure incentives so that they provide systematic motivation to practice fiscally conscious medicine that does not result in making individual treatment decisions based on their profitability for the physician. For example, decreasing the size of the disparity between reimbursements in the San Antonio HMO may decrease the incentive to put one's own financial gain before patient welfare. The losses incurred from dealing with complicated cases should be such that they prevent physicians from turning every case into an exception but not so great that they put prohibitively strong constraints on any exercise of discretion.

Similarly, many MCOs withhold a portion of a physician's salary until the end of the year in order to cover deficits in the fund of monies allocated for diagnostic tests, referral services, hospital care, and so on. Withholding large portions of a physician's salary and calculating the physician's expenditures at frequent intervals are two ways in which prohibitively stringent constraints are placed on the physician's ability to practice the craft of medicine. These are particularly Thrasymachean practices because of the Draconian manner in which they allow individual treatment decisions to jeopardize the physician's own financial interests. We can use financial incentives to encourage physicians to practice the craft of medicine before the craft of wage earning by placing smaller percentages of their salary in jeopardy or by calculating their expenditures over longer periods of time and taking account of larger numbers of patients (Orentlicher 1995). This allows the monies saved on patients incurring low costs to make up for those spent on those incurring higher costs. It also allows us to motivate physicians to provide cost-effective health care without appealing to their own financial advantage in a way that prevents the patient from appearing to be an adversary in competition with her doctor for the same scarce resources.

The point is a conceptual one: the fee-for-service environment and the practice of capitation as implemented by many MCOs encourage physicians to circumscribe their role as craftsman within the bounds of their role as wage earner. If our goal is to provide incentives for physicians to practice good medicine, then we cannot accomplish this by adopting a Thrasymachean view of medicine. If we accept this view—even tacitly—doctors will, in fact, compete with their patients, and Thrasymachus's claim that justice is a fool's game will turn into the claim that providing the best medical care is a fool's game as well. Doctors will be competing with their patients, and patients will see their doctors as competitors rather than as an ally. In both cases, the incentives are such as to encourage physicians to look after their own financial gain in their practice of medicine—thus confounding the relation between these two crafts.[15]

Setting Limits: The Interrelation of Crafts

So far I have argued that in Socrates's view of the craft of medicine, when a physician makes an individual treatment decision based not on the best interests of the patient but on the effect of a specific decision on his or her pocketbook, that physician is no longer practicing medicine and is instead practicing the craft of wage earning. Do not be misled, though. When I say this, I am not saying that we cannot practice medicine in an environment of fiscal scarcity. What I am saying, rather, is that medicine is not an isolated practice within our society. When we do not fully appreciate this fact, every attempt to curtail health-care expenditures looks like an attempt to put the wage-earning craft in control of the way we practice medicine. The tendency to reduce all economic influences on medicine to the influence of the wage earning craft pervades much of the debate concerning the need for cost containment in medicine. It is this largely unexamined assumption that lends an air of intractability to many of these problems.

The view of medicine that I have in mind, and that I want to reject as overly simplistic, is the view that Michael Walzer claims is latent in the way we treat the practice of medicine in society today. Very briefly put, Walzer sees medicine as a practice that occupies its own sphere of justice where in the distribution of medical resources is determined by the meaning of the goods that medicine provides. As such, he claims that the distributive logic inherent in our current practice of medicine "seems to be this: that care should be proportionate to illness and not to wealth" (1985, 86). By thinking of medicine as an isolated practice within our community, one that inhabits its own sphere of justice in which the allocation of resources is determined by medical need, Walzer effectively drives a conceptual wedge between health needs, on the one hand, and monetary concerns, on the other. Where the former are the lifeblood of medicine, the latter are at home in the market, and Walzer insists that the goods that are dominant in the market should not also dominate the sphere of health care.

This way of thinking about health care misrepresents the way the practice of medicine fits into our lives. It misrepresents, or perhaps fails to see, the sense in which the craft of medicine is subordinate to the art of politics or simply the political process. Both Plato and Aristotle were keenly aware of the relationship between the social practices of medicine and politics. Health is an important value in our lives. We value it in itself to the extent that, all things considered, we would rather be healthy than not. But it is not the only value in our lives and it is not necessarily the highest value. Rather, health is chiefly important because of the way it contributes to our ability to pursue the various projects and activities that give our lives a distinctive shape and meaning.[16]

For both Plato and Aristotle, politics is the discipline whose function assures that the structures of society are arranged in such a way as to allow individual citizens a fair opportunity to pursue those activities that make their lives valuable.[17] Because health is only one value among many in our lives, the craft that produces health—medicine—is not the most important craft in our lives. Health, then must not be pursued in such a way as to jeopardize our ability to pursue and engage in a panoply of other, perhaps more important, goals and activities. This means that the function of the political process is either to delegate or to oversee the delegation of resources to the various subordinate crafts according to the contribution each craft makes to the community's ability to pursue its most important goals. In other words, we each have an interest in seeing that our social resources are distributed in such a way as to preserve our ability to engage in whatever activities make our lives meaningful. We each, therefore, have an interest in ensuring that our health care reflects the importance we place on health in relation to the other goods our society values.

Because the political craft must ensure a proper distribution of resources within a community, it must set limits on the amount of money the community spends on health care. There are a number of ways this might be done. For example, the government might socialize medicine and set a fixed national health-care budget. Or it might delegate the task of curtailing health-care expenditures to companies in the private sector while maintaining oversight on the methods those companies utilize. Many important and difficult questions arise concerning the kinds of limitations that can be set on the practice of medicine and the methods that can be used to realize these limitations. For the moment I simply want to claim that the economic constraints on the practice of medicine growing out of these political realities must be distinguished from the pressures exerted on the practice of medicine by what Plato calls the craft of wage earning. In particular, the political constraints on the resources allocated to medicine can be justified by the way in which they reflect the place of medicine in the lives of the citizens. In the best possible case, decisions about the value of health care in relation to other social goods will be made by the citizens themselves. One function of the constraints that come from the practice of the craft of wage earning, however, is to ensure compliance with these general guidelines. As such, these constraints can only be justified to the extent that they succeed in maintaining compliance with the constraints set at the political level without forcing physicians to attend to their own advantage rather than the best interests of their patients.

We are now in a position to understand the sense in which the physician's role qua physician is to provide the most excellent patient care possible with available resources. In one sense, Levinsky (1984) and those with similar views are right to say that the sanctity of the physician's role as caregiver must not be violated. The doctor who does not make the most skillful use of the resources available for a patient's care is not fulfilling the physician's role as caregiver; each patient must receive skillful, knowledgeable, diligent care. However, we must not lose sight of the fact that the craft of medicine is rightly subordinated to the craft of politics and that, as such, we can justly place limits on the resources allocated to health care. This is the crucial point that Levinsky misses.

Clearly, there is a sense in which abundant resources are available for each patient—e.g., everyone with a head trauma can receive an MRI because the machine is just downstairs. In a more important sense, however, the resources available to the physician are not determined by physical proximity. As we have arranged our health-care system in the United States, the resources available to each individual patient are determined by the patient's entitlements. This is Morreim's point: "The resources owed to any particular patient are determined by the specific resource arrangement in force for that patient" (Morreim 1995, 87).[18] I am therefore arguing that a part of the doctor's role as a physician first is to determine what kind of resources are in force for a particular patient and then to make the most diligent use of those resources possible. Once we see that medicine is justly subordinated to politics, we can understand the reasons why the resources to which a patient is entitled are not simply a function of the patient's need. Rather, they are a function of the social and economic arrangements that an individual patient has undertaken for his own medical care and/or of the economic arrangements that we as a society have set up for those who cannot afford to make such arrangements.

The question as to what kinds of resources should be made available to each individual patient is, in large part, a question of public policy and, as such, I am not going to discuss it here. My point is that the new economic realities of medicine do not force us to give up our conception of doctors as craftsmen who scrupulously look after what is best for their patients. However, as Morreim points out, economic facts do force us to give up the idea that unlimited resources can be used for each individual patient. This, then, means that we must be careful about the way we understand the role physicians are going to play in the "rationing" of health care. Some argue that the resources available to physicians must be restricted by others so that the physician does not herself have to deny a patient the best possible care. As Morreim (1995, 58–60) argues quite persuasively, however, although this will work for some cases, it will not work for all. Physicians are going to have to make bedside determinations about where their medical resources can be most effectively used. But we should keep in mind that any sound rationing policy must be based on criteria of some kind.[19] In other words, although individual physicians may decide how to allocate scarce health-care dollars in particular cases, it is nevertheless necessary that these decisions be grounded in a general health policy framework of some sort. This means that we must consider general questions concerning under what kinds of circumstances what sorts of patients will be entitled to receive which treatments. Determining either what these criteria are or determining a procedure by which such criteria can be arrived at, even at the bedside, is a matter of public policy. Doctors are going to have to make bedside decisions in the sense that they are going to have to use their best medical judgment to determine which patients fit which criteria.

The point I want to stress is that in so doing, the physician is assessing whether or not a patient is entitled to receive a certain treatment modality based on precepts that have been sanctioned at a public policy level. Part of the physician's role as a craftsman requires him to ascertain the kind of resources available for a particular patient's care. Therefore, even if a public policy decision determines that physicians' use of some sort of cost-benefit analysis in deciding which Medicare patients are entitled to receive which treatments is appropriate, this should not be seen as asking physicians to violate the sanctity of their commitment to each individual patient. Even if physicians themselves must actually apply the cost-benefit analysis, they are being asked to use this method, along with medical criteria, in order to determine whether or not a patient is entitled to a certain treatment modality, given a specific policy of health-care rationing: the physician is being asked to ascertain which kinds of materials will be at her disposal in caring for a specific patient before going on to make a skillful use of those resources in treating that patient.

To say that the craft of medicine is subordinate to the art of politics is to say that medicine is not a self-sufficient social practice, isolated and unconnected from our larger social goals and activities. Rather, as Ezekiel Emanuel states, "a complete account of the purposes of the profession—a specification of its ends, a balancing of its internal ends, a balancing of its internal ends with nonprofessional ends—requires political philosophy" (1991, 29). That every physician must work always for the best interests of the patient is a value inherent in the practice of medicine itself. But in order to determine the kind of resources that will be available for the physician in a particular case, we must look to the superordinate discipline of politics. The amount of our available communal resources, the way in which they are made available, and the method by which they are distributed are questions of public policy that we each have a fundamental interest in deciding together.

This means that through the political process we must determine how health is to fit into our conception of human flourishing. How much of our resources are we willing to dedicate to health care? Under what sorts of circumstances are people to be denied certain forms of treatment? Similarly, we must ask ourselves whether MCOs should be able to make various kinds of restrictions in order to turn a larger profit. Should a global minimum of resources be available to everyone? These are political questions concerning the resources we are willing to make available for health care and the mechanisms by which these resources will be allocated or controlled. These are very different issues from the obligations that physicians have to their patients once those decisions have been made. Because we cannot formulate guidelines or policy statements that can be applied to individual cases, the judgment of the individual physician will likely play a crucial role in determining which patients are allocated which resources. Because this is true, that the framework in which they operate is just and that they make their judgments within this framework as physicians and not as wage earners is absolutely crucial. In order to ensure that physicians practice medicine within this framework, companies and government agencies will likely continue to employ incentives of various kinds. In doing so, however, we must ensure that these incentives encourage physicians to abide by the policies of the institution in question without encouraging a Thrasymachean conception of medicine.

I want to conclude by summarizing what I have said and then to close with a few remarks about self-interest. I have argued that understanding the physician's role, per the model of the classical conception of a craftsman, allows us to preserve the sense in which a physician's paramount concern must be the good of her patient while enabling us to understand the physician's place in the fiscal realities of contemporary medical practice. I have argued that politics is the discipline that determines how we are supposed to weigh our priorities in order to achieve the good life. As such, the craft of medicine is subordinated to it. Furthermore, public policy must determine questions regarding the level of resources that should be made available for health care and the kinds of restrictions that health-care companies should be allowed to place on the practice of medicine in order to make a profit. Within the practice of medicine itself, however, the physician must seek, above all else, to use the resources available to her to look after what is best for the patient. I have argued that although the resources available to a given individual patient may not be sufficient to fulfill all her medical needs, this does not mean that the physician betrays her role as caregiver if she does her best to make a skillful use of what is available to her.

I also argued, however, that we must be careful not to confuse the practice of medicine with the practice of wage earning when trying to motivate physicians to comply with these policies. I claimed that one of the motivating forces behind Thrasymachus's conception of the role of the politician as craftsman was his belief that we are each primarily self-interested beings competing for scarce resources. One of the main problems facing MCOs today is how to motivate physicians to comply with the new approach to medical care. As I argued, some of the mechanisms by which they have sought to achieve this goal force a Thrasymachean view of medicine on both doctors and patients. To the extent that doctors permit the pursuit of their own advantage to regulate their performance as physicians, they cease to function primarily as doctors and operate instead as businesspersons. I claimed that if we accept this view, doctors will, in fact, compete with their patients, and the claim that justice is a fool's game will turn into the claim that providing the best medical care is a fool's game as well. Doctors will be competing with their patients and patients will see a competitor in their doctor rather than an ally. Although the question I have been dealing with is separate from the question of the limits that should be placed on the powers of MCOs, these issues are not altogether unrelated.

One reason for the erosion in the trust between doctors and patients is the growing awareness on the part of patients that decisions are being made that do not have their advantage in mind but, rather, that of the doctor and his employers. The most pressing problem before us in this respect is twofold. First, we must make sure that safeguards are in place that prevent MCOs from putting unreasonable constraints on the practice of medicine. By encouraging physicians, patients, and MCOs to engage in an open and public debate about the place of health care in the good life, we can help ensure that the restrictions we place on our medical budgets are properly motivated and morally justified. Second, we must find means of motivating physicians to comply with the new ways they are being asked to practice medicine that do not presuppose a Thrasymachean view of medicine. I hope that understanding medicine and the role of the physician along the model I have suggested here will be a step in the right direction.[20]

Notes

1. All Plato translations are from Reeve (1992), although I have modified them in places for clarity and continuity.

2. The starkest example of this can be seen in the very idea that a company like American Medical Consumers is needed. Recently established in California by Dr. Vincent Riccardi, this company "plans to dispatch 'personal medical advocates' to negotiate for care on behalf of patients" (Larson, 1996).

3. The two primary discussions within the Hippocratic corpus of the sense in which medicine is a craft are *On Ancient Medicine* (Jones 1923, vol. 1, 1–64) and *The Art* (Jones 1923, vol. 2, 185–218).

4. I use "art" and "craft" interchangeably as translations for τέχνη. I also refer to the art of politics or the political craft but only for the sake of continuity. In no way does my argument rest on the assumption that politics is a craft or science, a question over which Plato and Aristotle themselves seem to disagree. For the present purpose, the notion of a political craft should be understood as an archaic way of referring to the "political process."

5. Aristotle *Nicomachean Ethics* I.1–3, 1094a ff. and Plato *Republic* 10, 601c–602a; see also *Meno* 97a–b, *Euthydemus* 290c–d, as well as Tiles 1984.

6. See *Nicomachean Ethics* I.10.1100b33–1101a5 where Aristotle says that good craftsmen are the ones who make the best use of the materials with which they are provided.

7. Annas (1981, 43) says that in claiming that no craftsman ever errs, Thrasymachus has merely made a "verbal move" that saves his position at the price of flouting our common beliefs about doctors, rulers, and other craftsmen.

8. For support for this reading, see Reeve 1988, 10–11 and Annas 1981, 40. For an alternative view see Nicholson 1974.

9. This argument presumes, of course, that the established rulers are, in fact, craftsmen. In both the *Gorgias* and later in the *Republic*, Socrates claims that none of the actual rulers practice the true political craft.

10. Reeve (1988, 19) claims that Socrates contradicts himself when he claims, first, that no craft can benefit its practitioner and, second, that the craft of wage-earning (μισθαρνητική) benefits the craftsman. I argue against this view at length elsewhere (London 1999). For the moment, let me simply point out that a craftsman may *receive* a benefit from practicing a craft even though in practicing that

craft he is *looking after* the advantage of something (or someone) else. Although the craftsman may receive a benefit, it is not because his craft *looks after* his advantage.

11. Bloom (1968, 333) claims that wage earning directs those crafts to which it is attached (see also Irwin 1977, 181) and that wage earning lacks a distinctive subject matter. Roochnik (1996, 143) recognizes that wage earning does not "direct" the other arts but nevertheless agrees that it has no determinate field of its own. I argue elsewhere against both of these views (London 1999). For the moment, let me simply make the following claims. First, to say that the craft of wage earning is conceptually different from the craft of medicine is just to say that one can learn and practice the latter craft without ever considering how one will make a living; one could practice medicine for free. Second, wage earning is a craft that deals with setting a price on one's goods or labor, advertising one's goods or labor, and perhaps other sorts of business concerns. As such, there is no reason to think that a physician could not consult an expert in this craft to learn how more effectively to structure the business end of a medical practice. Nor is there any reason to think that a craftsman could not practice the craft of wage earning for another in the sense that the craftsman might earn money for someone else rather than for himself.

12. Glaucon puts this forth as part of his elaboration and extension of Thrasymachus's argument, and it should be clear from *Republic* I that although he does not state it, Thrasymachus holds this view.

13. In the rest of Book I, Socrates goes on to argue that justice is a virtue of the soul (353e), that the soul too has a function (εργον)—namely, to live well (353d–e)—and therefore that the just soul and the just person live well. For now, suffice it to say that the reply to Thrasymachus is not complete without forceful arguments against his conception of human nature.

14. One alternative to financial incentives is to move to a fixed-budget system like the one in Great Britain. Under this system, physicians must conserve their resources in order to be able to treat all of those who need treatment. The advantages of a system such as this are defended in Orentlicher 1995.

15. I would also like to hold out the possibility of finding a set of effective incentives that do not appeal to a physician's financial interests at all. For example, perhaps MCOs could reward physicians who consistently perform within their desired parameters by allowing them to make treatment decisions such as patient referrals without much bureaucratic oversight. In other words, physicians would be given freedom from bureaucratic oversight so long as they continue to perform within acceptable limits. This may make it easier for the physician to practice her craft, free up more of her time to see other patients, and patients who receive expedited care might be happier with the health care they receive. I cannot say how such a system would work in practice. This is merely meant as an example of the kind of incentive I have in mind. After all, physicians value many things other than money and it may be possible to appeal to some of these other values in structuring incentives.

16. See Aristotle, *Nicomachean Ethics* I.7 1097a25–1097b6, keeping in mind that health is the excellence or virtue of the body; Plato *Republic* 357c; Daniels 1985, 19–35; and Callahan 1990, 105–110.

17. For Aristotle, "A state is a partnership of families and clans in living well for the sake of a full and independent life" (*Politics* III.5 1280b33–35), which then leads to the statement: "Now it is clear that the best constitution is the framework under which anybody whatsoever would do well and live in felicity" (VII.2 1324a23–25).

18. Morreim distinguishes what she calls the Standard of Medical Expertise from the Standard of Resource Use; the former represents the patient's entitlement to the physician's skill and attention, the latter her entitlement to medical resources. I am trying to outline the way in which these distinctions connect to the conception of the doctor's role as craftsman that I am presenting.

19. Among other things, a "sound" rationing policy is one that aspires to be as fair as possible. Whether a particular rationing policy is justifiable will depend on the amount of fairness it can achieve. The procedures or mechanisms of a "sound" rationing policy will thus be ones for which we can at least offer some moral justification. An unsound rationing policy would be one in which the procedures do not seek to be as fair as possible. Some might suggest that the rationing required under fiscal scarcity cannot be carried out according to broad policy guidelines. This may be true in the sense that we may not be able to formulate detailed and comprehensive sets of guidelines for making such decisions, either at a governmental or an administrative level. But it cannot be true in the sense that no rational procedures or criteria exist to guide such decisions. The reason is that these would not be rationing decisions at all. At best, they would amount to the arbitrary exercise of power on the part of those making the decisions; at worst, they would be the manifestation of mere prejudice.

20. I want to thank Cora Diamond and John Arras for the encouragement to pursue this topic and for the insightful comments they each made on various drafts.

References

Annas, J. 1981. *An Introduction to Plato's* Republic. Oxford: Clarendon Press.

Barnes, J., ed. 1984. *The Complete Works of Aristotle: The Revised Oxford Translation*. Princeton, N.J.: Princeton University Press.

Bloom, A. 1986. *The* Republic *of Plato*. New York: Basic Books.

Callahan, D. 1990. *What Kind of Life?* Washington, D.C.: Georgetown University Press.

Cross, R. C., and Woozley, A. D. 1964. *Plato's* Republic: *A Philosophical Commentary*. London: Macmillan Press.

Daniels, N. 1985. *Just Health Care*. Cambridge: Cambridge University Press.

Emanuel, E. J. 1991. *The Ends of Human Life*. Cambridge: Harvard University Press.

Hirshorn, M. W. 1986. "Some Doctors Assail Quality of Treatment Provided by HMOs." *Wall Street Journal* Sept. 16: 1, 21.

Irwin, T. 1977. *Plato's Moral Theory*. Oxford: Clarendon Press.

Jones, W. H. S. 1923/1972. *Hippocrates*. vols. 1 and 2, Loeb Classical Library. Cambridge, Mass.: Harvard University Press.

Larson, E. 1996. "The Soul of an HMO." *Time Magazine*, January 22.

Levinsky, N. 1984. "The Doctor's Master." *New England Journal of Medicine* 311(24): 1573–1575.

London, A. J. 1999. *Virtue, Wisdom, and the Art of Ruling in Plato*. Ann Arbor, MI: University Microfilms.

Morreim, E. H. 1995. *Balancing Act: The New Medical Ethics of Medicine's New Economics*. Washington, D.C.: Georgetown University Press.

Nicholson, P. P. 1974. "Unraveling Thrasymachus's Arguments in the Republic." *Phronesis* 19: 210–232.

Orentlicher, D. 1995. "Health Care Reform and the Patient-Physician Relationship." *Health Matrix: Journal of Law-Medicine* 5(1): 141–80.

Reeve, C. D. C. 1988. *Philosopher Kings*. Princeton: Princeton University Press.

Reeve, C. D. C. 1992. Plato, *Republic*, rev. of G. M. A. Grube trans. Indianapolis: Hackett.

Roochnik, D. 1996. *Of Art and Wisdom: Plato's Understanding of* Techne. University Park: Pennsylvania State University Press.

Tiles, J. E. 1984. "Techne and Moral Expertise." *Philosophy* 59: 49–66.

Walzer, M. 1983. *Spheres of Justice*. New York: Basic Books.

8

Potentiality and Persons: An Aristotelian Perspective

Christopher Megone

In much of the literature on the ethics of abortion, an issue receiving considerable attention is that of the moral status of the fetus. The question it asks is whether the fetus merits the same kind of moral treatment as a more developed human being (child or adult), or whether in virtue of differences between it and more developed members of the species, it deserves different moral treatment. Some writers (Harris 1985; Singer 1993) argue that a morally important distinction is relevant here—the distinction between the concept of a human being, which refers to a biological species, and the concept of a person that is not species specific in its application but can refer to a member of any species with certain characteristics. The sort of characteristics possessed by persons are usually said by these writers to include a capacity for pain and pleasure, a sense of self, a sense of time, and rationality. In this view, personhood is the morally significant category, fetuses are only human beings, not persons, and more developed children and adults are usually persons. This provides the rationale for treating fetuses differently from more developed humans.

Another consideration often introduced in discussing the question of abortion, and normally dismissed, is the potentiality of the fetus. Given the usual way in which potentiality is conceived today, arguments appealing to this consideration can be developed whether the fetus is thought of as a person or as a human being. Thus the appeal to potentiality is normally presented along the following lines (with the argument adapted for "person" in brackets):

At least the potential for a new human being {person} is then present [at conception] complete with its full genetic make-up and with all its uniqueness and individuality. And since the fertilized egg is potentially a human being {person} we must invest it with all the same rights and protections that are possessed by actual human beings {persons}. This we may call 'the potentiality argument' (Harris 1985, 11).

In this view, the fetus is a potential human being (or potential person) and has claims to certain rights and protections based on the premise that it will become a human being (or person). A standard reaction is to raise at least two objections to this position (Harris 1985, 11): first, that "the bare fact that something will become X is not a good reason for treating it now as if it were in fact X"; and secondly, that the unfertilized egg and the sperm are equally potentially new human beings (or persons), yet we would not wish to allocate them the rights and protections of a human being (or of a person). The fetus's potential, then, cannot be a morally significant factor.[1]

The aim of the treatment presented here is to reexamine both these issues from an Aristotelian perspective. In the first instance, the notion of potentiality in this context will be considered in the light of Aristotle's discussion of that concept, which will show that there are three relevant senses of potentiality. Furthermore this analysis will then cut across the debate concerning the distinction between persons and human beings. The Aristotelian understanding of the concept of potentiality casts doubt on the moral significance of this distinction because the Aristotelian approach identifies a novel sense (novel relative to the standard contemporary potentiality argument) in which the fetus's potentiality is morally significant. In this morally significant sense of potentiality, the fetus and the more developed human being share the same potentiality. Attention to this account of potentiality reveals that the notion of a person is, at most, of secondary moral significance, and may not be either morally significant or coherent.

Although discussion of both potentiality and the person/human being distinction is initiated here in the context of abortion, the Aristotelian approach, as developed, may also have wider implications for applied and systematic ethics. Insofar as the significance of the person/human being distinction is rejected, repercussions may occur for the discussion both of euthanasia and of the treatment of animals. Thus, attention to the morally significant potentiality of human beings may have implications for an account of death and dying; and the discussion may also imply that behaving in distinct ways to different species, on the basis of species difference, may not be objectionable. The main aim, however, is simply to identify a sense in which fetal potentiality is morally significant and to show that the relevant account of potentiality undermines the view that persons constitute a category of primary moral significance.[2]

Discussion begins by introducing the Aristotelian notion of essential or substantial potentiality and explaining its application in the human case. This initial account allows several points to be made. First, on this notion of potentiality, the fetus and the child or adult human share the same essential potentialities. Second, distinguishing this notion of potentiality from a second Aristotelian notion—that of material potentiality—allows the potentiality of the human egg or sperm to be distinguished from that of the fertilized egg, thus blocking the objection above that an appeal to fetal potentiality must allow that the unfertilised egg and the sperm are equally potentially new human beings. However, the concept of a person may still be introduced within this Aristotelian framework, but this concept is best understood in terms of a third Aristotelian concept of potentiality—state potentiality. This, then, accommodates the conclusion that from a moral point of view, an individual's essential human potentialities, not his state potentialities, are of primary significance.

The Potentiality Argument and Aristotelian Essential Potentialities

Aristotle was the first to examine carefully the concepts of potentiality and actuality. His work therefore provides a valuable resource for developing a critique of the widespread contemporary view of fetal potentiality described above. In elucidating his position, a starting point is his work on natural kinds, one of the areas in which his deployment of the potential/actual distinction was of particular significance. What follows is a brief overview, developed more fully elsewhere (Megone 1988).

In *Physics* ii 1, Aristotle investigates the distinction between natural substances and artifacts—an investigation that takes place in the context of his effort to produce an adequate explanatory framework for the changes that occur in the natural world. Natural substances are for him the primary constituents of the natural world, where the natural world's defining quality is that it is a world of change. The paradigm examples of substances in this world of change are animals and plants, that is, members of (biological) natural kinds. Natural substances are, for Aristotle, due to nature, which he clarifies by explaining that their distinguishing feature is that "each has in itself a source of change and staying unchanged" (*Physics* ii 1.192b8, 14–15). He goes on to observe that this feature is an inner source of change and is innate. Thus, a natural substance such as a cow or a rose is distinguished from an artifact in that it possesses an inner source of change. Furthermore, "anything which has a source of this sort has a nature" (*Physics* ii 1.192b33–34). In other words, a member of a natural kind is distinguished as natural by virtue of possessing a nature, and that nature is an inner source of change.

In the second half of *Physics* ii 1, Aristotle goes on to discuss whether this nature in a natural substance is to be identified with the substance's form or its matter. He has already established that a substance is informed matter—the possession of both form and matter is necessary to account for the possibility of change, and the natural world of which natural substances are the primary constituents is characterized as a world of change. Thus, both (substantial) matter and (substantial) form have a claim to constitute the nature of a natural substance, but Aristotle's discussion leads to the conclusion that form has the better claim (*Physics* ii 2.193b7–8).

Where does this identification of the nature of a thing with its form lead? In *Physics* ii 3, Aristotle states that the form is ὁ λόγος τοῦ τί ἦν εἶναι ("the account of what the being [the essence] would be"). This identification of the form with the essence is frequently made elsewhere in *Physics* ii 3 (ii 3.194b26–27; *Metaphysics* vii 7.1032b1–2 and vii 10.1035b32; see also Megone 1988). Aristotle has thus argued that nature is form, and form is essence; thus nature is essence.

This rapid survey suggests, then, that for Aristotle a member of a natural kind has a nature and that nature constitutes both its essence and an inner source of change. What exactly does this mean? (Once again, what follows has been argued in more detail elsewhere [Mourelatos 1967; Cooper 1982; Megone 1988].) Because Aristotle's objective is to produce an adequate explanatory framework for a world of change, when he talks of an inner source of change in a natural substance, he is referring to the fact that some of the changes that natural substances undergo can be explained in a particular way—a first key point. His view is that among the changes that natural substances undergo, some will be changes that occur regularly or for the most part—that is, are part of a regular cycle of change. Regularity here does not mean statistically most common. It refers to changes that occur repeatedly and cyclically (*Physics* ii 8.198b35–37; Cooper 1982). These constitute the cyclical changes of a successful or good member of a kind, where success here is associated with the survival of the kind. The inner source of change figures in the explanation of such changes.

Take the case of an acorn, which can undergo many changes. It can be eaten by pigs, it can be blown about in the wind, it can become manure, it can develop into a stunted sapling and then wither, and so on. Among these many possible changes, the ones Aristotle identifies as happening always or for the most part, that is, regularly and cyclically, will be those an acorn must go through (sapling, young oak, and so forth) if it is to develop into a full-grown, flourishing oak. Such changes, Aristotle claims, are "for something," that is, they are open to teleological explanation (*Physics* ii 8.198b10–12). What it means for changes to be open to teleological explanation is that among the changes an acorn can undergo are some that good or successful members of the kind undergo. A good acorn or oak is one that has grown, via an appropriate cycle, into a fully developed oak tree. Thus, changes explained by the inner source of change are changes that a good member of a kind undergoes.

To sum up this feature of Aristotelian natures: natural substances are distinguished in having a nature or inner source of change that plays a particular explanatory role with regard to some of the changes the substance undergoes: it figures in the teleological explanation of these changes in the sense just outlined. (Furthermore, the source of change is inner because these changes are open to this kind of change by virtue of what the substance is, and what it is depends on its nature not on any external determinant.) These ideas will be elaborated further in the light of Aristotle's notion of essential potentiality.

The second key point arises from the fact that the natural substance's nature is identified with its essence. Thus, the nature of a natural substance constitutes the property(ies) that make it what it is. In the light of the discussion of the teleological role of natures it follows that the changes that a good member of the kind undergoes are the changes by reference to which any member of the kind is identified as the thing it is. Furthermore, for Aristotle, the essential properties of a thing are its fundamental sortal properties—the fundamental properties by which we pick out the kind to which it belongs. The essence of a natural substance is also the essence of the kind to which it belongs. So when we pick out what a natural substance is, we pick out the kind of thing it is (*Meta.* vii 17.1041a20ff.). Thus, as well as playing an explanatory role, the nature of a thing, by virtue of being its essence, plays a classificatory role.

The natures of natural substances constitute, therefore, the intersections of Aristotle's classificatory and explanatory frameworks. On the classificatory side, the nature of a substance is comprised of the essential properties in terms of which we determine what a thing is, but these are the sortal properties for the kind, and those are the properties a good member of the kind exhibits. The classification of natural substances, and their definition, is therefore tied to the properties good members of the kind actualize. The possibility of classification depends on picking out natures in this way.[3] On the explanatory side, natures pick out certain properties (changes) whose occurrence is not fully explained unless it is explained as the behavior of a good member of a natural kind.

Having established these two features of the nature of a natural substance, the next step is crucial for present purposes. In *Metaphysics* ix, Aristotle elaborates the picture just described by characterizing the nature of a natural substance in terms of potentialities. This serves to introduce the first of his notions of potentiality.

Aristotle identifies a key sense of potentiality as "a starting point of change in another thing or in the thing itself *qua* other." He goes on to note that this potential may be a potential to act upon or to be acted on, an active or passive potential for change (*Meta.* ix 1.1046a8–18). One form of potentiality, then, is the potential to change (something else), or to be changed (by something else).

Having identified this potentiality for change, he proceeds to make a claim about the nature of a thing. It is, he holds, in the same genus as potentiality, for it is a principle of change—not, however a potential for change "in something else but, in the thing itself *qua* itself" (*Meta.* ix 8.1049b5–10). This link between a thing's nature and its potentiality needs clarification. What potentialities constitute the nature of a thing?

First of all is the idea that the potentiality in question is that which a substance has to change itself. This can be explained by reference to the idea that the thing's nature is its essence. In talking of the potentiality the natural substance has to change itself, Aristotle cannot mean that members of natural kinds will change themselves in certain ways irrespective of external circumstances. Clearly external factors affect any development of plants and animals. His view is clarified by a remark in *Metaphysics* ix 7. Members of natural kinds have this potential to change themselves in the sense that they will change themselves in certain ways "if nothing external hinders them" (*Metaphysics* ix 7.1049a8–15). The idea here is that the failure of a thing to change in this way must make reference not just to external circumstances but to the fact that such a substance has failed to behave as a (good) member of the kind does (bearing in mind that the behavior of good members of the kind is definitive of any member of the kind). Conversely, when a natural kind actualizes one of these potentialities, the explanation will be that this is what (a good member of) such and such a kind does. The thing changes itself in the sense that the change is explained by reference to what the thing is. The potentiality actualized is an essential potentiality. (This picks up again the sense in which the nature is an inner source of change.)

More light can be shed by noting a further claim made in chapter 8 of *Metaphysics* ix i.e., that the substance or form of a thing is its actualization (1050b2). Thus, since nature is form, the nature of a thing must also be in some sense its actualization. How can the nature of a thing be both potentiality and actuality? Aristotle's point concerns certain senses in which actuality is prior to potentiality (*Metaphysics* ix 8.1049b10–12). Most significant here is a general claim about the way in which potentialities are identified, the priority of formula or definition. As Gill 1989, 174 notes, "Potentialities [for change] ... are always directed to an end or goal—an actuality; and the potentiality is identified as the potentiality it is with reference to the actuality" (see *Metaphysics* ix 8.1049b4–17). Given that a potentiality cannot be defined without reference to the actuality brought about when that potentiality is actualized, identifying a thing's nature with (some of) its potentialities, implies a reference to the actuality those potentialities are directed toward.

This can now be linked with the earlier remarks about the changes that a thing's nature explains. The nature of a natural substance cannot be identified with whatever set of potentialities happens to be actualized as the substance undergoes change, but must be identified with another subset of its initial potentialities—that subset whose evolving realization, from the moment the set of potentialities exists, constitutes the behavior of a good member of the kind. In other words, the nature of a natural substance is an actuality only in the sense that the nature of any member of a natural kind is constituted by the potentialities that a good member of the kind actualizes.

An example may help. An acorn can be considered as a set of potentialities for change in the sense that it may undergo a huge variety of changes. If so, then its nature does not pick out those potentialities in fact actualized in the development of a particular acorn. A particular acorn may become manure, but such a change is not part of the cycle exhibited by a good acorn. Thus, such a change is not to be explained by reference to the kind of thing it is. It is not relevant to what it is. Therefore, this potential is not part of its nature. By contrast, a subset of the changes an acorn may undergo constitute the cyclical set that a flourishing acorn undergoes. Because these are the potentialities a flourishing acorn actualizes, this subset of potentialities constitutes the nature of every acorn. These are the essential potentialities of an acorn that figure in teleological explanation of its development.

Within this view, then, any member of a natural kind has a nature that is its essence, and the essential properties of that natural substance are a set of potentialities—the particular set that plays a role in the teleological explanation of the substance's behavior. In the case of any member of a species, what makes it the thing that it is—a member of that kind—is its instantiation of this set of potentialities. To clarify this point, the notion of instantiating potentialities requires elaboration. An acorn and a more developed oak instantiate the same essential potentialities in the sense that there is a set of potentialities, which a perfect oak actualizes, which each is in the process of actualizing, with greater or less success. This picture of essential properties as potentialities makes clear why a three-legged horse, say, is still a horse: such a horse still instantiates the crucial essential potentialities; it has just failed to actualize some of the more significant ones that would be actualized by a good member of the kind.

Now we can summarize the first Aristotelian notion of potentiality. Essential or substantial potentialities are those that constitute the nature of a natural kind. They are the potentialities that make a member of a kind the thing that it is, thus essential. And they are the potentialities that figure in teleological explanation of a natural substance's behavior in the sense that they are actualized by a good member of the kind. (Thus, as noted, Aristotle links identity conditions to the properties displayed by good members of kinds.)

Given this account, we may now return to the notion of fetal potentiality, considered in terms of the (Aristotelian) essential potentiality of a fetus. A fetus, as a member of a natural kind, that of human beings, must be the thing that it is by virtue of having a nature, by virtue of instantiating a subset of potentialities—namely, that set of essential potentialities whose actualization occurs in the life of a flourishing human being. (In Aristotle's view, these are the capacities actualized in the flourishing of a rational animal.) But in this respect, a fetus is no different from a child or an adult human being, since an adult, for example, is also the thing that it is in virtue of having a nature, and its nature, too, is that of members of the human kind, namely an instantiation of the relevant set of essential potentialities—those potentialities that play a role in the teleological explanation of human behavior.

Within this view of fetal potentiality, then, a fetus is not a potential human being; on the contrary, it is an actual human being by virtue of the potentialities it instantiates. And the criterion for it being a human being is exactly the same as that for an adult being a human being. Thus, this notion of essential potentiality blocks the first objection made to the potentiality argument outlined. (In fact, it also suggests that the appeal to potentiality made in that argument may be misconceived.) The fetus is not merely a potential human being, and there is no clear reason, on the basis merely of the kind of thing it is, to treat it differently from any other member of the kind.

The Potentiality Argument and Aristotelian Material Potentiality

What, though, of the second objection raised to the potentiality argument given at the outset? Can the Aristotelian account of fetal potentiality discriminate between a fetus and an unfertilized egg? In terms of the notion of essential potentiality so far presented, the answer to these questions really depends on the resolution of the following one. When is it plausible to say that a set of essential potentialities is instantiated and thus that a flourishing individual who begins to realize them is present? However, Aristotle's discussion of potentiality introduces a second notion that captures the pretheoretical view that an unfertilized egg is in some sense potentially a human, but allows it to be distinguished from the fetus.

Having introduced the notion of essential potentiality, in *Metaphysics* ix 6. Aristotle adds that another potentiality is the potentiality of matter to be a substance, of wood to be a statue, for example (*Metaphysics* ix 6.1048a25–b9, ix 7.1049a19–24; see also Gill 1989, 220–227). This is a distinct notion of potentiality, material potentiality. It is a potential that a natural substance has when conceived of only as (Aristotelian) matter. Thus a tree can be thought of only as wood, and, as such, a tree has the potential to be a statue or a table. However, whilst the actualization of its essential potentiality constitutes a natural substance's existence, the actualization of its material potentiality will usually occur when the substance has ceased to exist. The wood of a tree actualizes its potential to be a table (usually) when the tree ceases to exist.

Recognizing this second notion of potentiality thus leaves open the possibility that an unfertilized egg has human potential only in the sense that it has the material potentiality to become a human. The actualization of this material potential of the unfertilized egg (or the sperm) is compatible with the egg's ceasing to exist as an egg, and a new entity, a human being, coming into existence.

This appeal to material potentiality is not decisive since the question remains as to what purely biological change can most plausibly be associated with the instantiation of a new set of essential potentialities constituting a new human being. On the face of it, this biological change occurs at conception "when two cells with twenty three chromosomes unite and fuse to become a forty six chromosome cell, providing a unique genetic constitution, that new cell is the first stage in a dynamic and integrated system having nothing much in common with the individual male and female cells save that it sprang from them and will in time produce new sets of them" (Finnis 1974, 144–145).[4] Given this, it seems plausible that a human egg has a nature but that fertilization is not a further actualization of the essential potentialities constituting its nature. On the contrary, at that point the egg ceases to exist and realizes its material potentiality as the matter in which a new set of essential potentialities, constituting the nature of a different entity, are instantiated. This certainly seems to have been Aristotle's own view, and at the very least this second Aristotelian notion of potentiality puts the onus on an opponent to show that the unfertilized egg actualizes its essential potential, not merely its material potential, as a human develops (*Metaphysics* ix 7.1049a8–19).

The Ethical Significance of Persons

This Aristotelian discussion of the concept of potentiality shows that an appeal to fetal essential potentiality is not, therefore, open to either of the oft-repeated objections to the usual account of the potentiality principle. Crucially, in the Aristotelian view, the fetus's essential potentiality is what makes it an actual human being (and is to be distinguished from the mere material potentiality to be human of the unfertilized egg). At this point, however, the following objection may be made: what has been shown so far is that the fetus and the adult human are both human beings by virtue of instantiating a certain set of essential potentialities. But what matters for the ethics of abortion is the distinction between a human being and a person: it is persons that are of ethical significance—distinguishing the kind of treatment required for persons from that required for mere human beings is what is important and making this important distinction is still possible within the present framework. For, the objection continues, while it is true that both adult humans and fetuses share in instantiating a set of essential potentialities, it is possible to distinguish those human beings who have actualized some of their essential potentialities, who have certain actual capacities, from those whose essential potentialities remain unactualized. Those who have actualized some of their potentialities— who are actually self-conscious, capable of reasoning if they choose to, and so on, are persons—and, as stated, it is persons that matter from a moral point of view.

To reply to this objection examination of the supposed distinction between human beings and persons is necessary in the light of the resources provided by an Aristotelian discussion of potentiality. Consider first the initial motivation for the distinction between humans and persons. The basic claim (Singer 1993) is that when debating the treatment of a creature (in Aristotelian terms, a natural substance), an appeal to its species, the kind to which it belongs, is "speciesist" in a way that is analogous to sexism or racism. In this view, mere species cannot be a morally significant property. What matters is, on the contrary, what morally significant properties the entity in question possesses. Those morally relevant properties can be identified across species, and creatures that possess those properties can be distinguished as persons. Thus, the key claim in this view is that the concept of a person refers to morally significant properties, while an appeal to an entity's being human will be merely speciesist. This is what needs to be considered in the light of a fuller account of Aristotle's distinct conceptions of potentiality.

What is the basis for the view that the characteristics of persons are distinctive morally significant characteristics? Peter Singer (1993) begins arguing toward the importance of person characteristics, not those of humans, by appealing to a capacity not exclusive to humans. He endorses Bentham's claim that "the capacity for suffering [is] the vital characteristic that entitles a being to equal consideration" and continues with the claim that: "The capacity for suffering and enjoying things is a prerequisite for having interests at all, a condition that must be satisfied before we can speak of interests in any meaningful way" (Singer 1993, 57). In Singer's view, then, the basic characteristic that makes an entity morally significant is the capacity for suffering and for enjoying things. He goes on to note, however, that a difference obtains between being the sort of thing that has any interests at all and being the sort of thing whose life is valuable (Singer 1993, 61–2). At this point he introduces the concept of a person. A person is distinguished from a member of the biological species human being by virtue of having certain characteristics that give him special interests that are adversely affected by being killed. This is what makes the life of a person valuable while that of a human being as such (member of the biological species) is not.

In Singer's account, the core of the concept *person* is given by the characteristics of rationality and self-consciousness, though he notes other characteristics—"self-awareness, self-control, a sense of future, a sense of past, the capacity to relate to others, concern for others, communication and curiosity … [that] more or less flow from them" (Singer 1993, 86–7).[5] He then considers four possible reasons for giving special protection to the lives of persons—four explanations as to why the characteristics of persons have special moral significance. Thus, his argument has four bases: Utilitarian considerations ([1] of a classical-Utilitarian or [2] of a preference-Utilitarian sort); (3) a connection between these characteristics and the possession of rights; and (4) a connection between these characteristics and an appeal to the Kantian principle of autonomy (Singer 1993, 89–101; see also Tooley 1983). The discussion that follows will apply most obviously to the first three lines of argument since these rest most clearly on Singer's claim that persons have special interests that can be harmed by death.

An initial worry about the direction of Singer's argument concerns the fundamental claim that the criterion for having interests at all is possession of the capacity for suffering and enjoyment. If this is mistaken, some doubt may arise about the claim that persons, as defined by Singer, have special interests that are harmed by killing. Yet the fundamental claim does seem questionable. In the first place, living substances exist that do not, in any normal sense, have the capacity for suffering and enjoyment but certainly appear to have interests, namely plants. Thus, it seems pretheoretically acceptable to say that plants need various environmental conditions in order to flourish and it is in their interest to have such conditions. Furthermore, humans appear to have interests that are not obviously dependent on their having the capacity for suffering or enjoyment. They have an interest in certain kinds of physical development, so in health (as a noninstrumental good), and they have an interest in the attainment of goals, and in the achievement of understanding. While humans may enjoy some of these things, it is plausible that the enjoyment arises because they are in a human's interest rather than that the human capacity for enjoyment is the ground of their being a human interest.

If these pretheoretical views of the interests of humans and plants are plausible, then Singer's account of interests requires revision. An alternative view of interests can be developed at the same time as challenging directly the claim that persons are of special moral significance. Hursthouse 1987 has put forward such a challenge, but her argument will be developed here in the light of the Aristotelian discussion of potentiality. This development involves distinguishing the notion of essential potentiality already discussed from a third notion of potentiality, state potentiality.

Two Objections to the Supposed Ethical Significance of Persons

Hursthouse's objection begins with the observation that one of the motives for speciesism derives from a thought experiment in which humans encounter aliens very like themselves. The person theorist, who objects to speciesism, holds that it would be wrong for humans to treat the aliens quite differently simply on the grounds that they are aliens, not humans (Hursthouse 1987, 237). If this seems plausible, as it does, then one might hold that the crucial point must be that both the humans and the aliens are persons, and for that reason deserving of similar treatment. Being a person, not belonging to a particular species, is what matters morally. However, the thrust of Hursthouse's objection is that saying what sort of treatment is morally required for a person is impossible since "'person' has not been defined in a way that determines a sense for 'personal flourishing' or 'flourishing as a person'" (Hursthouse 1987, 248). Hursthouse develops this objection via two points. Singer's objective is to specify the concept of person by reference to nonanthropocentric characteristics (the objective being to avoid a supposedly speciesist morality, with the concept of a human being at its center). Both Hursthouse's points challenge this "thin" or nonanthropocentric specification of a person. First of all, she suggests that from a certain perspective the "thin" concept of a person is "simply a verbal trick." The relevant perspective is that "of a certain philosophy of mind (or of language) ... [according to which] ... it is only of creatures very similar to us in a vast variety of ways that it would even make sense to describe them as having a language, acting intentionally, having thoughts and desires ... and so on" (Hursthouse 1987, 251). In other words, though Singer identifies just two core characteristics of persons, rationality and self-awareness, only a creature that had all the other morally relevant human characteristics could be ascribed these features (Hursthouse 1987, 252).

According to this first point, then, any attempt to spell out the definition of (alien) persons (of the Singer variety) in such a way as to determine what their personal flourishing would consist in, and therefore what treatment is morally appropriate for them is bound to incorporate the whole package of morally relevant human characteristics. But this defeats the objective of having a "thin" nonanthropocentric concept of a person. And it suggests that the possibility that such a "thin" concept of a person is sufficient to determine morally appropriate treatment for persons is a delusion, one fed by the verbal trick.

Hursthouse's second objection rests on "contrary to what the [above-described] view in the philosophy of mind takes to be possible, [trying] to imagine and describe entirely 'inhuman' beings which fit some of the standard thin specifications of 'person' and see what our intuitions are about them." Thus she imagines a sort of creature that meets these thin specifications of "person" but has "the fewest conceivable emotions or emotional reactions. They do not feel anything about any other members of their species; they lead totally solitary lives; they are not frightened of death or pain or damage; nothing, not even the frustration of their own desires, upsets them; they are sublimely indifferent to everything." Yet they do pursue something with great vigor, and are prepared to go to great lengths obtaining, say, "the recently detached limb of a member of their own species." But if it is "physically impossible for them to achieve this objective, they do not mind." As a second example, she also imagines a species that has person characteristics but emotions entirely opposite to ours. Her claim, then, is that anyone who holds "that 'being a person' is all that matters must be prepared to say either (a) that there is not the slightest difficulty in regarding these two sorts of alien as 'part of our moral community' or (b) to provide a new specification of person, which while avoiding anthropocentricity, rules them out" (Hursthouse 1987, 252–3).

Hursthouse's thought is that option (a) is not tenable (and that any attempt at (b) will fail). So far as (a) is concerned, her point is that it is not possible to specify what treatment is morally appropriate for creatures so different from us as in the sort of examples she imagines. These creatures may be persons, but that fact provides an insufficient basis to guide moral conduct. In other words, her objection is again that it is implausible that a "thin" nonanthropocentric conception of a person is sufficient to determine the morally appropriate treatment of persons.

Aristotelian State Potentiality and the Objections to the Ethical Significance of Persons

Hursthouse's rejection of the claim that persons are of special moral significance can now be developed in the light of the Aristotelian discussion of potentiality. This involves calling upon a third Aristotelian notion of potentiality that can also be distinguished from the initial concept of essential potentiality. This third notion is that of state potentiality; a passage in *De Anima* serves to introduce it:

> For something is "a knower" in one sense (1), as we might say that a man is a knower because man is among the things that know and have knowledge; but in another sense (2), as we at once call a knower the man who possesses grammatical knowledge. And each of these is potential [but] not in the same way, the one (1) because his genus is such and his matter, the other (2) because when he wishes he is able to theorise, if nothing external interferes.... Now both of the first are potential knowers, but the one having been altered through learning and often changed from an opposite state [is a potential knower in one way], the other (2) from having arithmetical or grammatical knowledge but not exercising it to the exercise [is a potential knower] in another way. (Aristotle *De Anima* ii 5.417a21–b2, trans. Gill; see also Gill 1989, 175–181)

In this passage, Aristotle introduces two senses in which a human being may be the potential knower of a language. In one sense, any human has the potential to know a language, at whatever stage in its development, simply by virtue of being human—by virtue of the genus to which it belongs. This is an essential potentiality, and, in one sense, it is actualized when a human has learnt a language. A child that develops normally "is altered through learning" so as to change from one ignorant of language to one who knows a language. (A human being has this potential, actualized or not, throughout his life, by virtue of being human.)[6] But a human who has developed normally can also be said to be a potential knower of a language when he has that knowledge but is not exercising it. This is an agent who is in a state where he can use the knowledge if he wishes, if nothing external intervenes. (A human being only has this potential after having learned a language, and may lose it as a result of an accident, for example.) This is a state potentiality—a potentiality constituting the state a substance is in that gives it the potential to behave in certain ways. In the case just outlined, a human is in a state that gives him the potential to exercise his knowledge of a language. A plant that has developed appropriately might have the state potentiality to photosynthesize, that is, it might be in a state wherein it can photosynthesize when light shines on it. This contrasts with the essential potentiality to photosynthesize that all members of this species of plant have, by virtue of belonging to that particular species, at all times, whatever their development.

From an Aristotelian view, then, a human being might have both an essential potentiality for rationality and a state potentiality for rationality. Any human will have the essential potentiality by virtue of being human. A neonate or very young child will instantiate this potential, but because such humans will not yet be capable of reasoning about their beliefs or actions, they will lack the state potentiality for rationality. A human will only acquire such a state potentiality if development is normal (at least in this respect). To acquire this state is to be in a position to behave rationally, whether practically or theoretically, though one who is in the state may fail to exercise the potential through laziness or carelessness, for example.

Given this distinction, in these Aristotelian terms the core characteristics that Singer appeals to in order to identify persons, rationality and self-consciousness, are state potentialities. Singer's point is that these characteristics are not possessed by individuals by virtue of belonging to the species *Homo sapiens* (or by virtue of belonging to any biological species); they are characteristics that members of the human species can acquire if they develop normally (Singer 1993, 86–87). This point is now crucial in developing Hursthouse's criticism of the use of the concept of *person* in ethics.

A person theorist such as Singer holds that the concept of person refers to a kind, or genus, that can be found in different biological, or natural, species, where that kind of thing has morally significant characteristics that determine how such an entity should be treated, no matter what species it belongs to. In identifying the state potentialities of rationality and self-consciousness as the core characteristics of a person, Singer claims that identifying such a kind by reference to state potentialities is possible. However, within the Aristotelian picture, as has been seen, state potentialities are contrasted with essential potentialities, where essential potentialities are those that constitute the identity conditions for kinds and their members. Thus, it has been shown that a fetus and an adult human are the things that they are—members of the biological species human being—in the light of instantiating a set of essential potentialities—the set that a good member of the kind actualizes. By contrast, the state potentialities that a developing adult instantiates at any period in its development do not constitute its identity conditions.

Within this picture, the essential properties of a kind, and of any member of the kind, are those potentialities actualized in a regular cycle, the regular cycle that a good member of the kind would go through. Thus, to identify a natural substance as a member of the human species is not merely to identify its current condition as the actualization of certain potentialities but to suppose that this is a stage in a (more, or less, successful) attempt to actualize a cycle of potentialities. Therefore, the state potentialities instantiated at a particular period in the development of a substance cannot constitute the identity conditions for a substance. The identity conditions depend on the regular cycle of potentialities whose actualization the substance is attempting, as well as those state potentialities currently instantiated.

Thus, the person-theorist seeks to identify a morally significant kind but has produced identifying characteristics that cannot constitute the identity conditions for a kind or, therefore, for members of that kind. He has supposed the possibility of determining whether a thing is a person or not by considering whether it is instantiating certain state potentialities —rationality and self-consciousness—but the essential potentialities, not state potentialities, are the ones that serve to identify a kind of thing.

This Aristotelian framework can now be seen to underpin Hursthouse's first criticism of person-theorists, that the "thin" concept of a person is a verbal trick. From the Aristotelian point of view, though, the trick is that the person-theorist's characterization of "persons" is intended to identify a cross-species kind of entity. But the characterization appeals to state potentialities which, since they are not essential potentialities, do not identify a kind of thing at all. Because Singer has not provided identity conditions for personhood, the concept of a person is empty.[7]

The second closely related point is that the fact that persons are characterized in terms of state potentialities explains why stating what kind of treatment is morally appropriate for them is not possible. This is again because state potentialities are contrasted with essential potentialities. For, as has been indicated, the essential potentialities of a kind are those that a good member of the kind will actualize. In other words, it is by reference to a thing's essential potentialities that appropriate moral treatment is determined, since these are the potentialities that must be actualized if the thing is to be a good member of the kind (to flourish).[8] Thus, the fact that an entity currently instantiates the state potentialities of rationality and self-awareness can not determine appropriate moral treatment for the creature without information as to what cycle of essential potentialities it is attempting to actualize.

For example, there might be a kind of creature whose good members instantiate the state potentialities for rationality and self-awareness at a point only moments before they die. This could be contrasted with a kind of creature whose good members instantiate these state potentialities at a fairly early stage in their development, prior to forming the sort of relationships with other members of the species that are conducive to reproduction and thus the survival of the species. The differences in the essential potentialities of these creatures would determine appropriate moral behavior toward them, not the fact that they share the core characteristics of persons. Here the contrast between state potentialities and essential potentialities endorses and develops Hursthouse's second claim—that the "thin" concept of a person is too thin to determine adequately the appropriate moral treatment of persons.

The development of these objections in such terms is supported by the fact that pretheoretical beliefs endorse this Aristotelian view that essential potentialities, not state potentialities, are morally significant. Two examples will suffice here. First, the view that it is good to educate humans from an early age onward must rest on the fact that a child's essential potentialities determine his interests, not the state potentialities he instantiates when five. Similarly, the view that the life of a coma victim, or a significantly preterm neonate, is extremely valuable and that considerable medical effort and resources are worth expending on such beings cannot be explained by appealing to the state potentialities these humans instantiate. The explanation lies in their essential potentiality—that good medical treatment will enable these individuals to continue to realize their essential potential.

In addition, the importance of the essential potentialities of members of kinds endorses the development of an alternative account of interests to that of Singer mentioned earlier. In that account the basic criterion for having interests is the capacity for suffering and enjoyment. But in the Aristotelian view, if good members of kinds realize essential potentialities, and if the human essential potentiality is to be a rational animal, as Aristotle suggested, then it is in a human's interest to attain goals and achieve understanding, not merely to avoid suffering and gain enjoyment. Since plants are natural kinds whose essential potential is realized by good members, thinking of plants as having interests will also be appropriate. Thus this account is able to capture the pretheoretical beliefs about interests that raised objections to Singer's position on that matter.[9]

This aspect of the discussion can now be summarized. Aristotle's account of potentiality reveals a third concept, in addition to those of essential potentiality and material potentiality. In terms of these concepts of potentiality, the claim that persons are what matter morally comes to the claim that the state potentialities an individual instantiates are the morally significant elements, not its essential potentialities. In reply to this claim, I have argued that this is the wrong way round. State potentialities are not adequate to characterize a kind at all, and essential potentialities not state potentialities are of primary moral significance. (This position can allow that the state potentialities a substance instantiates can be morally significant indirectly in that the current state of a creature is relevant to what it requires if it is to actualize its essential potential in the future. But this only emphasizes that the essential potential is of fundamental moral significance.) Thus, the concept of a person is not morally significant but, rather, the essential potentialities that both fetuses and more developed adults share are what count morally.

Conclusion

The aim of this presentation has been to show that an Aristotelian discussion of potentiality has two significant repercussions for bioethics. It discloses an important sense in which the potential of a fetus is morally significant, and yet it suggests that the concept of a person, as developed by Singer and others, is not morally significant. Both these points have implications for other bioethical areas apart from abortion, such as euthanasia and the treatment of animals.

The Aristotelian analysis presented identifies three distinct notions of potentiality—essential potentiality, material potentiality, and state potentiality. In the light of this account, no defense has been offered for the contemporary argument that the fetus is a potential adult and thus morally significant. The argument states, however, that a fetus instantiates the same essential potentialities as any developing child or adult, and that these potentialities matter morally. By contrast, the material potentiality of an unfertilized egg to be human and the state potentialities used to characterize persons both lack moral significance.

A framework in terms of potentiality thus emerges for considering certain applied issues rather than answers to those applied issues themselves. For example, while rejecting the view that the instantiation of specific state potentialities is morally crucial, the framework can allow that different moral treatment will be appropriate for different stages in the development of a human being, as commonsense requires. However, the key claim is that the determinants of the morally appropriate treatment are instantiated by all members of the human species from the fetus onward. More generally, the aim here has been to provide an Aristotelian approach that casts doubt on possible impediments to clear answers to these questions rather than to settle the questions.[10]

Notes

1. This sort of appeal to potentiality has been discussed by various recent writers on abortion and rejected on the same grounds as in main text (Millican 1992; Singer 1993, 152–156; Tooley 1983, ch. 6). Hare 1993, ch. 10 adopts a different approach but still one not compatible with my exposition here.

2. None of the Aristotelian conceptions of potentiality allows the claim that a fertilized egg is potentially a human being (or person). Thus, while it is claimed that there is a sense in which foetal potentiality is morally significant, there is no defence of the standard contemporary argument given above.

3. An important further metaphysical question arises here, namely whether this classification simply reflects our (human) way of dividing up the world or is a result of natural divisions that we detect. This raises important issues about Aristotelian metaphysical realism but goes beyond the scope of the present discussion (see Irwin 1988).

4. This issue is also discussed by Ford 1988, 97: "Once fertilization has taken place the human sperm and egg cease to exist as distinct entities. A genetically human, new living individual cell is formed, a zygote, that has the proximate

potential to become a mature human person with the same genetic constitution." Ford, however, does not work with a very clearly worked-out notion of potential. See also Singer's mistakenly dismissive reference to the "never to be repeated informational speck" created at the fusion of sperm and ovum (Singer 1993, 155).

5. This characterization of a person is fairly representative. Tooley 1983 and Harris 1985 offer similar accounts.

6. This claim implies the view that such potentialities are not lost when they are actualized (see Gill 1989, 178–179).

7. As implied in Hursthouse's discussion referred to earlier in the chapter, the trick that there is such a thing as a "person," in the theorists' sense, works to the extent that the core characteristics identified actually bring along with them the whole package of human characteristics.

8. An implicit assumption here links good members of a kind with what is good for a member of the kind. This point, which is not elaborated here, has been discussed well by Whiting 1985.

9. Space does not permit a full discussion of the notion of interests here. My aim is only to gesture toward a position distinct from that put forward by Singer.

10. I am very grateful to audiences at the Cleveland Clinic Foundation, Rhodes University, and Stellenbosch University, as well as to David Charles, Roger Crisp, and colleagues at the University of Leeds, especially Roger White, for helpful discussion of previous versions of this investigation.

References

Charlton, W., trans. 1984. Aristotle, *Physics Books I and II*. Oxford: Oxford University Press.

Cooper J. 1982. "Aristotle on Natural Teleology," 197–222 in *Language and Logos*, ed. M. Schofield and M. Nussbaum. Cambridge: Cambridge University Press.

Finnis, J. 1972. "The Rights and Wrongs of Abortion." *Philosophy and Public Affairs* 2: 117–145.

Ford, N. M. 1988. *When Did I Begin?* Cambridge: Cambridge University Press.

Gill, M. L. 1989. *Aristotle on Substance*. Princeton: Princeton University Press.

Hare, R. M. 1993. *Essays on Bioethics*. Oxford: Oxford University Press.

Harris, J. 1985. *The Value of Life*. London: Routledge.

Hursthouse, R. 1987. *Beginning Lives*. Oxford: Blackwell.

Irwin, T. 1988. *Aristotle's First Principles*. Oxford: Oxford University Press.

Megone, C. 1988. "*Physics* II:1, Aristotle on essentialism and natural kinds." *Revue de Philosophie Ancienne* 6: 185–212.

Millican, P. 1992. "The Complex Problem of Abortion," in *Ethics in Reproductive Medicine*, ed. D. Bromham, M. Dalton, J. Jackson, and P. Millican. London: Springer-Verlag.

Mourelatos, A. 1967. "Aristotle's Powers." *Ratio* 8: 97–104.

Ross, W. D., trans. 1924. Aristotle, *De Anima*. Oxford: Oxford University Press.

Ross, W. D., trans. 1956. Aristotle, *Metaphysics*. Oxford: Oxford University Press.

Singer, P. 1993. *Practical Ethics*. 2nd edn. Cambridge: Cambridge University Press.

Tooley, M. 1983. *Abortion and Infanticide*. Oxford: Oxford University Press.

Whiting, J. 1985. "Aristotle's Function Argument: a Defense." *Ancient Philosophy* 8: 33–48.

9

Can Communitarianism End the Shrill and Interminable Public Debates? Abortion as a Case-in-Point

Mark G. Kuczewski

Much attention in the last decade has focused on the revival of Aristotelian motifs in contemporary practical philosophy. In particular, this interest has fostered the development of communitarian ethical and political philosophy. The names of Alasdair MacIntyre (1984; 1988; 1990), Michael Sandel (1982; 1984), and Charles Taylor (1989), to name only three, are readily recognizable not only to moral and political philosophers but also to many well-read people around the country. This line of thought has been popularized by Amitai Etzioni (1993) and, to a large extent, by the rhetoric of President Clinton and the work of Hillary Clinton (1996). The interest in communitarianism has a wide variety of sources, but we can identify some chief points of intrigue.

The tendency of our society to conduct its political and moral dialogue in terms of rights is generally less than satisfying. Although rights are important, there is surely more to morality than rights claims. Yet our political discourse sometimes seems to lack other shared moral notions. Furthermore, these arguments that turn on the rights of individuals are very shrill in tone and the debates seem never to end.[1] The abortion controversy provides a prime example.[2]

When one talks about abortion, the "r" word immediately begins to roll off the tongue. Some speak about a woman's *right* to choose, her *right* to have control of her body, her *right* to make reproductive choices, and her *right* of privacy. Similarly, antiabortion activists speak about the *right* to life of the fetus, the *rights* of the unborn, and so forth. To many who are not activists on either side of the controversy, this rhetoric has a hollow ring. Saying that a woman has a right to choose sounds like the beginning of a discussion on the morality of a choice to have an abortion, not the end (Callahan 1990). The assertion of a right to make a choice does not say anything about the morality of any particular choice. In some cases, a decision to indirectly terminate a pregnancy seems clearly appropriate—when, for example, to alleviate a grave threat to the life of the mother and the fetus could not successfully be brought to viability; in contrast, other cases seem clearly to be unethical—for example, abortion as a tool of gender selection. Even if the patient possesses a "right" in both cases, the right is irrelevant to the moral content of the choice. Similarly, discussion of the right to life of the fetus seems even "tinnier." It is hard to know in a pluralistic society how such a claim can be sustained and how to interpret it. So we translate this rights claim into terms such as the sanctity of life or the state's interest in preserving life.

Determining what such concepts mean in everyday life, how they apply, and how other moral considerations should be balanced with them are large and difficult tasks. These intuitions regarding the hollowness of rights and the need for more moral content have given the communitarian a foot in the door of the public debate. However, the need for genuine, thoughtful reflection on moral matters is seldom sufficient to promote much interest in a new movement. The communitarian really gains entrance onto the public stage because of the uncivilized nature of the debate over questions such as abortion.

One side shouts about the rights of women and the other side shouts about the rights of the unborn. These two rights claims are at loggerheads. A way to resolve the conflicting claims to the satisfaction of all the participants in the argument is lacking. In a sense, the Supreme Court's decision in *Roe* (1973) was a compromise between these two claims. The Court seemed to indicate that the rights of the woman were weightier in the first two trimesters whereas the state's interest in preserving life grows stronger later in the pregnancy. Although subsequent decisions have added nuances to the balancing of these conflicting rights and interests, the debate between the two opposing sides remains unimpeded. In fact, beginning with *Roe* and following upon each new subtlety that the Court adds (*Webster v. Reproductive Health Services* 1990; *Planned Parenthood of Southeastern Pennsylvania v. Casey* 1992), a new round of shrill public chatter begins, seemingly gaining impetus for its hostile tone from the subtle reasoning of the Justices. The communitarian promises to explain this phenomenon and, even more surprisingly, to bring it to an end.

The Communitarian's Explanation

As a good Aristotelian, the communitarian offers an explanation for the interminable shrill debates that characterize the public discourse in our society: We have lost a shared "something" that can be used to settle such questions. That something is variously characterized as a shared common understanding, a shared concept of the good, a shared concept of the good life, a shared hierarchy of goods, or a shared *telos* (end or goal). Although these terms and phrases are used somewhat promiscuously and interchangeably by most communitarians, the communitarian claim is clear. All we currently share is a notion of individual rights and this is too sparse to settle our debates. We must work together to come to share some richer moral conceptual apparatus (Emanuel 1991, 32–33). Communitarians sometimes try to outline mechanisms for arriving at these shared understandings.

This demand for a shared something presupposes that the communitarian reject the vision of the person embraced by our culture's underlying ethical and political philosophy and replace it with one of her own. Beginning with the Enlightenment, ethical and political philosophers despaired of producing widespread agreement, a shared common understanding, regarding the goods to be pursued in the good life. As a result, they left the choice of goods to the particular person, the individual. They argued that what is common to individuals is the ability to make choices about what good is to be pursued. The individual is determined by these choices. The rationale behind liberal democracy presupposes that the person is a being determined by volition, i.e., by will and choice. The person is described as the guardian of a sphere of her own private, opaque, self-contained interests and values. From this private realm spring choices that are beyond rational judgment and evaluation.

Beginning with Kant, the person is described as essentially beyond the purview of others. One's freedom is not a thing in the world that can be viewed like the person's body. The same is true of one's values and interests. These are not facts in the world that can be objectively evaluated;

they are subjective matters that only the individual can access for himself or herself. This self—one who lacks all objective determinations other than the power of the will, this "unencumbered self" (Sandel 1984, 83)— is cut off from others and is truly an individual. This self has no cooperative essence but is subject to a moral necessity to respect the individuality of other selves. It respects individual rights as long as they are compatible with a similar liberty for others. Such a being would have no special reason to seek genuinely cooperative relationships with others, only relationships that are coordinate. This self would be happy with voting rather than shared deliberation. In fact, voting may be the only means for settling conflicts because conflicts such as abortion stem from different fundamental values that cannot be reconciled. In the liberal democratic view, one's values cannot be part of a rational dialogue as they are the furniture of the private individual realm located beyond objective evaluation.

Communitarians believe, however, that this voluntaristic view of the self, the individual, is a fiction (MacIntyre 1984, 61). It is the attempt to answer moral questions from such a weak foundation that has produced our moral atrophy and the interminable debates we encounter. The communitarian asks that each member of the community enter into dialogue with the other members, believing that this is necessary because human beings are mainly cognitive animals who "discover" their values in interpersonal encounters. The communitarian view of the person sees the self as coconstituted by social roles, communal practices, and shared deliberative exchanges (Sandel 1982, 179–83). Thus, communitarians generally argue for mechanisms in the community that will permit the community members to come together to settle the fundamental questions of values and then proceed to deal with unsettlable issues. Of course, proposals regarding ways to do this vary. In order to see what promise these methods hold, I examine two that have received a good deal of attention.

Emanuel's Community Health Plan

One communitarian proposal that has received the attention of bioethicists is Ezekiel Emanuel's idea to divide health-care delivery into units of approximately 10,000 members who subscribe to a health plan. These Community Health Plans (CHPs) are based on the notion that the services offered are best determined by the members. His proposal presupposes a system committed to universal coverage of all citizens that, therefore, issues a voucher to each citizen (Emanuel 1991, 185). Citizens then form their own plans and make their own resource allocation decisions (Emanuel 1991, 178–9).

The Community Health Plan is formed in stages (Emanuel 1991, 179–82). Citizens first come together to determine their fundamental values. For CHPs that are forming based upon an existing religious or ethnic tradition (such as Orthodox Judaism), the fundamental value commitments might be fairly clear and their translation into services offered might also proceed rather smoothly. For those plans made up of citizens from less homogenous backgrounds, the stage in which fundamental value commitments are reached may take longer and involve consideration of cases in order to glean the values on which the members agree. Such plans would also need to take seriously ongoing refinement of services at various intervals since new cases may require further deliberation by the membership.

The Community Health Plan functions on the model of the New England town meeting (Emanuel 1991, 171). In this type of system, development of a core group that actually contributes most of the effort and performs the deliberations is likely. Generally, the majority are less involved and tend to register their approval or disapproval during open enrollment periods when they are allowed to change membership. Nevertheless, all citizens have an opportunity to develop their deliberative capacities and to engage their fellows in discussion regarding values and the translation of values into the everyday workings of a delivery system. One can discuss the values behind the delivery of abortion services and try to persuade one's neighbors about the range of services to be offered or prohibited in the CHP. However, if reasonable accommodations among the membership cannot be reached, it is probably a basic conflict of values, i.e., "fundamental disagreement" (Emanuel 1991, 168–169), and it would be better if the conflicting parties separated into different CHPs according to their fundamental values.

We see some surprising results. The communitarian is happy to create a system in which each person can develop his/her own deliberative capacities in order to discover his or her own values in concert with others.

However, the plan clearly reflects the liberal democratic belief that such endeavors will not be highly successful at producing harmony. As a result, the need arises to fragment society into smaller units, each with its own set of fundamental values. Will this solve the interminable and shrill debate on a question such as abortion?

At first glance, it seems highly unlikely. Prolife CHPs will occur with some frequency and no abortions will be performed within them. Will this make antiabortion activists content? Unlikely so. Because those activists do not want abortions offered anywhere, not only in their Community Health Plan. Thus, they will continue to be activists. Prochoice forces may be somewhat more sanguine about the CHP system since they do not insist that anyone have an abortion. They are not proabortion. Nevertheless, circumstances might arise in which prochoicers try to intervene in other CHPs. For instance, a case of rape or incest could undoubtedly arise in which a young woman had no access to abortion services because she was in a prolife CHP by virtue of her family's enrollment or values. This type of case would undoubtedly lead to calls for a universal guarantee of abortion services across CHPs.

Can this proposal be so easily foiled? Perhaps this system relies on additional presuppositions that are not apparent. Later I argue that these presuppositions are additional features of the communitarian theory of the person. I shall return to these after examining MacIntyre's mechanism for developing shared common values.

MacIntyre's Restoration of Tradition

Alasdair MacIntyre, perhaps the best-known voice among communitarians, also puts forward suggestions for dealing with the shrill and unceasing debates. MacIntyre argues that we must restore a shared hierarchy of goods to adjudicate value disputes. He believes that this shared hierarchy constitutes a vision of the good life. Thus, we must engage in a Socratic quest for a shared vision of the good life (MacIntyre 1984, 218–219). Such a grand project will be difficult to make operational.

MacIntyre suggests that the only way to develop a shared vision of the good life is by virtue of a reconstructed university (MacIntyre 1990, 230–232). He believes that visions of the good life are so disparate and their relative rankings of goods are so different that direct debate among them would simply mimic the shrill and interminable debates currently prevalent in society. So, each vision should be completed by like-minded scholars working together to conduct investigations within the particular tradition of inquiry in which the vision developed. These traditions will then compete for the public mind. Their relative abilities to make sense of life and to adapt to changing sociopolitical conditions, i.e., their ability to adapt to crisis, will prove the test among traditions (MacIntyre 1988, 366). Of course, one framework may simply be so comprehensive and adaptable that it assimilates the others into itself.

Once again, we see a surprising pessimism amidst an incredible optimism on the part of a communitarian thinker. MacIntyre is a pessimist in that he also shares the postEnlightenment belief that values are essentially untranslatable and incommensurable among people who do not share the same ones (MacIntyre 1990, 4). Although people are better off for joining in a communal quest for the good life, the endeavor is frustrating and hopeless unless they all begin by holding the same fundamental values. Like the Enlightenment philosophers he so disdains, MacIntyre presupposes that opposing values cannot be reconciled.

Nonetheless, he is remarkably optimistic regarding the ability of a restored tradition to resolve the shrill and interminable debates on particular issues. Is this warranted? Perhaps an example would help. Let us assume that some version of the Thomistic tradition (MacIntyre's own preference) and worldview is restored and becomes widely accepted as our shared understanding of the good life. Let us further assume that this restored tradition incorporates many of the classical elements of Thomism—for example, natural law theory, some version of personhood that is dependent on a theory of the rational soul, a doctrine of probabilism, a nuanced casuistry in applying these tenets, and so on. Exactly how wide a range of latitude this would give to abortion services is difficult to know with certainty. However, it is possible that such a shared tradition would condemn as immoral most of the abortions that currently are performed but would permit a certain class of them—for example, early-term abortions in which the life of the mother is threatened and the odds of bringing the pregnancy to term are small. Would the restoration of such a Thomistic tradition be sufficient to end the debate?

It would end debate if everyone were committed to accepting the consequences that follow from the values originally accepted as foundational. However, these values will be chosen by an elite in the relatively removed setting of a university, and enlisting everyone in that original agreement will be difficult. Furthermore, if one does not find the upshot of a fundamental value or principle acceptable, why not reject the value or principle? There is no evident reason why strongly prolife persons should accept the consequence that even a very small class of abortions will be permitted. Why would they not simply denounce the conclusions of the university as the propaganda of a liberal elite out to hoodwink people like themselves? Envisioning the arguments that would come from those on the opposite extreme is also a simple matter.

Like Emanuel's system, MacIntyre's can only be viable if we make some further presuppositions—presuppositions regarding the citizens' commitment to the conclusions of communal deliberation. These presuppositions merit further examination.

The Communitarian View of the Person Revisited

The communitarian approach to ethical problems seems to demand that people are willing to accept, or at least to tolerate, the outcomes of the communal deliberative processes. But why should they do so? The answer would seem to be because they will be persons of a certain type. They must come to value the processes of communal deliberation above the results; they are thus willing to live with the results rather than to threaten the process (Emanuel 1991, 168).

Citizens who value the process of communal deliberation above their own wishes must believe that something is gained by the process. In our liberal democracy, citizens value rights to the point that they are usually willing to put aside other convictions in order to avoid jeopardizing their own rights and those of others. This is clearly not sufficient, however, in the case of the shrill abortion debates; an appeal to the "American Way" does not stop people from infringing on each other's rights. Something more substantive must be gained from the process of communal deliberation. For the communitarian, that something is moral truth.

The communitarian sees truth as something discovered in the interpersonal encounter. Unlike the liberal vision of the person who makes moral truth a private matter of self-examination, the communitarian sees the person as reaching out to the other because truth is a matter of mutual self-discovery. One may have his or her own values, preferences, and moral knowledge, but the interpersonal testing of these personal holdings refines them and invites us to those commitments that make us who we are. This is a process that began at an indeterminate time in our past and continues into some indefinite time in the future as our legacy. In other words, we do not construct our personal narratives by ourselves but in collaboration with the community around us (Kuczewski 1997).

The communitarian notion of the person is reminiscent of the classical Socratic notion of citizenship and its relationship to philosophy. Socrates supposedly engaged in discussion with his peers in order that each might test his beliefs. This kind of self-examination helps to shape the character of the interlocutors. One's beliefs cannot be considered true until they are tested in the interpersonal arena of examination and crossexamination. Falsehoods are excluded and truth emerges as a function of this process. In Plato's dialogues, this process does not always please the interlocutor. However, the character of Socrates is happy to engage in these exchanges and believes that one must even engage the laws of one's state in this dialectical procedure. In the *Crito*, we see that Plato's Socrates believes that one must persuade the laws that they are unjust or obey them. He follows this conclusion to his own death.

When we discuss Socrates, we tend to speak in terms of the virtue of wisdom. In our modern idiom, however, we may look at these same attributes in terms of humility. Being part of a communal deliberative process means that I must begin with the supposition that I do not possess unqualified truth. If I believe I possess truth *simpliciter*, whether it be in the form of an absolute principle or a belief about the nature of reality, there can be no genuine mutual investigation of matters and no way for me to accept an alternative conclusion, no matter how well justified. But if I genuinely believe that I do not know everything and that I can benefit from the knowledge, experience, and vantage point of my neighbor, I may be willing to live with a consensus of the group, even if it does not presently seem correct to me.

Conclusion: What Communitarianism Contributes

A more theoretical way of summing up the insights we have gained is to draw a contrast between two methods of problem solving in communitarianism (Kuczewski 1997, 24–57). The whole tradition method of communitarianism emphasizes the need to restore an entire moral tradition in one move. Emanuel and MacIntyre offer strategies for how to restore such traditions. These strategies not only have their difficulties but are also unAristotelian in their philosophical presuppositions. They assume that a rigid dichotomy exists between facts and values. Unlike Aristotle, both Emanuel and MacIntyre are guilty of thinking that we cannot come to agreement on values from examining the matters at hand. In their pessimism, they more closely mirror the Enlightenment thinkers they decry than Aristotle. But, as we have seen, their whole tradition method also presupposes a more subtle notion of communitarianism that embraces a notion of the person as one who comes to discover himself or herself in dialogue with others. This is the method of communitarianism as mutual self-discovery. Such a method naturally asks how we can create the conditions under which a genuine dialogue among persons can take place in which they can discover and refine their values together.

According to the communitarians, resolving the shrill and interminable debates requires that these matters be part of an interpersonal process that goes much deeper than mere voting. Voting allows one to register transient whims based upon caricatures of reasoned positions. Communal deliberative processes demand that we each come to discover our deeply held values and commit to them operatively.

This emphasis on the process of mutual self-discovery, however, does not sort out how decisions about abortion are best made. It certainly implies that rights are too scant a moral concept to hold the entire truth about such an issue. How best, then, to handle this question is still an open subject, especially given the impracticality of the two communitarian schemes we have examined. They face a chicken-and-egg situation: their procedures require a certain kind of person but we only become that kind of person through a long process of adherence to their procedures.

In sum, we can draw two conclusions from our survey of communitarianism. First, the shrill and interminable debates will not end suddenly through the use of a communal methodology of deliberation. They will only end by a commitment to being a certain kind of person, one of humility who genuinely desires communal dialogue rather than interminable shouting.[3] Second, such persons are unlikely to want this communal deliberative process to be mainly a legislative process. Legislation in these matters is usually about establishing, broadening, or restricting the rights of one party or another.

The communitarian critique of the rights-based approach is telling. On both the personal and societal level, communitarianism calls us away from conversation-stopping assertions of rights and toward consideration of responsibilities. Communitarians seek ways to foster responsible decision making rather than "impulse buying." The main question becomes "How can the community encourage responsible decision making by its members?" Such responsible decision making will not inherently end the shrill debates. But it will begin to help people become the kind of persons who might engage in the kind of deliberative schemes we examined earlier.

Society will need to ask what role it could play in a genuine deliberative process. That is, how can it enhance the moral reflection of its members such that they truly come to understand their choices in light of their values and character development rather than as options from a menu of choices? How can this be done such that it contributes to a supportive environment for people faced with difficult choices rather than become a seeming punishment? It is likely that dialogue on such questions could lead to creating new options of assistance for those in need or taking measures that add to the appeal of certain options. The communitarian asserts that society need not remain neutral toward all choices, values, and conceptions of the good life. By what options it creates and fosters, society comes to know what it values. But it is not enough to pay lip service to certain values. Society must provide support to encourage actions congruent with those values in order to lay claim to those.

Communitarianism steers a middle way between the relativism of value neutrality and the value imperialism of whole tradition communitarianism. The vision of communitarianism as mutual self-discovery exhibits a faith in humans as a heuristic ideal, that is, when genuine communal dialogue takes place among persons of good will, people generally discover the right thing to do. In so doing, they begin to shape their character into being the kind of people who value such dialogue. Becoming such people is the sine qua non of ending the shrill debates. Conversely, moral deliberation and education break down when shouting replaces dialogue, blame replaces responsibility, and punishment replaces supportiveness. In this faith in the deliberative process, communitarianism echoes Aristotle's and Thomas Aquinas's belief that nature contains certain values that are discovered through ethical reflection. But, contemporary communitarianism eschews metaphysical formulations in favor of a phenomenology of deliberation. It seeks to find conditions that can help us become virtuous deliberators.

This point of view does not mean that legislation can never play a part in the life of a community. But, legislation that asserts rights seems unlikely to be a starting point in producing consensus. Working with professional organizations, community and civic groups, health care institutions, and religious organizations, that is, the places people turn for help and that foster virtue, is more likely to allow for a nuanced, nonthreatening approach to these matters in which citizens can learn from each other rather than talk past one another.

Notes

1. The terminology of "shrill and interminable" debates is borrowed from Alasdair MacIntyre. In *After Virtue* (1984, 8) he uses this phrase to describe the contemporary public dialogue on moral matters. MacIntyre's terminology may be unique to him but virtually every communitarian describes the current public dialogue in a similar manner.

2. Abortion is certainly the quintessential example. Asking what other issues are similar might also be useful. MacIntyre (1984, 6–7) identifies arguments concerning abortion, just wars, and equal opportunity as being similar in this manner. To readers in the United States, arguments about just wars seem remote because of the time that has elapsed since the divisive Vietnam conflict. However, MacIntyre's point about questions of equal opportunity is still very salient. Recent public debates in the United States concerning government entitlement programs, welfare reform, affirmative action, and so forth, can serve to illustrate his case.

3. This does not mean that some people will not end up with deep convictions that run counter to the societal consensus that emerges. The earlier example of Socrates is instructive. He does not give up his convictions. But, he accepts that under certain conditions, he must continue to respect his city's edicts.

References

Callahan, D. 1990. "An Ethical Challenge to Prochoice Advocates: Abortion and the Pluralistic Proposition." *Commonweal* 117(20): 681–7.

Clinton, H. R. 1996. *It Takes a Village and Other Lessons Children Teach Us.* New York: Simon & Schuster.

Emanuel, E. J. 1991. *The Ends of Human Life: Medical Ethics in a Liberal Polity.* Cambridge, Mass.: Harvard University Press.

Emanuel, E. J., and L. L. Emanuel. 1992. "Four Models of the Physician-Patient Relationship." *Journal of the American Medical Association* 267: 2221–6.

Etzioni, A. 1993. *The Spirit of Community: Rights, Responsibilities, and the Communitarian Agenda.* New York: Crown Publishers.

Kuczewski, M. G. 1997. *Fragmentation and Consensus: Communitarian and Casuist Bioethics.* Washington, DC: Georgetown University Press.

Lidz, C. W., P. S. Appelbaum, and A. Meisel. 1988. "Two Models of Implementing Informed Consent." *Archives of Internal Medicine* 148: 1385–1389.

MacIntyre, A. 1984. *After Virtue: A Study in Moral Theory*, 2d ed. Notre Dame, Ind.: University of Notre Dame Press.

MacIntyre, A. 1988. *Whose Justice? Which Rationality?* Notre Dame, Ind.: University of Notre Dame Press.

MacIntyre, A. 1990. *Three Rival Versions of Moral Enquiry: Encyclopedia, Genealogy, and Tradition.* Notre Dame, Ind.: University of Notre Dame Press.

Planned Parenthood of Southeastern Pennsylvania v. Casey 112 S. Ct 2791 (1992).

Roe v. Wade, 410 U.S. 113 (1973).

Sandel, M. J. 1982. *Liberalism and the Limits of Justice.* New York: Cambridge University Press.

Sandel, M. J. 1984. "The Procedural Republic and the Unencumbered Self." *Political Theory* 12: 81–96.

Taylor, C. 1989. *Sources of the Self: The Making of the Modern Identity.* Cambridge, Mass.: Harvard University Press.

Webster v. Reproductive Health Services, 492 U.S. 490 (1990).

10

Classical and Modern Reflections on Medical Ethics and the Best Interests of the Sick Child

Daryl M. Tress

The conjunction of ancient Greek philosophy and pediatric medical ethics may sound improbable. The historical distance alone of more than two thousand years that separates our world from that of classical antiquity may seem to provide insufficient ground for an intersection between them. For example, the advanced technology that today gives rise to many ethical dilemmas was, of course, nonexistent in the ancient world. Moreover, no medical specialty of pediatrics existed, nor was medicine itself practiced or conceived of in the same way we currently do. Philosophy, too, has been significantly transformed in the intervening millennia. Classical philosophy and pediatric medical ethics may seem an unlikely match for a dialogue.

In the last twenty years, however, several major works have appeared proposing a retrieval of classical philosophy for contemporary ethics. The ethical approaches and concepts of the ancient Greeks are identified and advocated in Alasdair MacIntryre's *After Virtue* (1981), in Albert Jonsen and Stephen Toulmin's *The Abuse of Casuistry* (1988), and in Martha Nussbaum's *Love's Knowledge* (1990), to name only several of the most important recent works. These ideas have been extended, in turn, to the field of medical ethics in Howard Brody's *The Healer's Power* (1992) as well as in many other works.[1] These books have generated a discussion so significant that the contemporary ethical debate has shifted. Classical "virtue ethics" or "eudaimonism"—ethics aimed at virtuous character, based on a conception of the desire for *eudaimonia* (happiness)—is no longer regarded as a foreign or outdated ethics. Now, virtue ethics stands alongside the standard modern ethical models of deontology (duty- or principles-based ethics) and consequentialism (ethics aimed at producing positive outcomes). Although these contemporary writers each make distinct cases for the revival of classical philosophy, I plan to show that they all view the ethics of Greek antiquity through a decidedly modern lens, resulting in the assimilation of classical and modern views. Because their turn to the ancient Greeks is prompted by a desire to resolve deep difficulties in modern ethical models, their adoption of classical ethical concepts is highly selective, reflecting modern needs far more than genuinely classical outlooks. Specifically, their emphasis on ethical particularism (the notion that ethical good is specific to particular situations or groups) and on a narrative method meant to support it (a method in which a story is constructed that is intended to include multiple subjective and situational elements of an ethical conflict) do not truly reflect the approaches of classical philosophy. Most importantly, these emphases obscure the real character of the ancient Greek philosophical outlook, which challenges the modern one and is therefore valuable to recognize today.

I affirm the real and important distance separating the classical and modern worlds. The ancient ideas of the Greek philosophers and physicians differ significantly from our contemporary modes of thought, as I hope to show, and their world may indeed seem foreign to us. This is not to say, however, that classical thinkers have nothing to offer. Rather, the lessons of their approach are not directly or easily accessible via modern issues; they need to be read on their own terms. In doing so, it is evident that particularism and its narrative technique are not characteristic of classical ethics. The resemblance is only apparent, arising from the perspective of modern ethics' deficiencies. Salient among these in medical ethics is the impersonality associated with both duty-based and calculus-of-goods ethical approaches, which particularism and narrative ethics are meant to counter. In contrast, classical ethics is distinctive in two respects: first, it is based on the enhancement of the ethical agent's virtue, that is, the development of excellence in the one who chooses and acts. Narrative ethical approaches, however, aim to be inclusive, extending the range of those who are ethically pertinent and offering a variable focus on one or another of them. Second, classical ethics sees the enhancement of virtue as involving transcendent factors in some way. (In ancient Greek philosophy, "the transcendent" refers to things taken to exist outside of spatial and temporal parameters, such as the essence of objects, mathematical figures and numbers, or the gods.) The enhancement of the virtue of the ethical agent—and in this discussion of pediatric ethics the agents are chiefly the doctors, nurses, and child's parents who chose and act—is particularly foreign to modern medical ethics, which is highly patient-centered.[2] The inclusion of transcendent factors is foreign to modern thought, which is largely naturalistic and pluralistic, and, in turn, alien to contemporary medicine, which is scientific in its foundations. As I will discuss, recent advocates of virtue ethics do not make the agent's virtue paramount because their revival of classical moral philosophy springs from exigencies in the contemporary situation and is intended to meet the current definition of our needs. In medical ethics, these are perceived to be chiefly the protection of the patient's rights and autonomy; in pediatric medical ethics they are chiefly the protection of the sick child when the course of treatment is in doubt and disagreement arises between parents and doctors. Therefore, although the turn to classical ethics by some of its recent advocates may seem to be an important change, it often remains largely dictated by modern values and requirements. Since the modern frameworks are acknowledged as faulty by the recent advocates of a classical approach, it is important to keep clear the distinctions between modern and classical ethics, and valuable to consider the contributions that an unmodified classical ethics might make.

The special field of pediatric medical ethics has been governed in recent decades by the best-interests-of-the-child guideline (the "best-interests" standard). This guideline, on its face, is unassailable insofar as it sets as a goal that those involved in the sick child's care act to serve the child's good.[3] On further probing, however, critics lately have found the guideline wanting in several ways, such as being unrealistic or vague as a standard in clinical decision making.

To examine these issues, this chapter is divided into four sections. The first section examines the best interests-of-the-child guideline as it is currently defined. After outlining what some critics claim are its shortcomings, I trace these shortcomings to the origin of the best-interests doctrine in the modern ethical models of both deontology and consequentialism. The current debate about best interests in fact illustrates the familiar dispute about and between these competing modern ethical models. Indeed, the character of the guideline is deeply modern, as can be seen in the emphasis it places on patient rights and quality-of-life considerations.

Can classical philosophy contribute to this deliberation? The second section presents the position of recent advocates of classical ethics (often referred to as neoAristotelians) that an important lesson taught by the Greek philosophers, especially Aristotle, is attention to the particularities of the situation in which the decision makers will determine the right course of action. This emphasis on the particular is meant to contrast with modern ethical approaches in which a universal rule or formula is imposed on the circumstances to determine the right course of action. These advocates recommend a narrative technique for gathering and holding the particulars and the local context in view, with the patient encouraged to tell his or her own story to lend continuity and meaning to the human factors involved in the course of the illness. I contend that ethical particularism and narrative methods are, at most, a hybrid of modern needs and some classical themes.

For both Plato and Aristotle, ethical knowledge is not attained from the artistic selection and arrangement of particulars, as in a story, but by finding the universal truth (or the essential *form* or the ethical *mean*) *in* the particulars. Subjective narratives cannot substitute for the inquiry and analysis—the examination of assumptions, opinions, and "stories"— that ground ethics in classical philosophy. Plato is especially concerned about the poets' stories which mesmerize both teller and listener, encouraging them to assume that they already possess the truth so that inquiry is discouraged.

In the third part of this essay I reflect on Sophocles's magisterial drama, *Oedipus the King*, showing that the limitations of stories in the realm of ethics—that is, the inability of stories to serve as a reliable guide for personal and public life—emerge even among the classical poets. *Oedipus* opens with the dark and moving specter of sick children and so is especially apt for this discussion. Finally, in conclusion (the fourth section), I offer a summary of what I understand to be the basis of the ethics of Plato and Aristotle and of how it might be brought to bear in pediatric ethics, suggesting two main topics. The first is the virtue of character, compared with a focus on autonomy or rights of the patient. Concentrating on the enhancement of virtue in those agents who are choosing and acting for the sick child acknowledges the child's vulnerability and incapacity and regards the agents' virtue in terms of their ability to determine and act for the child's good. Determining whose right to choose prevails, as in modern medical ethics, is no longer paramount. Because the agent's virtue develops over time, the classical approach alters the fundamental framework of contemporary medical ethics, moving away from resolution of discrete ethical problems that arise episodically, and toward the agent's quality of character. Furthermore, classical ethics, in contrast to modern ethics with its stress on acts from which agents should be restricted, allows for appreciation and commendation of the agents' excellence of character, constituted through their repeated good actions.

The second focus concerns the relations of "transcendent" elements to this inquiry. Because both classical philosophy and medicine integrate transcendent or spiritual elements, which they take to be crucial for a proper ethical orientation, they offer a response to the formality, abstraction, and impersonality associated with modern ethical models different from that attributed to them by neoAristotelians. Modern intellectual and social life largely debar the transcendent. Ethical particularism and narrative methods recommended by recent advocates of classical ethics are a substitute for the transcendent and, admittedly, are better adapted to the mentality and practices of our time. However, insofar as classical antiquity is alien to our modern assumptions, it is especially valuable in exhibiting those assumptions for us so that they can be scrutinized.

The Best-Interests Guideline

... the best-interests standard may seem vague if reasonable and informed people of good will cannot agree about how to use it. (Kopelman 1997b, 286)

"The best interests of the child" is the prevailing general guideline for decision making on behalf of children that is employed in both legal and medical contexts. It holds that "decision makers should try to identify the [child's] immediate and long-term interests and then determine whether the benefits of an intervention or procedure outweigh the burdens."[3] The guideline is meant to allow complex matters to be taken into account and difficult decisions concerning the child to be reached by involved and competent adults, usually the child's parents and doctors. An example of its use—perhaps an extreme example but one that is frequently called upon as a paradigm—would be in the case of a very young and seriously ill patient with a poor prognosis where life-sustaining treatment is causing pain and suffering. Is it in the child's best interests to have the treatment continued or not? In such circumstances, efforts would be made to assess the prognosis as exactly as possible and to make an objective, medical measure of pain so that these can be weighed and a decision made.[4]

While the guideline is quite simple and sensible at one level—that is, directing attention to the child and what serves the child best—its adequacy and even its ethical correctness are nonetheless open to objection in a number of ways. Let us consider three of these and inquire into the presuppositions that underlie them.[5]

First, some critics charge that the best-interests guideline, insofar as it sets the *best* as the aim, creates an unattainable and unrealistic demand. Therefore, the guideline is self-defeating and is of no practical help (Kopelman 1997b, 283). They point out that it is impossible for people to do what is best even in most ordinary instances, and in the kinds of situations where best interests is invoked, the difficult choice is usually between two or more undesirable options. The point the critics make, then, is twofold: first, "best interests" is perfectionist in that it sets too high an ideal, which people cannot be expected to attain; second, the interests in conflict in the ethical dilemma may not admit of a *best* or even a good but only of the least of several evils.

Its defenders, however, say that best interests is only a guideline and does not state an absolute duty, functioning often as an indication for intervention rather than as an ethical standard that would demand that doctors, parents, and others know and do what is absolutely the best thing for the child (Kopelman 1995, 360, and 1997b, 283). In the debate, the critics of the best-interests standard have detected the guideline's apparent reliance on an unstated, objective standard of goodness in invoking what is "best." Indeed, if such a standard were operating, it would grant best-interests its moral authority and save it from arbitrariness. But as noted, the critics hold that the *best* as a standard is perfectionistic and unrealistic; they thus conclude that best-interests is misguided. Defenders agree with the critics' argument that absolute standards are unattainable and undesirable; they seek instead to counter the critics' concerns with assurances that best-interests is neither absolute nor idealistic but, in fact, both minimalist with regard to ethical principles and pragmatic, allowing for a high degree of ethical adaptability to the particular circumstances and predicted outcomes. Here, both critics and defenders, in effect, reject a deontological approach in which ethics consists of binding obligations that rational agents can be expected to know and put into practice. On this point, critics and defenders share similar views about the character of ethics as pragmatic, the good as flexible, and the fallibility of human nature.

The second set of objections to the best-interests guideline arises from a very different group of critics, who hold that the weighing of interests the guideline involves is not an ethical process, particularly when it means predicting outcomes and calculating interests. These critics reject the very flexibility that others see as positive, supporting instead a "principles" approach, which, they hold, should govern medical ethics. (In one presentation of this approach, principles are discussed primarily in the context of deontological and utilitarian, or consequentialist, ethical theories by Tom L. Beauchamp and James F. Childress in *Principles of Biomedical Ethics*. The principles they present—autonomy, nonmaleficence, beneficence, and justice—in turn give rise to more specific rules.) This group of best-interests critics expresses the concern that in abandoning absolute moral principles (e.g., the fundamental worth of a human life and the duty to protect it), other, nonmoral factors (e.g., costs) and even immoral factors (e.g., selfishness or greed) will be legitimated in medical ethical decision making, and might then figure in the weighing of interests.

The concern about the potential for abuse when vital decisions are made not according to basic principles but rather to the calculations of surrogate decision makers projecting a quality of life concern led President Reagan and Surgeon General Koop in the 1980s to institute the "Baby Doe" rules. These rules prohibit the withdrawal of life-saving treatment from newborns except under clearly defined circumstances. They thus limit considerably the use of quality-of-life considerations while reaffirming a binding ethical principle (the duty to preserve life) governing such decisions. Koop (1989, 2–3) speaks unequivocally: "Nothing in medicine —and nothing anywhere else in our Western, Judeo-Christian tradition— enables one person to make a judgment about another person's 'quality of life.'"

Critics in this second category, like Dr. Koop, implicitly object to the consequentialism that best-interests implies (Kopelman 1995, i 360, and 1997b, 284–285). That is, they deny that ethics amounts to trying to maximize the good outcome, to produce the greatest good for the greatest number. Defenders of the best-interests guideline argue, however, that using it as an absolute rule deprives parents and doctors of their autonomy by rigidly imposing an abstract, impersonal principle upon them in complex circumstances. Unlike the first category of objections, in which critics and defenders share a conception of ethics, here the basic conceptions of critics and defenders are in opposition. Even here, however, critics and defenders have roughly a common notion of human nature as fallible, but they respond to that fallibility in different ways. Critics like Dr. Koop restrict freedom of choice and preference in the belief that allowing the inclusion of a myriad of factors obscures the principles that truly constitute ethics. Best-interests guideline defenders, in contrast, preserve an extensive range of potentially relevant considerations for the decision makers so that in constructing their decision they can make as suitable a decision as possible.[6]

A third criticism of best-interests bears a curious relation to the previous two. It holds that best-interests is too individualistic. Critics here maintain that best-interests directs the surrogate decision makers to consider exclusively the sick child's interests, thereby denying legitimacy to others' interests, such as other children in the family, whose needs should be taken into account in serious decisions.[7] Some of these critics may voice their objections, as the first group does, from a consequentialist vantage point. They notice and react against the rule aspect of best-interests, with its strong demand that decision makers protect the single, vulnerable individual (i.e., the sick child) without regard to others' needs. They are concerned to keep in view the wider field of ethical considerations and the multiplicity of interests. Other critics on this point, however, may voice their objections from a more deontological point of view. This group, maintaining a principles approach, might posit the family rather than the individual alone as the appropriate ethical decision-making unit and insist on strong obligations to protect it.

The presence of different subgroups of critics using conflicting rationales for their objections signals the instability in this third claim and, by extension, the vagueness of best-interests generally. In this case, expanding the range of individuals whose interests are ethically pertinent is in inverse proportion to guaranteed protection for the sick child, insofar as these individuals' interests are weighed against one another. Indeed, when the critics who favor strong principles have complained that the best-interests guideline is open to abuse in just this way, defenders have replied, as the U.S. President's Commission did, by reaffirming its sole focus on the patient, stating that "This is a very strict standard in that it excludes considerations of the negative effects of an impaired child's life on other persons, including parents, siblings, and society."[8] But such exclusivity may appear undesirable, even impossible, in some situations. Beyond this dispute, however, is a deeper problem: best-interests does not seem to underwrite in any way exclusive attention to the sick patient, nor does the guideline provide justification for giving ethical weight to family members and circumstances. Searching in vain for a philosophical warrant for one or the other course is a reminder that best-interests can function only as a very general guideline and is open to different, even conflicting, interpretations.

The impasse between defenders and critics of best-interests mirrors the impasse between consequentialist and deontological ethics, the two major modern approaches to ethics. The deontologist, on the one hand, objects that the consequentialist, with a focus on outcomes, allows any and all factors to weigh in decision making, under the misapprehension that somehow these can be tallied up to yield an ethical decision. The consequentialist, on the other hand, objects that in a deontological scheme principles govern too rigidly, too impersonally, and too abstractly. The impasse reflects as well, no doubt, the contemporary circumstances in which much medical ethical decision making is undertaken, that is, in the institutional setting of the hospital, with complex technology available, among a team of doctors, many of whom are specialists and may be strangers to the patient and his or her family, and so on. In such circumstances, any patient, and a sick child most of all, is small and vulnerable and may be urgently in need of protection. Consequentialists and deontologists both sponsor the protection of the patient, albeit in widely different ways, and behind sponsorship of protection is an assumption common in the medical ethics literature of opposed interests, or potentially opposed interests, among the medical team, the parents, and the sick child. Many, if not most, of the discussions of best-interests present just such problems of conflict between doctors' recommendations and parents' wishes, with best-interests introduced to resolve dilemmas about what to do and who should decide.

The dispute between the two modern approaches, as expressed in the criticisms of the best-interests-of-the-child guideline and more generally, gives the strong impression of being unresolvable. New advocates of classical ethics attempt to break the impasse by introducing, or reintroducing, virtue ethics, usually making *phronesis*—"practical wisdom"—central to it. They also address the recurring issues of impersonality (of principles and rules) and inconclusiveness (of context and circumstances) by way of a narrative emphasis, claimed to be part of classical ethics. The next section examines their proposals and how the primacy of their aim to overcome the failures of modern ethics leads to a misrepresentation of classical philosophy.

The NeoAristotelians

The idea of our being large is inconceivable. . .
We have a growing appetite.
For littleness. . .
Mark Strand, "Dark Harbor" 1998

The title of Eric B. Beresford's valuable paper, "Can *Phronesis* Save the Life of Medical Ethics?" gestures to an earlier important paper, "How Medicine Saved the Life of Ethics," by Stephen E. Toulmin.[9] Toulmin observes that when ethics was called upon in recent decades to grapple with particular problems and specific cases as they arise for hospital ethics committees and other institutional and governmental bodies attempting to set ethical policy for medicine, the old, interminable conflicts between the ethical theories faded well into the background. Surprisingly, participants in these meetings frequently reached consensus on their ethical recommendations. Toulmin's explanation for the unexpected agreement is that these groups began their deliberations with a close scrutiny of particular cases rather than by trying to agree at the start about a theory (such as deontology or consequentialism) or about general principles (e.g., human life must be preserved under all circumstances) that would then be applied to the individual patient's case. The lesson is that ethics—medical ethics as well as ethics generally, in Toulmin's view—needs to proceed from the particular and concrete, not from the general theory, principle, or rule in order to move beyond its endless disagreements.[10] In order to shift from theory to an ethics of interpreting particular situations, a special skill is required, and Aristotle's *phronesis* is proposed as this skill.

It is with a widely shared sense of dissatisfaction about the current state of ethics that scholars such as Alasdair MacIntyre and Martha Nussbaum have sought to offer an alternative to modern models. Like Toulmin, they see that turning to the particularities of concrete cases rather than to the generalities of theory provides a way to bypass disputes that are unresolvable at the theoretical level. Toulmin recommends "casuistry," a case-based ethical approach with origins in late Greek antiquity that flowered in the Middle Ages. MacIntyre and Nussbaum focus more strictly on Greek antiquity. They see classical philosophy as giving primacy, in different degrees, to particularities, to local tradition, and to *phronesis*. In their retrieval of Greek philosophy, these scholars' accounts of classical ethics—especially *phronesis* and its relation to a narrative approach—are instructive.

MacIntyre's landmark book, *After Virtue* (1981), begins with a parable that conveys the current crisis he sees in ethics: like survivors of a terrible disaster, we continue to use ethical terms and to talk about "good" and "bad" with only the most fragmentary and inadequate sense of what they mean and what they might refer to. People hold ethical principles, of course, but strong conflicts exist among them as well as serious difficulties in the application of general principles to situations of choice. Rules, too, which are more specific than principles, face many of the same difficulties of application and "fit" with particular situations. How else, and how better, might we know what to choose and what to do? MacIntyre's recommendation is *phronesis*—practical moral judgment that operates in, and *within*, lived situations. For MacIntyre, there is no detached, external place where we can stand and apply objectively known and universally valid principles to solve our moral quandaries. Rather, human beings are always situated within a tradition that construes the choice and the options for how it is to be made. (Thus his parable about our dire state of affairs in the modern Western world, where we no longer recognize our tradition.) Nor does a neutral place exist where conflicting principles or theories or traditions themselves can be fully measured against one another and adjudicated. MacIntyre's appropriation of *phronesis*, then, is marked by an emphasis on incommensurability: first, the incommensurability of theories implies that ethics must necessarily turn from the general to the particular to do its work; second, incommensurability implies that particular situations may each be unique and in need of being judged uniquely.

Toulmin, as noted, was inspired by the broader possibilities for agreement, and thereby resolution of moral conflicts, to be accomplished via the casuist procedure of starting deliberation from particular cases rather than from moral theory. So, too, MacIntyre is motivated importantly by his aim to delineate an effective, workable moral philosophy, given the starting conditions of incommensurability. Thus, a strongly pragmatic drive pervades MacIntyre's work, as well as Toulmin's and Nussbaum's, in contrast to the speculative or intellectual thrust of classical thought, which presses to define and distinguish. The emphasis these recent advocates of a classical approach place on resolution of moral conflicts and the means of achieving consensus marks them as modern in two ways. First, they are attuned to the broadly pragmatic sensibility of much twentieth-century philosophy, both Continental and AngloAmerican, that tries to be guided by what people actually do or say or experience rather than by theoretically established ideas. Taking actual practice, personal or communal, as a basis or norm in philosophy has seemed to many twentieth-century philosophers (in the face of the sorts of difficulties examined in section 1) to be more promising than modern theories have been.[11] Second, the urgent need to find efficient procedures of resolution and to reach social consensus on moral issues is symptomatic of a pluralist, secular modernity. A society without shared moral authority or values must have another method in order to carry on. Toulmin, MacIntyre, and Nussbaum, in their own ways, are motivated by this need, and their work may be viewed as offering a means of reaching satisfactory moral resolutions under difficult modern conditions.

Certainly ancient Greek philosophy is concerned with putting moral philosophy into practice: Socrates in Plato's dialogues persistently asks whether virtue can be taught and what forms of education best lead to virtue; Aristotle remarks famously in the *Nicomachean Ethics* i

3.1095a5 that the purpose of ethics is not just to know the good but to help men to *do* good. A salient difference, however, arises between modern and ancient aims, primarily in that the classical philosophers saw speculative inquiry as a prerequisite for more practical recommendations. In particular, some understanding of the Good or of the human *telos*—the proper perfection of a human life—is necessary, in their view, for directing practical philosophy and for cultivating *phronesis*. Toulmin sees such overarching, universal matters as impeding discussions that would lead to consensus; MacIntyre sees them as being in such deep dispute in our day that understanding can only be hoped for "locally," within a given tradition. Nussbaum, too, avoids general claims about *the* good, which she associates with Plato, and favors instead a plurality of goods, determined locally for the most part, a view she associates with Aristotle.

These modern scholars share, to a greater or lesser extent, a modern sense of futility about speculative knowledge and its implications for the moral domain. This pessimism, however, was not the shaping outlook of the classical philosophers. For them, metaphysics formed either an intrinsic part of ethics, as in Plato's notion of virtue as knowledge of the transcendent Forms, or it played a crucial role in identifying the best human happiness, as in Aristotle's delineation of it as the most godlike activity (that is, contemplation of the changeless things), which then serves to order all other human activities and virtues.

One step in releasing ethics from its modern impasses and making it "work" is to cease trying to establish a single, common idea of goodness and human life to which everyone would or should agree—in other words, to relinquish the expectation of demonstrating ethical truth. Recent advocates of classical ethics take this step, intending it as a departure from the standard modern models and their apparently doomed, and sometimes dangerous, ambitions for universality. Toulmin, MacIntyre, and Nussbaum thus echo the critique of reason in its modern form that has been a central theme of philosophy for well over a century. Kant and his skeptical predecessors had already called for philosophy to stay within the bounds of human experience, but the hopes that Kant maintained for preserving some universality have steadily eroded. Reason, for the most part, is no longer thought capable of establishing ideals and norms; nor can it be trusted not to become tyrannical. With reason, or theory, deemed thus incapable, many contemporary philosophers have turned to human practices as an alternate basis and guide.

The turn to human practices and away from theory as a basis for philosophy and ethics in view of the perceived failures of reason is typical of twentieth-century philosophy, but not of Platonic and Aristotelian philosophy. This is especially the case since modern skepticism, with its distrust of reason, constrains modern ethical theory to abandon the teleology that the ancients posited as fundamental to their speculative inquiries. In the classical world, teleology lent coherence to the very notion of virtue at the heart of its ethics. It included a universal human nature structured toward a common goal of *eudaimonia*—happiness. In Aristotle's ethics, *eudaimonia* is defined as activity of the soul in accordance with virtue (*Nicomachean Ethics* i 7.1098a13–18, i 8.1098b30–1099a5, and x 7.1177a12–14). The key virtues concern reason, the capacity marking what is superior in human beings and fundamental to the best human life. But classical teleology has not survived into the modern scientific era, and it is inconsistent with current demands that reason refrain from positing universals. Moreover, teleology is based on hierarchy, and the ranking implied in it is in disrepute today. For these reasons, teleology cannot function in the contemporary retrieval of classical ethics. Commentators who now champion ancient Greek ethics need another means of establishing coherence and making moral life intelligible. A narrative approach furnishes a substitute for teleology.

The turn to narrative in ethics is consistent with this trend in twentieth-century thought and in particular with the criticisms of the modern ethical models to which it gives rise. Narrative, which gives structure to acts and events across a broad spectrum, from the personal to the social, fills the philosophical void left with the diminution of the authority of reason and teleology. Narrative ethics recommends the inclusion of stories in moral life in a variety of ways: telling or creating stories out of the particularities of personal experience as a way to give that experience coherence and moral meaning, reading stories for moral edification, comparing them with one another, or bringing techniques of literary analysis and criticism to bear in the moral domain (Nelson 1997, x–xii). In its variety of expressions, narrative ethics eschews the normativity central to modern ethical models of deontology and consequentialism; reason cannot be counted on to achieve moral answers, as modern ethics expected, and moreover the universalist and impersonal norms reason establishes for morality appear both unrealistic and undesirable. What is especially important is that stories are humanly constructed. We must rely on our own devices, ethically speaking, because we do not have an operative teleology or dependable speculative reason or providence, and so forth, to provide direction. Narrative as human invention is thus in keeping with the current predicament.

Nussbaum's advocacy of the narrative approach to ethics, which she attributes to Aristotle, takes into account another difficulty in modern ethics observed in connection with the best interests standard. That problem is the impersonality and abstract nature of modern ethical reasoning. Many recent critics object that deontology and perhaps, to a lesser degree, consequentialism employ abstract principles or rigid rules that cannot comprehend human personalities and predicaments. Narrative, however, can counter these difficulties.

In Nussbaum's view, ethical judgments are made first and foremost *in* concrete circumstances, taking into account all of the particularities and the uniqueness of the situation. Stories can capture these in a way that modern reasoning processes in ethics do not. One should not proceed deductively from general principles to their application in a given situation. She uses Aristotle's ethical and political writings to present arguments against the notion that practical reasoning is scientific in this way, holding that Aristotle's position involves "an attack on the ideas that all valuable things are commensurable; an argument for the priority of particular judgments to universals; and a defense of the emotions and imagination as essential to rational choice" (Nussbaum 1990, 54–5). Ethical decisions cannot be derived deductively from preestablished principles because these may not encompass the unique goods of the concrete situation, and because, as she says Aristotle holds, the virtues themselves are defined by human beings in their concrete, historical circumstances (Beresford 1996, 213).

Nussbaum's nontraditional portrait of Aristotle is a most humanistic and naturalistic one throughout. Transcendence, attention to which pervades the philosophy of Plato and Aristotle, is trimmed to human scale in her work.[12] For the Greek philosophers, however, the transcendent is beyond the ordinary human domain. Thus, in Plato, for example, the

Form of justice is a real, timeless standard for recognizing and judging incidents of justice and injustice. Aristotle retains significant elements of this way of thinking in two major ways: first, in his concepts of formal and final cause whereby essences and ends are real and found universally in ethics; second, in his positing of divine activity as a standard of human happiness. In Nussbaum's version of Aristotle, however, transcendence in the ethical field is, in effect, human growth with a marked psychological and experiential emphasis that is characteristic of the temper of the twentieth century. In keeping with her humanistic interpretation of Aristotle, narrative emerges as the appropriate, indeed the obvious, method for ethics: human storytelling about human experience.

In summary, contemporary motivations shape the efforts of Toulmin, MacIntyre, and Nussbaum to retrieve ancient ethics via particularism and narrative in numerous ways: in the urgency of their need to find a workable ethics to meet the conditions of the late twentieth century, in their desire to move beyond sterile disputes about ethical theory, in their effort to develop a model by which persons could supply the missing basis of moral coherence in their experience, and in the desire to acquire an ethics that could be truer to subjectivity and its circumstances.

Two issues may be identified for further inquiry: (1) is it accurate to refer to particularism and the narrative method as *classical* philosophical approaches? and (2) do these constitute the path to good ethics? Concerning the first issue, the full case against identifying these contemporary approaches with classical ethics involves lengthy scholarship and so cannot be pursued here.[13] The point, however, is not to refute these treatments but to clear the way for ideas more truly characteristic of classical thought. To do so, we rely on an indirect route showing that the match between the motivations for and the outline of ethical particularism and its narrative method, on the one hand, and the central concerns and major tendencies of twentieth-century philosophy, on the other, suggests that they more likely spring from modern rather than ancient Greek soil.

Before pursuing these questions further, let us take a brief look at particularism and narrative—specifically in medical ethics, through the contribution of Howard Brody—one among the growing number of medical ethicists who see a value in the narrative approach. Advocates of narrative in medical ethics represent a spectrum of views: at one end, narrative is seen as a supplement to conventional, modern modes of ethical decision making; at the other end, as a replacement for them.[14] According to those taking the milder view of narrative's usefulness, literature adds a sensitizing dimension to medicine and medical education, teaching lessons about the human predicament and alerting decision makers about pertinent nonmedical factors. More importantly, the patient or the patient's surrogate is encouraged to tell the story of the illness as it unfolds, plot-wise, with a beginning, middle, and end. Again, the narrative form is held to help elicit potentially important medical and human elements that will factor into the application of principles or the weighing of interests (Marta 1997, 199–200 and Chambers 1997, 172–175). The patient-centered and problem-resolving approach characteristic of recent medical ethics remains in place: the doctor and other medical personnel are instructed to listen to what is important to the patient so that a better resolution of the ethical conflict at hand can be reached. According to those taking a stronger view, however, stories replace applying principles and/or calculating interests because such procedures are viewed as ethically invalid. An extension of the story model regards the entire practice of medicine as being deeply literary and interpretive so that, for example, the patient is said to be "read," like a text (see the discussion in Cooper 1994). Brody himself adopts the more moderate model of narrative as supplement.

Brody's discussion of narrative medical ethics reveals how very much it is a reaction against and meant as a constructive response to modern medical conditions. Brody, like others, sees the need for significant changes in medical ethics away from the "engineering" model (the formalized, modern rights-and-rules approach) and toward a "conversation" model that retains some role for principles and formal reasoning. (He acknowledges Toulmin's work in this connection, adding that it must, however, be stripped of any residual components of natural law, presumably because natural law would seem implausible to many people in this day, or because it violates that tenets of contemporary pluralism.)

Brody's recommendation results primarily from the growing awareness of significant power discrepancies today between physician and patient. The physician controls the expertise, the technology, the hospital, the office, the medicines, and so forth. Brody also identifies numerous other subtle variables that favor the doctor's (appearance of) power, such as her charisma and social status. He is not at all the first to identify this imbalance in medicine; the emphasis in medical ethics over the last twenty to thirty years on the patient's autonomy and rights bespeaks the perception of the patient's sense of growing powerlessness. However, the deontological and consequentialist theories aimed at protecting the patient have the shortcomings already pointed out.

Further, in Brody's view, the potential for arbitrariness and inconsistency in the rights-and-rules ethical models—perhaps most tellingly in connection with patients where best-interests decision making is involved—point up our society's need for *some* shared values around life and death (Brody 1992, 162). Brody expresses these concerns in his evocation of Dostoyevsky's Grand Inquisitor scene in his medical narrative chapter, "The Chief of Medicine." His hope is that as the story of the illness is shared, the power divide between doctor and patient is bridged somewhat. Power and its distribution, particularly its unequal distribution, is an animating theme of much twentieth-century thought, both in philosophy, politics, and the social sciences. Evident in Brody's work, as well, is a narrative conception of a human life. He writes, citing MacIntyre's influence: "One can speak of the virtuous person when one views human lives as integrated narratives, from birth to death, and asks what standards of excellence can shape such narratives" (Brody 1992, 253).

Introducing a narrative conception into ethics is meant to supply the integration and coherence to a life, over time, that is missing in the piecemeal, "conflict-resolution" approach of modern ethics, and missing, too, in any shared way in a pluralistic and secular society. It has the advantage of preserving personal experience in the midst of an impersonal and sometimes bureaucratic medical process, thus empowering the patient and redressing the power imbalance with the physician. We might notice, first, that even when narrative is introduced in its more moderate version, it can be far-reaching, affecting the very framework within which we conceive of ourselves and others. Second, these features of the narrative approach—its ability to lend coherence by giving a narrative structure to events that occur over time, to preserve subjective experience, and to correct, to some extent, the power differential—are merits relative to contemporary conditions and needs. For just such reasons Brody endorses a role for narrative in medical ethics.

Brody's recommendation of narrative does not hinge on any claim by him that this is a specifically classical ethical approach, although his work is clearly influenced by scholars who do make this identification. In the next section, I suggest that the identification of particularism and narrative method as classical is incorrect and discuss a second issue identified earlier, namely, whether particularism and narrative comprise a *good* path to ethics. I suggest the contrary by showing, through the timeless Sophoclean drama *Oedipus the King*, that even the classical poets were cognizant of the ethical limitations and risks of stories—that is, of their restricted ability to direct our lives. Plato and Aristotle, who saw philosophy as distinct from and often in opposition to epic, tragic, comedic, and other poetic forms, can hardly be expected to accord them great moral importance than the poets themselves did.[15] In the next two sections, I indicate some of the shortcomings of the contemporary models, shortcomings that are evident from the perspective of classical philosophy.

Sickness and Stories in Ancient Greece

Ah! my poor children, known, ah, known too well
The quest that brings you hither and your need.
Sophocles, *Oedipus the King*, ll. 58–59

The classical world's archetypal story of Oedipus sheds some light on what the ancient Greek storytellers and philosophers often conveyed about the limitations of stories. We see, in addition, the distance between classical and modern mentalities as well as classical and modern conceptions of illness and its treatment. It is striking, too, that Oedipus's perilous course of self-discovery, from the story about himself to the truth about himself, has its dramatic initiation at the behest of sick children.

The very first word of Sophocles's *Oedipus the King* is "Children" (*ho tekna*), as Oedipus addresses the sick children of Thebes assembled in front of his palace. They are there as supplicants seeking his help with the plague that is destroying them and everyone around them. The play thus opens with Oedipus (the great, "the world-renowned king") emerging onto the scene from behind the massive doors of his palace to confront the throng of pathetic children. The reason why they have come is explained to him by the old priest who accompanies them. In Greek tragedy, children themselves usually remain silent. (The dramatic convention of children's silence emphasized their vulnerability to danger and their helplessness, and they are often portrayed as being unable to understand what was happening to and around them [Sifakis 1979, 69, 72].) The old priest tells of a blight on the land, of women dying in childbirth, and that "the God of Plague/Hath swooped upon our city emptying/The house of Cadmus, and the murky realm/Of Pluto is full fed with groans and tears" (27–30).

The plot of the well-known Oedipus story does not require retelling. It was familiar to Sophocles's audience, too, prior to his dramatization. The plague that marks the beginning of Sophocles's play was not, however, a part of the traditional story of Oedipus and its appearance there would have startled the ancient audience.[16] Why did Sophocles include it? Answering this question yields aspects of the historical context of ancient medicine and its distance from modern medicine.

One likely possibility for Sophocles's introducing a plague at the start of the play is that it was written just a few years after Athens suffered its first outbreak of a devastating plague in 430 B.C.E. Those in the audience would remember and respond to its dreadful evocation (Griffith 1996, 39). From the account of the illness given by the Greek historian Thucydides, one can well imagine the terror to which even the memory of it would give rise:

Suddenly and while in good health, [they] were seized first with intense heat of the head, and redness of inflammation of the eyes, and the parts inside the mouth, both the throat and the tongue, immediately became blood-red and exhaled an unnatural and fetid breath. In the next stage sneezing and hoarseness came on, and in a short time the disorder descended to the chest, attended by severe coughing. And when it settled in the stomach, that was upset, and vomits of bile of every kind named by physicians ensued, these also attended by great distress; and in most cases ineffectual retching followed producing violent convulsions, which sometimes abated directly, sometimes not until long afterwards. Externally, the body was not so very warm to the touch; it was not pale, but reddish, livid, and breaking out in small blisters and ulcers. But internally it was consumed by such a heat that the patients could not bear to have on them the lightest coverings or linen sheets, but wanted to be quite uncovered and would have liked best to throw themselves into cold water—indeed many of those who were not looked after did throw themselves into cisterns—so tormented were they by thirst that could not be quenched; and it was all the same whether they drank much or little. They were also beset by restlessness and sleeplessness which never abated. (Thucydides, *History of the Peloponnesian War* II. 49.1–6)

This, then, or something very much like it, is what the children are asking Oedipus to save them from.[17]

Modern medicine has an enormous array of effective measures against illness; even when it cannot cure, it can often meliorate illness and palliate suffering. As Thucydides makes clear, however, the Greeks were utterly helpless against this illness. There was, of course, no cure, and nearly nothing could be done to relieve the afflicted. Nor did physicians or others who cared for the sick have any protection for themselves, given that the Greeks did not have a concept of infection. In a moving passage Thucydides writes:

> And the most dreadful thing about the whole malady was not only the despondency of the victims, when once they became aware that they were sick, for their minds straightway yielded to despair and they gave themselves up for lost instead of resisting, but also the fact that they became infected by nursing one another and died like sheep. (Thucydides, *History of the Peloponnesian War* II. 51.3–5)

A second relevant but no doubt surprising factor in explaining the presence of the plague at the start of the play is that Sophocles himself had a serious interest in disease and healing. As Griffith 1996, 39–40 writes:

> He held the priesthood of the healing hero Amynus, the "warder off of evil" (*Vita Sophocles* T.A. 11 *TrGF* emend. Koerte; *codicum lectio* Halonos) and his house evidently doubled as a shrine to that hero. This was no passing interest on the poet's part, for when the worship of Asclepius [hero and god of healing, whose cult for several centuries practiced forms of spiritual or ritualized healing] was introduced into Athens several years after the probable date of *Oedipus the King*, and before a temple was built for his worship, he was 'entertained as a guest' by Sophocles in his own house (Plutarch *Numa* 4.6, *Etym. Magn.* s.v. Dexion).

Two points seem pertinent here. Sophocles's involvement with healing comes as a surprise because we are accustomed to thinking about medicine as a distinct profession, requiring extensive training and full-time engagement, and because we often presume an opposition between the artistry of drama and the science of medicine (as in C.P. Snow's "two cultures" of art and science).

Thus, we may be surprised to realize that a dramatist of Sophocles's stature had the time or ability or inclination to be involved with matters of health and illness. In the classical world, however, medicine was not yet professionalized. In ancient Greece, anyone could practice medicine and it appears that many did, including, for example, a number of ancient philosophers; the ancient world does not exhibit the compartmentalization of interests and pursuits typical of our modern and more technical disciplines. In ancient medicine, there was no licensure, no organized profession, no readily identifiable expert mainstream in contrast to which other forms of healing were automatically viewed as suspect. With medical knowledge still rudimentary, many different modes of treatment were proffered by ancient healers. Nor was healing driven by complex technology. For all these reasons, much less of a gap existed between physicians and their patients; many ordinary people were informed and held opinions about health and illness. When the Hippocratic school began the practice and advocacy of "rational medicine," that is, a more empirical and naturalistic approach to disease and its symptoms— the forerunner of modern scientific medicine—it had to establish itself in this medically pluralistic setting.[18]

Further, we see that Sophocles was a healer of the traditional kind, that is, he was affiliated with cult or ritual healing, the predominant approach to treating illness and disease in early antiquity prior to the ascendancy of Hippocratic rational medicine. Chief among the healing cults was that of Asclepius, said to be the son of Apollo. Asclepius's temple was an important healing center, and a "guild" of Asclepiads carried on the traditional healing techniques. The best known of the ritual modes of healing was *incubation*, in which a patient was brought to the temple grounds and, after engaging in a series of purification rites, descended into an underground chamber or cave for a sacred sleep that produced healing visions and dreams.[19] (We might note, too, that Aristotle's father was an Asclepiad and served as the physician to the Macedonian royal family.)

Even while the Hippocratic school championed the new, more scientific view of illness and healing, it still incorporated many of the more traditional cult elements in its practice.[20] What is notable is that the spiritual dimension of healing had a long history in ancient Greece and aspects of it were retained even within the newer, rational medicine. Thus, we see something of the contrast between ancient and modern medicine in these three respects: (a) ancient healers had no remedies for serious illness and few treatments to alleviate suffering; (b) medicine was nonprofessionalized and nonstandardized, with diverse healing modes and practitioners; and (c) spiritual or ritual aspects largely constituted ancient healing and persisted even with the introduction of Hippocratic medicine. We will revisit these points in section 4.

To return to *Oedipus the King*: in the opening scene, Oedipus enters his palace courtyard where he is surrounded by sick children. The contrast at the start between his stature and vigor, on the one hand, and their small-ness and affliction, on the other, presages the "suffering, recognition, and reversal" pattern that makes this drama *the* model of tragedy for Aristotle (*Poetics* 11 and 14–16). That is, as Oedipus discovers the truth of his own sick childhood (his parents, afraid of the prophecy about him, pierced his ankles to cripple him and abandoned him to die on a wild mountain-side), the greatness of his world comes precipitously undone. In the end, it is not the children, as he believed (l. 58), but he who is the most pitiful of human beings, as Teiresias prophesies (427–428).

The classic turning point in tragedy is the recognition, the discovery of the truth, and in *Oedipus* true self-discovery is set against the fabricated stories about Oedipus and his origins. Indeed, the progress of the drama involves the steady shearing away of the stories he was told: he is not a foreigner from Corinth but a Theban native; he is not the son of Polybus and Merope but of Laius and Jocasta; and so forth. The stories confound his life so that, for example, on learning as a young man from the oracle that he will kill his father, he flees Corinth to avoid committing this crime—but in fleeing, commits it because the story that he has been told and believes is that Polybus is his father. Oedipus's famed cleverness, especially at solving the Sphinx's riddle, is no defense against false and dangerously misleading stories. His only protection is his relentless deter-mination to know the truth—and, to help, that is, to know Laius's killer in order to rid the city of the miasma and so end the plague.

In Sophocles's view, just as the plague has supernatural rather than nat-ural sources (an oracle, not a doctor, must be consulted about eliminating it), so, too, the truth about Oedipus is divinely established rather than humanly invented or produced. Oedipus's task of ridding the pestilence in the city is accomplished by ridding himself of illusions. He must discover a truth that is preordained; Sophocles suggests that this is the nature of truth (even if it is not the nature of human *lives* to be preordained). There is no technique or procedure for discovering this truth, nor could any human invention or production substitute for it. In this respect, the classi-

cal mentality contrasts with that in later eras that emphasizes human ingenuity and inventiveness. While the truth for Oedipus is quite terrible,
Sophocles gives dramatic approval to its discovery by depicting Oedipus's
noble demeanor in his abject state (see Segal 1981, 247–248).

A central message of *Oedipus the King* is that, whether impelled by
external or internal imperatives, the truth must prevail. And the truth, in
contrast to stories, is not of human making. Rather, the truth is prior to
human beings, perhaps dictated by the gods in the manner of fate, and is
unlike stories invented by humans that can be variously, perhaps endlessly,
altered and interpreted. Stories, in the final analysis, do not have this power.

Having considered the ethical limits of narratives by way of this classic
drama, a brief closing word is in order about particularism, poetry, and
classical philosophy. As mentioned, Aristotle regards *Oedipus* as the pre-
eminent tragedy, and drama is estimable insofar as it speaks of what is universally true. He writes: "Hence poetry is something more philosophic
and of graver import than history, since its statements are of the nature of
universals, whereas those of history are singulars" (*Poetics* 9.1451b4–5).
In telling their stories, poets affix names to their characters, he continues,
but the characters and their actions are important only in that they
illustrate the patterns and possibilities in human nature. According to
Aristotle, these are the truths that are philosophically significant, and they
are prior to the stories that, at their best, might exhibit them. Thus,
Aristotle's reasons for valuing stories are contrary to those of the recent
particularists who support a narrative ethics because it gives importance
to subjective elements and individual circumstances.

Another Look at Classical Ethics

For it is not as a human being that one lives thus [in complete happiness], but
in that something present in one is divine. (Aristotle, *Nicomachean Ethics* x
7.1177b27)

What would ancient ethics look like, unmodified for modern times? And
what lessons might it have today for pediatrics and ethical decisions concerning children?

We begin with a summary description of the Greek mind, using as a
rough guide the following list of classic Greek values:

(1) a habit of seeing the world in terms of unchanging, objective absolutes rather than subjective, constantly fluid relatives; (2) the belief that human nature is constant over time and space; (3) the insistence that word match deed; and (4) the conviction that culture, not race, is supreme with its corollary that not all cultures are equal. (Willett 1999, 93).

With respect to the absolutes of the first point, these are found in the written laws—such as those that Socrates obeys to the death and in unwritten ones, such as those that Antigone obeys to hers—governing human beings and the world. Greek cosmologists and mathematicians endeavored to formulate the unitary patterns of nature, and Plato and Aristotle, each in his own way, sought for the timeless forms that order the multiplicity of reality.

Regarding item (2), the stability of human nature: this idea arises from the basic notion expressed in the first, namely, that a real basis exists for regularity, pattern, stability, and order—which the philosophers, scientists, lawmakers, architects, and artists of Greece sought in different ways to express. This is not to say that the Greeks held a uniform view of human nature. Greek tragedy gives a fairly dark picture of the unresolvable difficulties of human existence where noble actions are nonetheless deserving of admiration. Although the poets and philosophers do not subscribe to a single, shared picture of human nature, they found instantly recognizable a representation of human nature as poised between the godly and the bestial, with powerful tendencies toward the latter. Human beings are not naturally good, but can learn to be so, according to Aristotle and perhaps according to Plato. Furthermore, all human beings naturally desire to know and to achieve *eudaimonia*, Aristotle holds, and humans have what today would be considered utterly remarkable abilities both to intellectually grasp reality and to achieve a life of sublime happiness. Item (3)—that words must match deeds—shows that Greek thought is rooted in realism, that is, in the notion that standards of conduct are real in advance of any individual (e.g., Plato's forms of virtues, or Aristotle's "mean" which must be found in ethical deliberation) rather than being humanly established. Item (4)—in holding that not all cultures are equal, speaks of the persistent Greek idea (challenged by Sophistry) that ideals or standards are real and can be brought to bear in comparative judgments. Evident here, as well, is teleology at work in the nature of things, permitting hierarchies.[21]

Even this limited list is at odds with the particularist and narrative-based interpretations of Greek ethics referred to above, namely those of Toulmin, MacIntyre, and Nussbaum. Particularism, whether case-based, situational, or local-traditionalist, proceeds on a small scale whereas Greek thought characteristically looks at the universal and the unifying principle amidst multiplicity. Narrative-based ethical methods, which are intrinsically multiple and variable, depend upon human creativity and selectivity, whereas Greek realism sees the world asserting itself quite apart from the making and preferences of humans.

Noting the differences between classical and modern medicine helps to explain, in part, what has made particularist ethics and a narrative approach attractive recently to ethicists. As noted, the limited knowledge and resources for healing in classical antiquity contrasts with the vast increase in the powerful capabilities of physicians in the twentieth century; in turn, that rise in power engendered the era of bioethics in the later part of the twentieth century, shaped by deontological and consequentialist ethical models, to protect the patient's autonomy and other rights. When those models proved wanting, alternatives were sought. But neither classical medicine, which was not powerfully equipped to cure, nor ancient Greek ethics, which arose from asking about what the good is and what the good life is, originated from circumstances or needs similar to those of our time. Further, the smaller scale on which the ancient Greek healer practiced, without the hospital or any centralized medical system, meant that a different and probably less formal interaction between physician and patient was possible. Given the variety of healing modes available then—and it was not uncommon for persons to avail themselves of several different ones—a variety of interactions could certainly occur, and the sick were not necessarily exclusively dependent on any one physician.

Finally, the persistence of a spiritual dimension in healing in the ancient world seems to have spoken to an important human need for meaning and coherence. This need is generally neglected within the framework of strictly scientific medicine and neglected, too, within the secularist assumptions of modern ethics.[22] Particularism and a narrative approach appear to be the acceptable, contemporary substitutes for aspects of the healing experience that were routine in the classical era and absent now.

Some of the drawbacks of particularism and the narrative approach already have emerged in this discussion: particularist ethics without a foundation in universal truths (which in ancient Greek philosophy would be speculatively derived) has neither ethical footing nor safeguards at its disposal. Further, it is not necessarily a significant departure from consequentialism. It may have similar difficulties both in identifying what is *morally* significant in a situation and in avoiding relativism.

Plato worried quite a lot about the poets' stories, especially their tendency "to flatter," as he put it, to tell what the audience wishes to hear rather than what it needs to know, and to inflame the emotions (*Republic* ii–iii, and most famously x 595a–608b). Aristotle realized that storytelling can do some psychological good (through *katharsis* or purgation of pity and fear), but he asserts that stories are philosophically instructive to the extent that they are concerned with the universal truth, not the particularities of circumstance, which in themselves are not significantly revealing (*Poetics* 9).[23]

Let us consider again two features of ancient Greek ethics that distinguish it importantly from deontology, consequentialism, and from the motivations that impel particularism and narrative-based ethics: the primacy of the ethical enhancement of the agent and the determination of the good by way of transcendent factors. If these features were to be incorporated in contemporary medical ethics, they would significantly alter it, shifting medical ethics from a problem format and a patient's rights or interests orientation. This would yield at least two results to which we are unaccustomed: (a) allowing for—indeed, requiring—the recognition and praise of the worthy actions and decision efforts of doctors, nurses, and parents in the pediatric setting, and (b) allowing the routine caring activities they perform to be recognized as ethically relevant. That is, the province of ethics would become the everyday work of caregivers and decision-makers, in contrast to the current definition of "ethics" in medical ethics as episodes of crisis and the need to resolve dilemmas to which they give rise. And in such a province, praise as well as blame would be accorded.

First, the ethical agent has an intrinsic desire for his own virtue. A key notion for Aristotle is the natural desire of human beings for *eudaimonia* —for happiness, which is the highest good. Ethics, then, as the inquiry into what is good and what is its practice, is in service of this central human aim. The study of ethics involves the necessary analysis and sorting of different views of what the human good really is—that is, what kind of life best leads to human happiness. Study and deliberation about what is good activates the rational dimension of the soul and so are virtuous and commendable activities in themselves.[24] The practice of ethics includes nonstudy activities that express the moral virtues (such as justice, courage, temperance).

How virtue is achieved immediately sets the classical approach to ethics apart from modern, problem-based ethics that aim to settle the question of what I should do here and now. Rather, Aristotle's ethics places that sort of question in a context: What is the good human life? The answer is determined by human nature: everyone agrees that the good life is a *eudaimon* life, a happy life. In the *Nicomachean Ethics*, of the many different things that human beings want and that they believe will please them, Aristotle shows that virtue best leads to *eudaimonia* (*Nicomachean Ethics* i 7, especially 1098b30). When things go well in life, that is, when basic human needs are met and major mishaps are avoided, moral and intellectual virtue can lead to the most sublime *eudaimonia*—the contemplation of those realities that transcend the ordinary conditions of change as well as activity described as divine. When things do not go well in life and disaster strikes, virtue aids in withstanding the hardships. Thus, a person who is aware of these basic ethical parameters tries to enhance her virtue, in other words, tries to act in accord with reason at all times, knowing that such action is virtuous, helping to form a moral character capable of *eudaimonia*.

Clearly the agent is the focus of ethical attention in the classical ethical approach, and the agent's choices arise from character and the ongoing cultivation of virtue. Thus, it is unlike modern approaches that accentuate ethical dilemmas, calling upon the decision maker to know and make the right choice episodically, using the principles or the calculus of goods or, in the contemporary alternative, by creating a story to reach resolution. A focus on the agent exchanges resolution of problems for ethical depth, in that the agent's aim is to develop virtuous character over a lifetime. Incidents of choice are set in the context of the agent's life but without the suggestion that the life should be identified with the story about the life. In another respect, too, the contrast of ancient Greek with modern medical ethics is plain in the use of narrative ethics, in which the patient or the illness may have a story but the physician's moral character or that of the parent, who is a decision maker in pediatric settings, is not taken into account.

For Aristotle, the very experience of morally choosing is different, too, in that the intellectual effort brought to bear in analysis, discussion, and deliberation is itself dignified and perceived as humanly fulfilling, rather than woefully inadequate to the dilemma. In these and other respects, then, moral character with its capabilities for deliberation and discerning insight in situations of choice, won over time through training and experience, departs from the procedures of problem solving or crisis resolution that are paramount in modern ethical models and persist in medical ethics, even within particularist and narrative-based revisions.

Seeking the rationale for such an ethics brings to the fore a second feature of classical ethics: its grounding in the transcendent—that is, in a reality, according to the Greek philosophers, that is nonmaterial and unchanging, perfect, and exemplary. In Greek drama, this often takes the form of fate or divine decree. In Greek medicine, even in its rational modes, it means an acknowledgment of the gods.[25] For classical philosophers, goodness in human existence is established by transcendent reality, whether by the Forms in Plato's philosophy or by ungenerated and unchanging forms "within" natural things in Aristotle.

Transcendent reality is neither subjective nor socially constructed. For Aristotle, *phronesis*, practical wisdom, mediates in human situations by knowing both the particulars and the universals, thereby aiding in practical decision making. Nonetheless, *phronesis* is subordinate to *theoria*, contemplation of divine or timeless things, as the best happiness of which human beings are capable.

Human beings develop and enhance reason (*logos*) or the mind (*nous*) in order to know realities so that they may serve as a guide in all respects. Because ethics necessarily includes the rational processes both of knowing the end or aim and deliberating about the proper means to it, it has first an intellectual, speculative dimension and then a practical one. Intellectual efforts are oriented to the order of reality that Plato and Aristotle both take to be ordained by (even if not created by) what is good. In this connection, too, the transcendent nature of what is good saves the self-regarding feature of classical ethics from becoming harmfully selfish. Plato and Aristotle maintain that everyone benefits from such a priority of virtue, not the agent alone, since it is of the essence of excellence to benefit.[26]

For medical ethics and pediatrics, the approach of the ancient Greeks implies a very different perspective from that of the strictly patient-centered and problem-centered one that has been dominant in our society for several decades, a perspective from which the decision maker's ethical character (although not, of course, his or her personality) is largely invisible.[27] According to classical virtue ethics, the physician's virtue and the parents' virtue—their personal excellence that, paradoxically, is their least self-seeking aspect—is central. Further, virtue ethics not only shifts ethical attention from the patient to the agent(s); it also acknowledges as praiseworthy actions nobly undertaken and performed. This facet of commendation correlates with the emphasis of virtue ethics on the long-term development of the agent's moral character, serving *eudaimonia*. The commendation aspect also distinguishes it from modern models aimed at achieving correct outcomes in situations of choice where the agent (merely) avoids wrongdoing.

Because virtue ethics does not take a problem approach or crisis perspective, ethics itself is more broadly conceived, and the actions to be praised include the day-to-day, ongoing work pediatric doctors and nurses do in caring for sick children as well as the daily work of the parents in their caring. This attitude relinquishes the drama associated with difficult cases and extreme dilemmas often presented as paradigms in medical ethics textbooks that might play into the narrative method by heightening interest and suspense.[28] Praiseworthy acts also include, in the classical view, the *action* of ethical deliberation when dilemmas and crises do, in fact, arise, quite apart from the many difficulties of resolution that may present themselves and apart from how successful the resolution may appear to be. Deliberation itself is praiseworthy action because, as noted, it engages human rationality and because discerning the good is both possible and most valuable.

Just as Oedipus's parting words and thoughts in Sophocles's play are for his children,[29] so they must be here because it is crucial to know what the shift in outlook and attitude toward the decision makers implies for sick children. The ancient Greeks emphasized the extreme vulnerability of children. Indeed, sick children were at high risk not only of succumbing to their illnesses but of the social practice of exposure, abandoning of the sick or malformed or unwanted, and leaving them to die (as Oedipus himself was left). The lesson classical antiquity offers is that children are deeply dependent—upon their parents and, when they are sick, upon their doctors.

Useful comparisons could be made with today's attitudes and assumptions about children that tend to favor their capability and autonomy. Although protective rules and policies of rights are valuable, as stories might be, too, as aids in some difficult circumstances, from the viewpoint of classical ethics, the protection that the vulnerable sick child needs primarily is the virtuous integrity of doctors, nurses, and parents in providing properly for the child. Their virtue is signaled by their ability to communicate well and cooperate for the well-being of the child; this includes their willingness and ability to engage in deliberation about well-being and how it is best promoted. Socrates and Aristotle would see the needed virtue as a combination of wisdom and goodness. That is, virtue combines some understanding of the nature of the good and some sound practical judgment that finds the means to it in the circumstances at hand (*phronesis*). Virtue is not assured; rather, it must be assiduously inquired into and sought after. But its achievement is, after all, possible.[30] For classical philosophy, virtue—and the aspiration toward it—is what the sick child ultimately depends upon.[31]

Notes

1. Howard Brody is notable for thoughtfully considering the lessons of this recent turn in ethics and applying them to issues in medical ethics; see his *The Healer's Power* and *Stories of Sickness*. Other recent examples of introducing ancient concepts, such as *phronesis*, into the medical ethics discourse include Davis 1997, Scott 1995, and Schultz and Carnevale 1996.

2. Brody (1992, 253) writes: "The 'new' medical ethics has been dominated by a rights-and-rules approach in which problems are taken one at a time and specific, observable behavior is recommended by way of resolution. What sort of person the physician is, how consistent his views and attitudes are over a lifetime, and the intentions and reflections that accompany his problem-resolving behaviors are all pushed aside as of little ethical interest." (Brody continues: "It has now become more common to include some mention of virtue in medical ethics.")

3. Kopelman 1995, 360. The guideline also functions as a test in legal matters; see Holder (1985).

4. Kopelman 1995, 360, and Kopelman 1997a, 217, for example. As Silverman (1996) points out, the notion of best interests, in some circles, has been used to underwrite physicians' interventions.

5. Brody (1992, 167, n6) writes: "A helpful observation is made by Welch (1989), who notes that the concept of best interests first emerged in those areas of property and estate law where the items in dispute could be measured in monetary terms. It is therefore easier to see how the concept of best interests could convey, to the legally informed observer, an aura of objectivity that it does not possess when transported into the medical arena." Kopelman (1997b) lists a number of objections made to the best-interests doctrine and replies to them.

6. Although not specifically on pediatrics, the discussion of this topic in Brody 1992, ch. 10 is helpful.

7. See Downie and Randall 1997, Kopelman 1997b, 283–284, and *Encyclopedia of Bioethics* 1995, i 360.

8. U.S. President's Commission, 1983, 219, quoted in *Encyclopedia of Bioethics* 1995, i 360; see also Buchanan and Brock 1989.

9. Toulmin 1982 and Beresford 1996; I am indebted to Beresford's analysis for the second section of this essay.

10. Beresford 1996, 209–210; *Encyclopedia of Bioethics* 1995, i 344: "Today the word ['casuistry'] might be defined as the method of analyzing and resolving instances of moral perplexity by interpreting general moral rules in light of particular circumstances"; see also Jonsen and Toulmin 1988.

11. See Page 1987, who gives a good analysis of the pragmatic trend in connection with the problems of reason and rationality in modernity. Also of interest is Vattimo 1997.

12. Nussbaum writes, "Philosophy has often seen itself as a way of transcending the merely human, of giving the human being a new and more godlike set of activities and attachments. The alternative I explore sees it as a way of being human and speaking humanly." She continues, "But as 'Transcending' argues [referring to a section of her book], there are ways of transcending that are human and 'internal,' and other ways that involve flight and repudiation" (Nussbaum 1990, 53).

13. Scholars differ in their views of the extent to which Aristotle's ethics differ from the other branches of knowledge he recognizes (i.e. the theoretical and productive branches). In one view widely held today, ethics differs significantly from other kinds of knowledge in that it does not allow for *episteme* and does not have the character of a science with universal first principles. Nussbaum, for example, represents this perspective. The more traditional position I favor is that ethics, according to Aristotle, is distinct but is like other sciences in which, for the most part, things can be truly known. Reeve (1995) gives an excellent exposition and analysis of this reading; see also Kraut 1989.

14. See Introduction to Nelson 1997, and Brody 1992, ch. 15.

15. Plato is famous as a harsh critic of the poets; Aristotle may, by contrast, seem to be sympathetic.

16. On the matter of the plague and Sophocles's interest in medicine, see Griffith 1996, 39–40.

17. A great deal of speculation remains concerning the identity of the disease Thucydides describes; it may have no modern counterpart. Poole and Holladay 1979 summarize many of the proposals; also of interest is Parry 1969.

18. See Lloyd 1979, ch. 1, on the competing medical modalities in the ancient world.

19. On ancient Greek "incubation" healing and its connection with mysticism and prophecy, see Kinsgley 1999, 79–81 in particular; also Zaidman and Pantel 1992, 128–132.

20. Hippocratic treatises such as *On the Sacred Disease*, in which the author vigorously argues against the traditional ideas and cult assumptions of divine involvement in medical disorders, do not tell the whole story of the relation between traditional cult and Hippocratic rational approaches to sickness. As Lloyd (1979, 45) explains, cult healing often included rationally sound recommendations and the new Hippocratic medicine often included religious elements. This is not to deny that Hippocratic medicine was a highly significant innovation: "It was the Greeks who first evolved rational systems of medicine free from magical and religious elements and based upon natural causes. The importance of this revolutionary innovation for the history of medicine can hardly be overstressed" (Longrigg 1998, 18; see also Longrigg 1993). On the religious Asclepiadic and secular Hippocratic approaches to healing that existed side by side in the fifth century B.C.E., see Carrick 1985, 4 and Lloyd 1979, ch. 1.

21. Some of these examples appear in Hanson and Heath 1998, ch. 2.

22. For contemporary work that counters the secularist trend, see Pellegrino and Thomasma 1997, 6. Examples of the more standard approach to pediatric medical ethics may be found, for example, among the papers collected in *Seminars in Perinatology* 1998, 22 (3) and in *Clinics in Perinatology* 1996, 23 (3).

23. For further discussion of the philosophical problems associated with narrative approaches, including antirealism and relativism, see Cooper 1994.

24. "Study" in the classical sense should be taken to include solitary reflection as well as interpersonal discussion and exchange.

25. Even the Hippocratic Oath, for example, begins with the physician or physician-apprentice swearing by Apollo; see Longrigg 1998, 101.

26. On the good as generally beneficial, see, for example, Plato, *Timaeus* 30a and Aristotle, *Politics* III.

27. Brody (1992, ch. 16) points out the problem and discusses the physician's character but not in the manner of ancient Greek philosophy.

28. See Brody 1992, ch. 4, 56–61, in particular, on the importance of primary care medicine as the paradigm for medical ethics rather than intensive care or emergency room care. His rationale concerns the various power relations between physician and patient that occur in these different settings.

29. Oedipus's closing words (l. 1523): "Rob me not of these my children."

30. Aristotle, for example, urges that virtuous individuals, *phronimoi*, be regarded as ethical models for others to imitate. His approach in this regard is suggestive for the teaching of medical ethics, especially in clinical settings.

31. I thank Professor Hilde Nelson and Ms. Valeri Banfi for their help, and Rev. Joseph Koterski, S.J., Prof. Adrienne Fulco, and Prof. Ronald Polansky for their comments on an earlier draft. The Earhart Foundation supported time for research on this paper, and I am grateful to the Foundation for its assistance. My special thanks to George Lister, M.D., Chief of Pediatric Critical Care; Richard Ehrenkranz, M.D., of the Division of Perinatal Medicine; and Dr. Alan Mermann, all of the Yale University School of Medicine. They generously met with me and explained their reasoning processes regarding ethical matters. This discussion, above all, led me to think about how classical ethics could illuminate and commend the ethical practice of medicine that they, and many physicians, exemplify.

References

Barnes, J. ed. 1984. *The Complete Works of Aristotle*. Princeton: Princeton University Press.

Beresford, E. B. 1996. "Can *Phronesis* Save the Life of Medical Ethics?" *Theoretical Medicine* 17: 209–224.

Bloom, A. 1968. *The Republic of Plato*. New York: Basic Books.

Brody, H. 1988. *The Power of Sickness*. New Haven: Yale University Press.

Brody, H. 1992. *The Healer's Power*. New Haven, CT: Yale University Press.

Buchanan, A. E., and D. W. Brock. 1983. *Deciding for Others: The Ethics of Surrogate Decision-Making*. New York: Cambridge University Press.

Carrick, P. 1985. *Medical Ethics in Antiquity: Philosophical Perspectives on Abortion and Euthanasia*. Boston: D. Reidel.

Chambers, T. 1997. "What to Expect from an Ethics Case (and What it Expects from You)," in Nelson 1997.

Cooper, M. W. 1994. "Is Medicine Hermeneutics All the Way Down?" *Theoretical Medicine* 15: 149–180.

Davis, F. D. 1997. "*Phronesis*, Clinical Reasoning, and Pellegrino's Philosophy of Medicine." *Theoretical Medicine* 18: 173–195.

Downie, R. S., and F. Randall. 1997. "Parenting and the Best Interests of Minors." *Journal of Medicine and Philosophy* 22: 219–231.

Griffith, R. D. 1996. *The Theatre of Apollo: Divine Justice in Sophocles' Oedipus the King*. Buffalo: McGill-Queen's University Press.

Jonsen, A. R., and S. E. Toulmin. 1988. *The Abuse of Casuistry: A History of Moral Reasoning*. Berkeley: University of California Press.

Hanson, V. D., and J. Heath. 1998. *Who Killed Homer?* New York: The Free Press.

Holder, A. 1985. *Legal Issues in Pediatrics and Adolescent Medicine*. New Haven: Yale University Press.

Kingsley, P. 1999. *In the Dark Places of Wisdom*. Inverness, Calif.: The Golden Sufi Center.

Koop, C. E. 1989. "The Challenge of Definition." *Hastings Center Report* January–February 2–3.

Kopelman, L. M. 1995. "Children: Health-Care and Research Issues," in *The Encyclopedia of Bioethics*, ed. W. T. Reich. New York: Simon and Schuster Macmillan.

Kopelman, L. M. 1997a. "Children and Bioethics: Uses and Abuses of the Best-Interests Standard." *Journal of Medicine and Philosophy* 22: 213–217.

Kopelman, L. M. 1997b. "The Best-Interests Standard as Threshold, Ideal, and Standard of Reasonableness." *Journal of Medicine and Philosophy* 22: 271–289.

Kraut, R. 1989. *Aristotle on the Human Good*. Princeton, N.J.: Princeton University Press.

Lloyd, G. E. R. 1979. *Magic, Reason and Experience. Studies in the Origins and Development of Greek Science*. New York: Cambridge University Press.

Longrigg, J. 1993. *Greek Rational Medicine. Philosophy and Medicine from Alcmaeon to the Alexandrians*. New York: Routledge.

Longrigg, J. 1998. *Greek Medicine: From the Heroic to the Hellenistic Age. A Source Book*. New York: Routledge.

MacIntyre, A. 1981. *After Virtue*. Notre Dame: University of Notre Dame Press.

Marta, J. 1997. "Toward a Bioethics for the Twenty-First Century: A Ricoeurian Poststructuralist Narrative Hermeneutic Approach to Informed Consent," in Nelson 1997.

Nelson, H. L. ed. 1997. *Stories and Their Limits: Narrative Approaches to Bioethics*. New York: Routledge.

Nussbaum, M. C. 1990. *Love's Knowledge: Essays in Philosophy and Literature*. New York: Oxford University Press.

Page, C. 1987. "Axiomatics, Hermeneutics and Practical Rationality." *International Philosophical Quarterly* 27: 81–100.

Parry, A. 1969. "The Language of Thucydides' Description of the Plague." *Bulletin of the Institute of Classical Studies* 16: 106–118.

Pellegrino, E. D., and D. C. Thomasma. 1997. *Helping and Healing: Religious Commitment in Health Care*. Washington, D.C.: Georgetown University Press.

Poole, J. C. F., and A. J. Holladay. 1979. "Thucydides and the Plague at Athens." *Classical Quarterly* 29: 282–300.

Reeve, C. D. C. 1995. *Practices of Reason: Aristotle's Nicomachean Ethics*. New York: Oxford University Press.

Schrag, F. 1995. "Children: The Rights of Children," in *The Encyclopedia of Bioethics*, ed. W. T. Reich. New York: Simon and Schuster Macmillan.

Schultz, D. S., and F. A. Carnevale. 1996. "Engagement and Suffering in Responsible Caregiving: On Overcoming Maleficence in Health Care." *Theoretical Medicine* 17: 189–207.

Scott, P. A. 1995. "Aristotle, Nursing and Health Care Ethics." *Nursing Ethics* 2: 279–285.

Segal, C. 1981. *Tragedy and Civilization: An Interpretation of Sophocles.* Cambridge, Mass.: Harvard University Press.

Sifakis, G. M. 1979. "Children in Greek Tragedy." *Bulletin of the Institute of Classical Studies* 26: 67–80.

Silverman, W. 1996. "Medical Decisions: An Appeal for Reasonableness." *Pediatrics* 98: 1182–1184.

Strand, M. 1998. "Dark Harbor" in *The Best of American Poetry, 1988–1997,* ed. H. Bloom. New York: Scribner Poetry.

Toulmin, S. 1982. "How Medicine Saved the Life of Ethics." *Perspectives in Biology and Medicine* 25: 741.

Willett, S. J. 1999. "Can Classicists Think Like Greeks?" *Arion*, Winter, 84–102.

Zaidman, L. B., and P. S. Pantel. 1992. *Religion in the Ancient Greek City.* New York: Cambridge University Press.

11

Facing Death Like a Stoic: Epictetus on Suicide in the Case of Illness

Christopher E. Cosans

And man has learned speech and wind-swift thought and the temper that rules cities, and how to escape the exposure of the inhospitable hills and the sharp arrows of rain, all-resourceful. He meets nothing in the future without resource; only from Hades shall he apply no means of flight.
—Sophocles, *Antigone*, 354–361 (Lloyd-Jones trans. modified)

In spite of our differences, we have one thing in common about which we are all aware: all humans are mortal. With the remarkable powers it has acquired over life and death during the last century, Western medicine has not changed this fact. It has, however, obtained the ability to postpone the timing of our demise. Today some physicians wonder if medicine should seek even more control over the timing by complementing its new-found powers with a rather old procedure: suicide. When medicine cannot cure a terrible disease or injury, they hope that it can at least help provide the patient with a less gruesome ending. Engelhardt 1986, 312 argues, for example, that:

Even if pain can be controlled, the various debilities consequent on disease, ranging from anal and urinary incontinence to exhaustion, may make any further life unacceptable. Suicide may be the most reasonable choice under such circumstances, and the aid of others may be needed.

Today, some would thus extend the mission of medicine beyond the traditional promotion of health to include even the destruction of life in order to avoid the ravages of disease and pain. As medicine ponders taking this step, I would like to reexamine some philosophical work on suicide by one of the philosophers most dedicated to applying philosophy to the daily decisions we make in the course of human life. The Stoic philosopher Epictetus has some especially complex insights on the subject.

Born as a slave around 50 A.D., when Roman emperors and soldiers dominated the Western world, Epictetus has much advice to offer on how we should handle events that seem beyond our control. Although he did not write a book himself, one of his students, the historian Flavius Arrian, recorded his words in two works: the magnum opus *Discourses*, of whose eight books four survive, and a compact manual, the *Encheiridion*, which offers a more concise treatment of the human condition. Epictetus advances a tough-minded philosophy that stresses our capacity to make reasoned judgments freely. In his ethical system, the key to happiness rests on our effort to focus entirely upon our thoughts, which lie totally within our control, while living in peace with all the other events that we cannot control. By adopting such an attitude, the individual gains independence and freedom. In articulating his ethical system, Epictetus displays a fierce intellectual independence, which draws out the implications of his ideas even when these might sound extreme or put him at odds with other philosophers. Epictetus's independent spirit manifests itself in especially interesting ways in the case of suicide.

With the example of suicides from such prominent Stoics as Zeno (the school's founder), Cato, and Seneca, the Stoics are well known for endorsing suicide as the best action in several circumstances.[1] Diogenes Laertius reports: "They [the Stoics] say that the wise man will commit a well-reasoned suicide both on behalf of his country and on behalf of his friends, and if he falls victim to unduly severe pain or mutilation or incurable illness" (Diogenes VII.30).[2] Although as Rist 1969, 254 points out, some controversy takes place within the school on suicide and "no single Stoic theory of suicide" holds, Diogenes seems to represent the "mainstream" Stoic view. The Stoics consider virtue the only true good and vice the only evil; they thus view death, and many other things, as an "indifferent" (ἀδιάφορα). If a virtuous act, an intrinsic good, results in a person's death (an indifferent), the Stoic sage would accept the consequence of death. Both Cato (see Plutarch 1895, 441–442) and Seneca (Englert 1994, 75–86) committed suicide as ways to express the importance of freedom in face of political tyranny, and thereby to help their cause. In his writings, Seneca is especially enthusiastic about suicide for giving the individual the freedom to escape the vicissitudes of fortune (Englert 1994, 77–78).

The reasons many Stoics endorse suicide in the case of illness is more complex. Most believed that some indifferents could be preferred and nonpreferred because "they are capable of activating impulse (ὁρμῆς) and repulsion" (Diogenes VII.105).[3] Although an "indifferent," a quick death could be preferred to a nonpreferred painful terminal illness and thus provide a Stoic a good reason for choosing a quick exit.

Epictetus seems more torn on the ethics of suicide. Although he teaches that one should refuse to commit evil or dishonorable acts even if threatened with death by a tyrant (thereby passively committing "political suicide," so to speak), he pulls back from advocating actively killing oneself, especially in the case of illness (*Discourses* III.20.14). Even when he indicates that suicide might be less objectionable than lamenting about difficult circumstances, he falls short of saying that it is a good or virtuous option.

In the discussion that follows, I argue that this difference with his Stoic colleagues stems from Epictetus's greater emphasis on the moral distinction between events that do not strictly arise from us and those things that we freely will. Insofar as he explicitly claims that our impulses (ὁρμαί) are under our control (*Encheiridion* ch. 1), indifferents would carry less weight in a decision to commit suicide than they might in the ethical systems of other Stoics.

The Problem of Suicide

According to Epictetus, a self-respecting human being should face death with the courage of Sarpedon. He reasons that since death is ineluctable, and we have a moral capacity to avoid true evils (τὰ κακά), we must not view death as an evil (*Discourses* I.27.7). He does not even mention the possibility of considering death a nonpreferred indifferent, as it was by other Stoics. Rather than worry unduly about what we cannot avoid, Epictetus argues that a noble person lives like Zeus's son Sarpedon, who fights in Homer's *Iliad* either to achieve an honorable victory or to allow his opponent the same honor if he is fated to die (XII 310–328). With his constant focus on the inevitability of our death, Epictetus treats the very state of being a mortal human as a terminal condition. In the *Encheiridion* (ch. 3) he goes so far as to recommend that "if you kiss your own child or wife, say to yourself that you are kissing a human being, for when it dies you will not be agitated (ταραχθήσῃ)."[4] Although you cannot do anything to avoid death, you still can control how you think about it. If we can train ourselves not to fear death, then we can maintain some calmness and peace of mind no matter what challenges we face. Epictetus claims that "it is not death or hardship that is a fearful thing, but the fear of hardship or death," and praises an unknown tragic poet for saying: "Not death is dreadful, but a shameful death" (*Discourses* II.1.13). By accepting our mortality, we free ourselves to face the challenge of acting nobly and avoiding shame regardless of the cost.

When death approaches, rather than being despondent, as if it were a terrible event, Epictetus advises you to think to yourself that "it is now the right time (καιρός) for the matter from which you are constituted to be restored to those elements from which it came" (*Discourses* IV.7.15). As parts of this universe, we live as members of an organic whole in which events occur in due measure, including our own demise. We can thus seek some consolation by viewing this restoration of our body as serving an essential role in the greater life of the cosmos:

The paltry body (σωμάτιον) must be separated from the bit of spirit, either now or later, just as it existed apart from it before. Why are you grieved, then, if it be now? For if not now, it will be later. Why? So that the revolution of the cosmos may be accomplished; for it has need of the things that are now coming into being, that shall be, and that have been accomplished. (Epictetus, *Discourses* II 1.17–20)

Many Stoics, like Epictetus, see the universe as proceeding in an everlasting cosmic cycle between periods in which fire consumes everything in a universal conflagration and periods in which an ordered system unfolds (Long and Sedley 1987, i 274–279). By giving our body's demise a context in the greater course of the cosmos, Epictetus seeks to transform death from a meaningless ending to a vital player in the cycle of life. When we think about death in this context, we can look beyond the disintegration of our paltry flesh toward the wondrous good of the universe as a whole.

If Epictetus makes death no great tragedy, one would think that he would have little objection to our bringing about our own demise. At several places in the *Discourses* he alludes to suicide euphemistically and seems seriously to entertain it as a virtuous death. He occasionally refers to the grave as a door that stands open, which could be interpreted as implying that we can enter it at our convenience. For example, in arguing that we should not fear hardship, Epictetus explains:

The poor flesh is subjected to rough treatment, and then again to smooth. If you do not find this profitable the door stands open; if you do find it profitable, bear it. For the door must be standing open for all situations, and then we have no trouble. (*Discourses* II 1.19–20)

In this passage, the mere *possibility* of suicide offers a guaranteed refuge that helps us to face any circumstance without being troubled. Elsewhere he likens life's hardships to being in a smoky house, pointing out that "whenever you wish, you walk out of the house, and are no longer bothered by smoke" (*Discourses* IV 10.27; see also *Discourses* I 25.18–20). On first consideration, Epictetus would seem to have little reason to find suicide objectionable, since he focuses ethics on the internal life of the mind, viewing the body as an object outside of our control and therefore not of primary moral concern. He hardly bestows upon the body enough significance to in any way hinder us from acting according to good reason. Hence, in discussing how humans can endure anything but the irrational, Epictetus asserts that "whenever someone feels that it is reasonable (εὔλογον) he goes and hangs himself" (*Discourses* I 2.3). The case of suicide thus offers perhaps the most striking instance of how humans may do things antithetical to their bodily existence for the sake of reason. While this passage indicates that suicide is understandable in some circumstances, it leaves open the question of the conditions under which Epictetus would consider hanging oneself the best course of action.

Xenakis 1969 interprets Epictetus as giving suicide an unqualified endorsement and even being in favor of "mercy-killing," which was endorsed by some other Stoics. He argues that Epictetus believes that suicide affords us a good escape from this life's pains and that "Epictetus would say ... a preconception ('Suicide is bad') can cause or increase suffering" (Xenakis 1969, 18). Epictetus's blunt talk about the ever-present availability of suicide does indeed often sound like a sanction. Nonetheless, to remind us of the possibility of suicide and to say that we should actually commit it are two quite different things. I contend that a closer scrutiny of the text reveals a complex attitude toward suicide, indicating Epictetus's view that the decision to commit suicide is not the most virtuous course of action, and may perhaps be bad, in many difficult circumstances. Although Epictetus uses the possibility of suicide to inspire confidence in facing hardship, this falls far short of an outright endorsement of the actual act. Indeed, at one point he characterizes suicide to escape hardship as a childish behavior:

But to sum it all up: remember that the door has been thrown open. Do not become a greater coward than the children, but just as they say "I won't play any longer," when the affair does not please them, so do you also, when things seem to you to have reached that stage, merely say, "I won't play any longer," and take your departure; but if you stay, stop lamenting. (*Discourses* I 24.20)

In this passage, Epictetus uses suicide rhetorically, as a way not only to instill courage, but also to condemn excessive lamenting about the things outside of our control. It seems that he considers losing one's peace of mind a greater evil than death. His use of the metaphor of a child quitting a game he is about to lose in order to shame excessive lamenting hardly puts suicide in a flattering light. Epictetus explicitly compares children unfavorably to philosophers when attributing their irrational fear of death to a lack of education (*Discourses* II.1.15–7 and IV.7.32). Suicide may be better than complaining, but that does not make it more virtuous than toughing it out like a brave man or woman. Indeed, if fear motivates a "childish" escape from a difficulty, death may be tainted with some of the shame that Epictetus finds truly dreadful.

Epictetus raises serious concerns about suicide when he considers whether we should end our lives without a sufficient reason. He considers hypothetical students who, being persuaded by him that the spirit gives them a kinship to the gods while the body is an object of indifference that fetters them to all the problems of this world, ask for the sanctioning of their suicide (*Discourses* I.9.12–15). Epictetus replies:

Men, wait upon God. When He shall give the signal and set you free from this service, then shall you depart to Him; but for the present endure to abide in this place, where He has stationed you. Short indeed is this time of your abiding here, and easy to bear for men of your convictions. For what tyrant, or what thief, or what courts of law are any longer formidable to those who have thus set at naught the body and its possessions? Stay, don't depart irrationally (ἀλογίστως). (*Discourses* I 9.16–17)

By claiming suicide irrational in this case, Epictetus explicitly rejects the notion that his philosophy itself provides a pretext for killing oneself. The students, it seems, have misunderstood Epictetus's message about suicide. He teaches that we should view the body itself as an indifferent not so that we can readily cast it away but so that we are better able to bear its wounding by slings and arrows. With strong philosophical convictions, a person can endure virtually any hardship. Indeed, following Socrates's example in Plato's *Apology*, he speaks of life as analogous to a military assignment in which we have a duty to remain where God has stationed us. Arbitrarily deserting our position with no good reason would be an irrational violation of our duty to the greater order of things.

Elsewhere Epictetus considers the case of a friend who "with no cause made up his mind to starve himself to death" (*Discourses* II.15.4) and was unwilling to entertain arguments against his decision. Epictetus initially asserts that he would even aid the suicide *if* his friend has good reasons for it, which Xenakis 1969, 17 interprets as implying that he is "clearly in favor of mercy-killing." Yet, the quip about helping would seem to be only rhetorical in light of Epictetus's two further elaborations—his claim that his friend indeed lacks a good reason and his ensuing remarks in opposition to suicide in this case. Once again, Epictetus sets up a presumption against suicide:

Without any cause you are taking out of this life, to our detriment, a human being who is a familiar friend, a citizen of the same state, both the large state and the small; and then though in the act of murder (φόνου), and while engaged in the destruction of a human being that has done no wrong, you say that you "must abide by your judgments." (*Discourses* II.15.10–12)

As with the students, Epictetus suggests that the friend should reconsider his judgment in light of the role his life plays within the greater order of things. Given his relation to others, an unjustified suicide could be a shameful flight from duty. Indeed, by taking an innocent human life without a good reason, even if it is his own life, the friend would violate the human political order with an unjust act of murder no less wicked than an unfair judgment by a capricious tyrant. Insofar as the "large state" refers to the greater cosmos, Epictetus implies that he sees unjustified suicide as an unnatural violation of the universe's greater order (*Discourses* I.9.16). If there is a "right time" (καιρός) for our death in the course of the greater state, we need to consider the full meaning of our demise before bringing it upon ourselves.

Epictetus's various references to suicide offer us a murky picture. He sometimes sounds as if he accepts the Stoic doctrine in general but fails to identify particular instances where he would apply it. While he bluntly asserts that we can always leave the house if it is too smoky, since he makes these remarks in the context of arguments for courage, they can also be interpreted as largely rhetorical ploys against excessive lamenting and fear. Furthermore, he cautions that we should have a good reason for such an action and argues against suicide in the two specific circumstances considered above. Perhaps suicide serves as the atomic bomb of Epictetus's philosophy, whose best use lies not in its actual deployment but in serving as the ultimate deterrent against whining.

Some dispute emerges in the scholarship on how to interpret Epictetus's comments on suicide. While Xenakis 1969, 16–9 portrays Epictetus as almost enthusiastic about suicide's possibilities, Rist 1969, 251 argues that Epictetus finds the act extremely problematic and that his "distance from Seneca is immense." In his consideration of Epictetus's theory, Bonhöffer 1996, 65 concludes that "suicide is moral in the full sense only when it is based on a clearly recognized call of god." To shed further light on Epictetus's views of suicide, I examine their place in his overall philosophy and then consider the implications of his reflections within the medical context. In the case of illness, at least, Epictetus makes a significant break from Stoics like Seneca and considers patient endurance to be the most virtuous response to disease.

An Ethical System Based on Reasoned Choice

Epictetus's work endures as one of the most systematic efforts to apply philosophy to everyday life. He presents the primary benefit of philosophical wisdom as empowering the individual to maintain peace of mind no matter what happens. Thus Socrates, the paradigmatic philosopher, does not wail and lose his composure when his opportunities for leisurely study are abruptly halted by his arrest and death sentence; as a philosopher, he makes his goal in life "to be serene, to be unhampered, and to be unhindered" (*Discourses* IV.4.22) so that he can maintain his *proairesis*. Just as it takes time to master a bull, "man does not become noble at once, but must undergo winter training, to prepare himself and not plunge recklessly into inappropriate things" (*Discourses* I.2.32).

Annas 1995, 247 characterizes the notion that virtue is a skill requiring practice for development as "one of the most prominent theses in

Stoicism." Epictetus's philosophy demands constant work to free one-self from the passions. For example, he suggests that "occasionally when you are very thirsty take in cold water and spit it out, and tell no one" (*Encheiridion*, ch. 47). The philosopher thus seeks mastery not only over bodily desires but also over any proclivities toward bragging about such mastery, which should be pursued for its own sake. One strives for the serenity and freedom of Socrates by training oneself to accept the limits of one's personal action. Hence, Arrian opens his handbook of Epictetus's philosophy with a key distinction:

Some things are up to us (ἐφ' ἡμῖν), while others are not up to us. Up to us are conception, impulse (ὁρμή), desire, aversion, and in a word, whatever are our deeds, not up to us are the body, property, reputation, office, and in a word what-ever are not our deeds. (*Encheiridion*, ch. 1)

One undertakes the study of philosophy in order to focus one's attention upon what we can control while learning to be indifferent about events outside of our control. Long 1989, 80 points out that by holding that "happiness consists solely and entirely in ethical virtue," the Stoics advance an ethical system in which the individual holds securely in his power the freedom to obtain happiness. In the case of Epictetus, we exercise this liberty by vigorously maintaining our proper judgment. We cannot control what external impressions (φαντασίαι) we receive from the sensory faculties that we share with animals, but as rational beings we have a choice of what to think about them. For "the gods have put under our control only the strongest faculty of all that dominates the rest: the capacity to correctly use external impressions" (*Discourses* I.1.7 and 20.5). Failure to employ our rational faculty and to follow instead the animal whims of our senses destroys our humanity.

In his lucid analysis of Epictetus's theory of love, Stephens 1996, 199 points out, "each person's misfortune and unhappiness are self-imposed on Epictetus' view, and result from making wrong judgments about things—judgments contrary to nature." Hence, Paris was not ruined when the Greeks assaulted Troy, but "when he lost his sense of shame, faithfulness, respect for hospitality, propriety (κόσμιον)" (*Discourses* I.28.23), and seduced his host's wife. Rather than being carried away by his passions, the philosopher exercises, strengthens, and lives by his reason. Epictetus claims that students studying philosophy should end up "enduring, cooperative, dispassionate, undisturbable (ἀταράχους), having some such provision for the journey of life, so that being anchored with it they are able to bear nobly whatever happens, and derive honor from it" (*Discourses* III.21.9). While Xenakis 1969, 12–16 characterizes Epictetus's ethics as treating life as a game whose main objective is happiness, Epictetus also concerns himself a great deal with honor and shame. If things outside of one's control go wrong, a philosopher should honorably face the adversity with courage.

Epictetus bases ethics on man's capacity to make free reasoned choices. In order to make one's life good, the moral agent must concern himself with προαίρεσις (*proairesis*), which has been translated in a philosophical context by such terms as "choice," "intention," "will," and "moral purpose" (Dobbin 1991, 113n8).[5] In his analysis of Epictetus's psychology, Long 1991, 112 characterizes *proairesis* as "our capacity to give or withhold assent" to judgments we might make about sensory impressions. At times, Epictetus even identifies *proairesis* with one's true self (see *Discourses* I.1.23–4, and IV.5.12). Dobbin 1991, 118 argues persuasively, I think, that Epictetus gives such prominence to *proairesis* as a response to critics who claim that Stoic fatalism makes no room for human freedom. Epictetus is indeed quite passionate about freedom: as Oldfather 1925, xvii notes, he uses the terms *free* and *freedom* no less than 130 times, which gives them a much greater relative frequency in his writing than in contemporary texts of the *New Testament* or Marcus Aurelius.

Such a stress on freedom places greater emphasis on human responsibility than it receives in the accounts of other Stoics. Epictetus claims that "the essence (οὐσία) of the good is a kind of *proairesis*, and that of evil is also a kind of *proairesis*" (*Discourses* I 29.1): "straight judgment" (δόγματα ὀρθὰ) concerning externals makes your *proairesis* good, while "twisted and distorted" judgment makes it evil (*Discourses* I 29.3). Long 1991, 116 argues that morally bad judgments follow from the agent's failing to "fit representations of particular circumstances to preconceptions" of what would be living well. Epictetus believes that we have complete control over our *proairesis*, since no one but us can determine how we think. Indeed, when responding to a hypothetical tyrant's threats against his person, he claims that "you can fetter my leg, but not even

Zeus himself has power to overcome my *proairesis*" (*Discourses* I.1.23). Forschner 1981, 112 claims that *proairesis* gives man a realm so free of restrictions that "herein man himself is divine i.e. a part of God."

Maintaining a good *proairesis* turns out to be decisive in the human struggle to give the best, and most virtuous, response to difficult situations such as facing death. In considering the sweep of man's free choice, Epictetus alludes to suicide and remarks: "What is it that destroys the whole man, sometimes by hunger, sometimes by a noose, sometimes by hurling him over a cliff? *Proairesis*" (*Discourses* II.23.17). By grounding the suicide in *proairesis*, Epictetus stresses the extent to which it is a free act for which the individual bears full responsibility. If the focus on *proairesis* is unique to his approach to Stoicism, as Dobbin argues, this may explain why he might subject suicide to greater scrutiny than his Stoic colleagues. Before taking one's own life, one should make sure that this does not bring about the shameful death that Epictetus considers dreadful. For it to be the best course of action, suicide must engender good in the internal realm of things that are up to us. Impatience or fear would not be good reasons for suicide; to determine the extent to which pain might justify suicide, we need to examine Epictetus's ideas on how we should treat the body.

In contrast to our free choices, externals (τὰ ἐκτά), such as the body, lie outside of our control and are morally indifferent. While most Stoics approach some indifferents as things preferred and others as not preferred (Englert 1994, 69; Long and Sedley 1987, i 354–359), Epictetus downplays any distinctions among indifferents. Throughout the *Discourses*, he insists that indifferents are neither good nor bad and makes no mention of indifferents being preferred or notpreferred (*Discourses* I.30.3–4 and II.9.15, 13.10, and 19.13). They serve as mere materials, which a good or evil *proairesis* uses for its end. A person's virtue rests in her ability to make good use of *whatever* externals she faces. Given the unbounded nature of human resourcefulness, a particular external could not be designated in a principled way as preferred or dispreferred in Epictetus's ethical system. Hence an external "is neither good or bad, but the use which I make of it is either good or bad, and that is up to me" (*Discourses* II.5.8). Although they may appear valuable, upon reflection material objects, like the body, ultimately derive any importance as tools of our own free will; in themselves such objects are not of any consequence. When the destruction of property distresses one person, Epictetus bluntly responds: "are you a piece of crockery, then? No, but *proairesis*" (*Discourses* IV.5.12). You should strive not to worry about controlling externals, so that you do not lose sight of the internal goods of your mind.

Placing undue value on externals gives them power over you and subjects your serenity to life's vicissitudes. Since we can control our wishes but not the external world, Epictetus advises: "seek not for things to happen as you wish, but wish for things to happen as they happen, and your life will flow well" (*Encheiridion* ch. 8). If we abstain from unduly worrying about the course of an illness, we can guarantee our peace of mind. By training ourselves to be indifferent regarding externals so they cannot distress us, we may be free to flourish regardless of our external circumstances. For example, James Stockdale relates how his previous study of the *Encheiridion* helped him to retain and defend much of his freedom even while being tortured as a POW in Vietnam (1981, 45–46). He argues that the challenges of stress, however unpleasant, can drive humans to push their spirit to its greatest limits and to induce the fullest development of the mind (1981, 49–51).

Rather than opposing and bemoaning events beyond our control, Epictetus urges that we should keep our *proairesis* in harmony with nature. He believes that freeing ourselves from the whims of externals allows us to pursue a higher purpose in life:

Each of the animals God makes, one to be eaten, another to serve in farming, another to produce cheese, and yet another for some similar use; to do these functions what need have they to understand external impressions and to be able to differentiate between them? But God has brought man into the world to be a spectator of Himself and of His works, and not merely a spectator, but also an interpreter. Wherefore, it is shameful for man to begin and end just where the irrational animals do; he should rather begin where they do, but end where nature has ended in dealing with us. Now she did not end until she reached contemplation and understanding and a manner of life harmonious with nature. (*Discourses* I.6.18–20)

There is much more to the life of a human than the life of a cow. Long 1991, 113 reads Epictetus's claim that man must live as an interpreter as implying that well-functioning humans "need to reflect on and evaluate the appearance that the world and our internal states generate in us."

With our intellects, Epictetus sees us as being able to look beyond sense impressions and appetites so as to apprehend and follow a divine force in nature. Indeed, at one point he quotes Stoicism's founder Zeno as remarking that "man's end is to follow the gods, and the essence of the good is the proper use of external impressions" (*Discourses* I.20.15). Since Epictetus believes each person has a free *proairesis*, he sees God as having left the outcome of the internal struggles between good and evil in the hands of the human soul.

Unlike animals that live in the world of the senses, our greater understanding and freedom bestows a duty (τὸ καθῆκον) to treat humans properly: "For I ought not to be unfeeling (ἀπαθῆ) like a statue, but should preserve my relations, both natural and acquired, as a pious person, a son, a brother, a father, a citizen" (*Discourses* III.2.4).[6] Far from calling for a dulling of all sentiments, Epictetus directs the philosopher to focus his *proairesis* on fulfilling his moral obligations to the greater wholes to which we belong. Insofar as striving to respect others leads to the realization of one's fullest potential as a living human being, the effort to do one's duty carries its own reward. Blundell 1990, 234 argues that by serving the common good, the Stoic sage preserves "his rational self, which is perpetuated by his contribution to the cosmos as a rational whole." Although attachment to others might seem excessively emotional for a Stoic, Stephens 1996, 195 points out that such affections for Epictetus "are natural human feelings which are compatible with what is reasonable, and so he does not consider them to be 'passions' (πάθη)." Epictetus sees our struggle to fulfill our duties and live as good people as analogous to maintaining a post in a difficult military campaign at which God, acting as general, has stationed us (*Discourses* III.24.34–35). In order to help us stay at our post no matter what happens to externals like our body, God has given us the virtues of endurance, great spiritedness, and courage (*Discourses* II.16.14). For Epictetus, Socrates is his model of a good soldier. He especially admires Socrates's brave decision to continue speaking on behalf of justice even when Athens threatened his death (*Discourses* I.9.22–26). By always acting justly no matter what course the external events of the world take, the philosopher transcends his local human government, acknowledges a certain kinship with the gods, and lives as "a citizen of the universe" (*Discourses* I.9.1; see also II.10.3).

Enduring Illness and Facing Death

With its emphasis on issues arising from human mortality, Epictetus's ethical system offers a perspective on medicine. Although medicine has made dramatic progress since his time, it has not changed the fact that every human being ultimately dies, and often events occur in the course of life that are beyond our control. While physicians can often alleviate illness, a follower of Epictetus would be careful not to stake his or her happiness on the accomplishments or failures of the medical profession. Since they are states of the body, health and disease are externals, which should not determine how we maintain our *proairesis* or threaten our peace of mind. If you think of an ailment as limited to the indifferent realm of the body, then you better enable yourself to preserve the freedom and tranquility of your inner spirit no matter what happens. When considering pain, Epictetus explicitly declares: "I am not saying that it is not permissible to groan, only do not groan from within" (*Discourses* I.18.19). While medical care may offer some relief for the body, the patient must look to his soul and bear the illness well so as:

Not to blame God or man, not to be oppressed by what happens, to await death well and nobly, to do what is enjoined upon you; when your physician comes not to be afraid of what he will say, nor to be overjoyed if he says "you are doing splendidly"; for what good to you lay in that remark? (*Discourses* III.10.13)

Epictetus finds nothing wrong with seeking and following a physician's advice so long as one does not expect too much and maintains an independent attitude proper for externals. Worrying excessively about the course of an illness disturbs one's peace of mind. If this occurs, no one is to blame for this wretchedness but oneself.

When confronted with an affliction, Epictetus argues that we should not be too anxious either for our recovery or for our demise, but should pledge simultaneously, "I will not flatter my physician, I will not pray for death" (*Discourses* III.20.14). Epictetus seems to advise a modest approach in the human battle with disease, in which we neither take dramatic measures that may be futile nor actively bring an end to our ailment with death. If we desire to control the state of our body too much, then we sacrifice our freedom and become slaves to our bodies and medical technology. In the human struggle with disease, Epictetus places greater value upon internal goods like courage, personal integrity, and peace of mind than on health. By facing our disease bravely, we can assure ourselves of victory no matter what happens to our bodies. Indeed, if we treat a difficult affliction as a trial and use it to build good character, "it is possible to derive advantage from illness" and even from death (*Discourses* III.20.4–5).

As an external, the body serves as a tool for *proairesis* that should be *used* properly. As with any fine tool, a person should take a respectful attitude toward the human body. Epictetus recommends, for example, maintaining proper hygienic practices such as brushing your teeth "in order that you may be a human being, and not a beast or a pig" (*Discourses* IV.11.11). While the body itself falls into the realm of indifferents, how we decide to treat or maintain it remains up to us and falls squarely in the moral realm. On some level it would be unseemly, if not disrespectful, to try to contemplate and interpret God's works while maintaining one's body in an unnaturally filthy and poor manner. Since humans live as citizens of a state, we should keep our bodies clean if only as an act of consideration for those around us. As a good citizen you should think "that your body has been entrusted to you like a horse; wash it, rub it down, make it so that nobody will turn his back on you or move aside" (*Discourses* IV.11.17). The body sick or well requires some care.

In considering one particular situation, Epictetus gives significant weight to a proper respect for the integrity of the body. He considers the case of an athlete who owing to an injury faced the choice of having his genitals removed or risk death, a tragic dilemma that athletes of our day are fortunately spared thanks to antibiotics and protective cups. When asked if the person made his ultimately fatal decision to forgo treatment acting as an athlete or a philosopher, Epictetus replied: "As a man (ἀνήρ), indeed a man who had been proclaimed at the Olympic games and had striven in them, who had been at home in such places, and had not merely been rubbed down with oil in Bato's wrestling school" (*Discourses* I.2.26). In addition to making an allusion to the nature of the operation in question, the word "man" (ἀνήρ) is often associated with courage and the quest for honor.[7] Epictetus seems to admire the man for his decision to face the course of his injury with his body intact rather than having it dramatically altered in an effort to save his life, risking both life and health because of the high value he placed upon maintaining his body's integrity. Given that the body was the tool with which the man gained honor on the athletic field, he may have felt a duty to treat it with such respect that he would risk his life before seeing it mutilated. Since ancient athletes competed in the buff, the alteration of the man's anatomy would be quite noticeable in any future competitions. Epictetus considers this case as a paradigm of holding "regard for one's proper-character (πρόσωπον)" (*Discourses* I.2.28); he likens the man's resolve to that of Helvidius Priscus, a Stoic senator who was executed because he spoke out for what he believed was right despite the Emperor's threats. In his analysis of this passage, Stephens 1997 suggests that Epictetus would recommend people allowing, and perhaps even seeking, a death as consistent with their πρόσωπον as possible.

If he accepts and even admires someone's decision to forgo potentially life-saving treatment, the question arises why Epictetus claims that a sick person should "await death well and nobly" (*Discourses* III.10.13) and not even pray for death (*Discourses* III.20.14). Epictetus, seems to make a moral distinction between passively forgoing medical treatment and actively bringing on one's own death. In one case, a person peacefully accepts whatever consequences follow from not attempting to alter a course of external events; in the other, he worries about externals and tries to control them by ending the life of his body. Indeed, physician-assisted suicide may be viewed as analogous to the amputation declined by the athlete, since by this act, physicians alleviate pain by mortally harming the body. Insofar as praying for death involves asking the gods for a different course of events, the supplicant assumes the gods do not know the best course of things; if she goes beyond prayer and terminates life, then she could be breaking out of her human character (πρόσωπον) and playing god. When deciding whether to take one's own life, one must consider if the measure stems from a good and just *proairesis*. Insofar as Epictetus considers sense perceptions like pain neutral externals, about which we can make any judgment, they would weigh less in a decision to destroy a living body than in the ethical systems of the other Stoics, like Seneca, who express stronger preferences among indifferents. Given that humans can benefit in unforeseen ways from conscious reflection upon the trials faced on the deathbed, as Tolstoy has illustrated, the best course of action might be to endure an illness to the natural end.[8]

Epictetus suggests each person seek solace by seeing his or her illness and death not as isolated instances but as parts of the greater course of things:

Now if you regard yourself as a thing cut off, it is natural for you to live to an old age, to be rich, to enjoy health. But if you regard yourself as a human and as a part of some whole, on account of that whole it is fitting for you now to be sick, and now to make a voyage and run risks, and now to be in want, and on occasion to die before your expected time (ὥρας). Why, then are you vexed? Do you not know that as the foot, if cut off, will no longer be a foot, so you too, if cut off, will no longer be a human? For what is a human? A part of a state; first of that state which is made up of gods and men, and then of that state that is a small copy of the universal state. (*Discourses* II.5.25–26)

As citizens of the universe, humans have more to live for than the sensory experience of the body. Since we are neither beasts nor gods, humans play a unique role in this cosmic order. In contrast to beasts, each human is afforded the opportunity by the events in his or her life for contemplating and praising a divine arrangement in the cosmos. In order fully to do this, Epictetus believes that we should be at peace with whatever death we are fated to have, finding solace that it is the right time (καιρός) even if it is not the expected time (ὥρα). Given the nature and limits of human foresight, he argues that we should wait patiently at our post to the end:

The philosophers well say that if the noble and good knew what was going to happen, he would help on the processes of disease and death and maiming, because he would realize that this allotment comes from the arrangement of the whole, and the whole is more sovereign than the part, and the state than the citizen. But since we do not know before hand what is going to happen it is our duty (καθήκει) to make the more natural choice, since we were born for this. (*Discourses* II.10.5–6)[9]

In this passage, Epictetus explicitly rejects the Stoicism of Seneca by arguing that we should not use artificial means to expedite the processes of death and disease. In contrast to gods, humans never fully know the events throughout the world and in the future. Hence the virtue, and even duty, for humans to abstain from efforts to control external events while focusing on deciding how to think about them. With this move, Epictetus advances Stoicism in an interesting direction. In her analysis of the Stoic attitude toward suicide as articulated by Seneca, Nussbaum 1994, 97 claims that "in a crucial way it is internally incoherent," since by deciding to kill oneself in response to some event, the Stoic entangles herself in the world's evils no less than if she gives any other such dramatic response. Yet

Epictetus accords with the indifference of external events to the point of making patient endurance the most virtuous response to an illness.[10]

If we see our death as part of the role we play in the greater cosmic order, we can find something meaningful even in a wretchedly painful bodily demise. At one point in his handbook, Epictetus claims that all the world is a stage:

> Remember that you are an actor in a play, the nature of which is what the Playwright wants; if He wishes it to be short, it is short; if long it is long; if He wishes you to play the part of a beggar, act even this role adroitly; and so if your role be that of a cripple, an official, or a private man. For this is your task, to play the character (πρόσωπον) given to you well; but the selection of the role is Another's. (*Encheiridion* ch. 17)

In Epictetus's view of life, even our very last scene may have something special to offer. Rather than fearing your death, Epictetus argues that you should "make it your glory, or an opportunity for you to show by deed what sort of person a man is who follows the will of nature" (*Discourses* III.20.13). After noting that "I cannot flee death," Epictetus rhetorically asks: "instead of fleeing fear of it, will I die in lamentation and trembling?" (*Discourses* I.27.9–10). By accepting the ineluctability of death, the philosopher frees himself to focus on maintaining his peace of mind. When considering his own mortality, Epictetus hopes that "death would overtake me occupied with nothing but my own *proairesis*, trying to make it tranquil, unhampered, unconstrained, free" (*Discourses* III.5.7).

As an assault on the external closest to our true being, the degeneration of the body in illness poses the greatest threat to our *proairesis* of any event that is not up to us. If we fight this battle philosophically, and take no desperate measures either to hold onto or to give up life, we can focus upon and strengthen our *proairesis* even as our body weakens and dies. Human virtue lies not in the maximization of bodily comfort, but in nobly struggling to meet life's many challenges. By bravely staying at our post to the end, no matter what happens, all of us can win honor for a battle well fought.[11]

Notes

1. Bonhöffer 1996, 239–244 and Englert 1994, 69–75 provide detailed accounts on how most Stoics tended to favor suicide.

2. Translations of Diogenes Laertius are from Long and Sedley 1987, vol. 1.

3. An exception was Aristo of Chios, an unorthodox pupil of Zeno who denied any intrinsic preference between indifferents (Diogenes VII 160). As we proceed, we will see that Epictetus also placed little stress on expressing preferences concerning indifferents.

4. I will use Oldfather's translations of Epictetus with modification.

5. Dobbin 1991, 129–34 offers rich analysis of the many layers of meaning that *proairesis* has for Epictetus.

6. Long 1989, 92 characterizes καθήκοντα (proper functions) as "a set of rules for 'living in agreement with nature,'" which humans are in a unique position to follow as rational beings.

7. Stephens 1997 argues that Epictetus sees one's gender as important enough to one's identity to warrant risking one's life and notes that Epictetus himself claims he would let a tyrant cut off his head before agreeing to shave off his beard, which can be viewed as not only symbolizing his vocation as a philosopher but also his masculinity.

8. Tolstoy offers an especially rich exploration of the spiritual possibilities of living the life of the deathbed to its fullest in *The Death of Ivan Ilyich*.

9. The most plausible case for which Epictetus might recommend suicide in the medical context would be a disease that threatened one's sanity, and thus could be viewed as a threat to *proairesis*. An example from the ancient context would be the case of someone who was bitten by a rabid dog. I believe that the best evidence, however, indicates that Epictetus might still admire an effort to endure the disease with the modest use of medicine. First, the Greeks held that they had some medicines effective enough against madness to offer some hope, even in the case of rabies (Galen, *Sect. Int.* ch. 8, 18–19). Second, and on a deeper level, as a Stoic, Epictetus might be reluctant to concede the possibility that a living and conscious human be could be entirely devoid of *proairesis*. In *On the Doctrines of Hippocrates and Plato*, Galen attempts to use the case of insanity as evidence against the Stoic theory that we have one unified rational faculty (τό ἡγεμόνικον) (*PHP* iv 5.23). Epictetus could thus not concede that bodily disease can somehow destroy *proairesis* without giving ground to the opponents of Stoicism. In his analysis of suicide in the case of illness, Bonhöffer 1996, 56 concludes that "Epictetus regarded suicide as justifiable only in the most extreme of all cases of physical misery."

10. While it is outside of the scope of this discussion to explore in detail whether Epictetus would advise suicide in cases where it fulfills some duty to one's country or preserves personal honor, the present analysis of the case of illness does not rule this out as a possibility. Since how we act in the realm of human politics is up to us, suicide could be the most virtuous course in some situations. Bonhöffer 1996, 59 suggests, for example, that suicide would be honorable in the case of a military commander whose entire army has been destroyed and that the enemy tries to capture alive.

11. I would like to thank the many people who have discussed with me the various ideas of this essay. W. Stephens, D. DeGrazia, E. Asmis, M. Higuera, M. Mahowald, E. Pellegrino, A. Cosans, and an anonymous referee read previous drafts and offered many helpful suggestions. I received helpful comments when I read an earlier version at the meeting of the Society for Ancient Greek Philosophy at Binghamton, N.Y., on 25 October 1997. My discussion also owes much to the people who showed me, when I spent time as a volunteer at VITAS Hospice in Chicago, the extent to which humans can face a terminal illness bravely and peacefully.

References

Annas, J. 1995. "Prudence and Morality in Ancient and Modern Ethics." *Ethics* 105: 241–257.

Annas, J. 1989. "Naturalism in Greek Ethics." *Proceedings of the Boston Area Colloquium in Ancient Philosophy* 4: 149–171.

Blundell, M. W. 1990. "Parental Nature and Stoic Οἰκείωσις in Epictetus." *Ancient Philosophy* 10: 221–242.

Bonhöffer, A. 1996. *The Ethics of the Stoic Epictetus*. Trans. W. Stephens. New York: P. Lang.

Dobbin, R. 1991. "Προαίρεσις in Epictetus." *Ancient Philosophy* 11: 111–135.

Engelhardt, H. T. 1986. *The Foundations of Bioethics*. New York: Oxford University Press.

Englert, W. 1994. "Stoics and Epicureans on the Nature of Suicide." *Proceedings of the Boston Area Colloquium in Ancient Philosophy* 10: 67–96.

Forschner, M. 1981. *Die stoische Ethik*. Stuttgart: Ernst Klett.

LLoyd: Jones, H. trans., *Antigone, the Women of Trachis, Philoctetes, Oedipus at Colonus*, Loeb Classical Library, vols. 1 and 2. Cambridge, MA: Harvard University Press.

Long, A. 1991. "Representation and the Self in Stoicism," in *Psychology* ed. S. Everson. Cambridge: Cambridge University Press.

Long, A. 1989. "Stoic Eudaimonism." *Proceedings of the Boston Area Colloquium in Ancient Philosophy* 4: 77–101.

Long, A., and D. Sedley. 1987. *The Hellenistic Philosophers*, 2 vols. Cambridge: Cambridge University Press.

Nussbaum, M. 1994. "Commentary on Englert." *Proceedings of the Boston Area Colloquium in Ancient Philosophy* 10: 97–114.

Oldfather, W. trans. 1925. Epictetus, *The Discourses, Fragments, Encheiridion*. Translation and Greek text, Loeb Classical Library vols. 1 and 2. Cambridge, MA: Harvard University Press.

Plutarch. 1895. *The Lives of the Noble Grecians and Romans*. vol. 4. Trans. John Dryden, rev. by A. H. Clough. Boston: Little, Brown.

Rist, J. 1969. *Stoic Philosophy*. Cambridge: Cambridge University Press.

Stephens, W. 1996. "Epictetus on How the Stoic Sage Loves." *Oxford Studies in Ancient Philosophy* 14: 193–210.

Stephens, W. 1997. "Epictetus on the Irrationality of Fearing Death and Reasons for Suicide." Meeting of the Society for Ancient Greek Philosophy, Binghamton N.Y., 26 October 1997.

Stockdale, J. 1981. "Education for Leadership and Survival: The Role of the Pressure Cooker." *The Ethics of Citizenship*. Dallas: University of Texas at Dallas.

Tolstoy, L. 1995. *The Death of Ivan Ilyich*. Trans. R. Edmonds. New York: Penguin Books.

Xenakis, I. 1969. *Epictetus Philosopher-Therapist*. The Hague: Martinus Nijhoff.

12

Euthanasia and the Physician's Role: Reflections on Some Views in the Ancient Greek Tradition

Georgios Anagnostopoulos

At the most basic level, euthanasia is the termination of a life by an act that interferes in some way or other with the natural or normal course of events as far as the continuation of life is concerned.[1] Looked at in this way, human euthanasia has some common features with suicide, and thus it raises all the familiar problems associated with actions that aim to end the life of a human being. Human euthanasia, however, in its paradigmatic cases is the termination of the life of some person by another person or persons. Thus, one might distinguish at least three kinds of questions relevant to suicide or euthanasia:

(1) Ethical questions about terminating life.
(2) Ethical questions about terminating one's own life.
(3) Ethical questions about terminating someone else's life.

These questions are clearly interrelated. Any answer or answers to question (1) are bound to affect possible answers to (2) and (3). Yet it is also clear that these questions are to some extent distinct. At least from the perspective of the type of theory of virtue that Plato and Aristotle hold, the kinds of acts relevant to each of these questions may fall under different virtues. As we shall see, Aristotle argues that the kind of act described in (2) raises questions about courage and on some occasions about justice, but the same need not be the case with the kind of act described in (3).

I am, of course, aware that euthanasia is not merely the termination of one person's life by another person. If it were, then all homicides would be cases of euthanasia. Further, contrary to typical dictionary definitions that are often based on etymology, euthanasia is not a quiet and pleasant death. Again, if this were the case, all homicides carried out in a quiet and pleasant way, for example, by first administering anesthesia or some kind of tranquilizer to the victim, would be cases of euthanasia (Foot 1983).

What seems essential to euthanasia is that the termination of the life of an individual is for the good of that individual. Understanding euthanasia in this way introduces several other types of questions and problems:

(a) Under what circumstances is the death of a person a greater good for that person than any other alternative?
(b) Who is to make the determination as to whether the termination of life is the greater good for a particular person?
(c) How is the determination to terminate a life to be made?
(d) Who is to terminate a human life?

My concern here focuses primarily on questions (b), (c), and (d), although some of what I discuss in this essay bears also on question (a). In particular, I wish to explore some recurring arguments and prevalent conceptions in Greek philosophy with regard to any possible role the physician might have in *determining* whether termination of life is the best course of action in certain situations and whether the physician should have a role in *terminating* a life. These questions are neither merely theoretical nor trivial; on the contrary, they are practical and of great importance—they are, literally, questions of life and death. Most of all, none of them is easy, despite some recent claims to the contrary.

I begin by raising some doubts about the primacy of autonomy in questions about the termination of life and suggest that much remains to be determined about the rightness or wrongness of decisions about terminating life even if autonomy is given its appropriate place. I then discuss the Pythagorean Oath's injunction against any role of the physician in terminating life and argue that, contrary to some recent claims, this injunction reflects a deep-seated conviction that the goals of medicine, ideally construed, limit the physician's role in deliberations, decisions, or actions that concern termination of life. This conviction is supported by an essentialist conception of medicine and its goals that Plato and Aristotle expound—a conception that views medicine as necessarily aiming at health and the improvement of life and excluding other considerations from influencing the aims of medicine and its practitioners. This is true, I argue, even though Plato and Aristotle defend a view of authority, based on expertise, that seems to give unlimited authority to medical experts on matters of health. However, these philosophers set definite limits to the authority of the physician by defending the view that deliberations about termination of life fall within the scope of different expertise—that of ethical and political knowledge.

Euthanasia and Autonomy

Many contemporary philosophers argue in favor of the primacy of individual autonomy, insisting that a necessary and sufficient condition for a justified act of terminating a human life is the exercise of autonomy in the decision process by the person whose life is to be terminated. They argue that decisions regarding termination of life must be made by the one whose life is to be ended and that every individual has a right to terminate his/her life. They thus speak in support of voluntary euthanasia and find nothing wrong with such a practice (see, e.g., Rachels 1983; G. Williams 1978; and Dworkin et al. 1998).

The importance of autonomy should not be underestimated. Autonomy might not be as foundational to ethics as Kant claims or as indispensable to political theory as liberalism insists. Clearly, however, it is central to the conception we have of a person as an agent who deliberates and chooses without external coercion or interference (Rawls 1993). In the legal sphere, autonomy is most important in creating and protecting a "space" within which an agent can make the choices he/she wishes to make. What is also clear is that, by assigning the highest priority to autonomy, one can answer easily some of the questions raised above, especially (2) and (b).

Yet not all of the questions mentioned above are easily disposed of by merely assuming autonomy. It is not clear whether or how the exercise of autonomy affects the moral character of a choice or act and whether all likely cases of euthanasia are cases in which autonomy has any meaningful role to play. Many, if not most, cases of euthanasia are cases in which the subject whose life is to be terminated is not in a position to determine anything at all. Insisting that one should have made a determination with regard to the termination of one's own life prior to becoming incapacitated, and thus prior to becoming unable to make any decisions regarding one's own life, is not a strong argument because in some cases, humans are born without the relevant capacities for making such decisions, or they lose these capacities before they are developed to the degree required for making the kind of judgments pertaining to matters of life and death.

Some have raised doubts as to whether autonomy is meaningfully exercised about matters of death even by those who possess fully developed faculties. They doubt, that is, whether ordinary human beings can be sufficiently detached and objective when confronted with the awesome and irreversible decision of terminating a life, especially when the life is their own (see, e.g., Kamisar 1978, Beauchamp and Childress 1994, and Kuhse 1998). Aristotle himself points to the difficulty of making a rational decision while in the grip of pain or suffering, even for those who are considered objective and detached observers of matters of life and death—the physicians themselves: "Doctors themselves call in other doctors to treat them when they are sick, and trainers call in other trainers when they are exercising, their assumption being that they are unable to judge truly because they are judging about their own cases, and while in pain" (*Politics* iii 16.1287a41–b3).

Proponents of strong autonomy might attempt to circumvent this difficulty by restricting euthanasia only to cases where the right of autonomy can be meaningfully exercised. According to these proponents, since autonomy is a necessary condition for euthanasia, termination of life without the exercise of autonomy could not be euthanasia. Yet this only shows that autonomy cannot be a necessary condition of euthanasia, for it rules out the possibility of meaningfully applying the term "euthanasia" to acts of terminating the life of nonhumans.

Although autonomy may not be a necessary condition for euthanasia, it could still be a sufficient condition. Yet this does not seem correct either, and admitting autonomy does not help much insofar as finding answers to several of the questions raised above is concerned. Exercising one's autonomy or one's right to Φ does not necessarily imply that it is right to Φ—even in the rare cases where Φ-ing does not affect anyone else. For example, one may have the right to smoke whenever doing so does not adversely affect others; it does not follow from this, however, that smoking is the right thing to do. Similarly, one may be said to have a right to terminate one's own life if one decides to do so, but it does not follow from this alone that suicide is the *right* course of action. Proponents of autonomy argue at times that even a right to be or to do wrong exists. But by insisting on such a right, one is tacitly admitting that the exercise of autonomy does not determine the moral character of the act, for if one's autonomy can be exercised in doing wrong, then clearly the rightness or wrongness of the action is not a consequence of autonomy. If the action in relation to which autonomy has been exercised is right (wrong), it is right (wrong) for reasons that may have nothing to do with autonomy.

The reasons that agents are likely to appeal to in deliberating about or justifying the rightness of terminating a life can be quite complex. The most prominent of these reasons must be those pertaining to the good or well-being of the person whose life is to be terminated. It is unlikely that considerations of autonomy play any role in deliberating about or justifying the rightness of terminating a life. Such considerations may weigh much in our decision whether to interfere with an individual's choice to terminate his/her own life but, clearly, this is a different matter and does not determine the moral character of the choice itself. This is seen more easily, and perhaps more clearly, in the case of smoking. Our decision to abstain from interfering in the exercise of someone's autonomy to smoke —another form of choosing to terminate one's life, albeit slowly—says nothing about the rightness of the choice.

Of course, these considerations do not show that circumstances could not arise in which the good that figures in our deliberations may be autonomy itself—the securing, maintaining, or increasing of autonomy. Yet, although reasons might exist for treating autonomy itself as a good, perhaps a highly important one (see Johnston, 1994), and not merely as something exercised in relation to goods, it cannot be the good that figures in deliberations about or justifications of acts aiming at terminating lives. Such acts do not typically aim at nor do they result in securing, maintaining, or augmenting the autonomy of the person whose life is being terminated. Cases may arise, however, where termination of someone's life is believed to result or actually results in securing, maintaining, or increasing someone else's autonomy, and it is the bringing about of such an outcome that motivates the termination of the first person's life. Such cases, however, cannot be standard cases of euthanasia since they do not aim at the good of the person whose life is terminated. An act to terminate one's own life for the sake of the autonomy of others may, of course, proceed from the exercise of one's own autonomy. Yet the autonomy of the act may not, others things being equal, make it a case of euthanasia. If A makes the autonomous choice to have his own life terminated for the sake of securing, maintaining, or increasing B's autonomy, then A is, strictly speaking, sacrificing himself for the sake of B. If A's act is to be at all considered a case of euthanasia, it must, in addition to being A's autonomous choice, proceed from a deliberation that includes substantive reasons that may have nothing to do with autonomy—either A's own or that of others.

Moreover, it is doubtful that autonomy contributes much toward answering question (d). The exercise of my autonomy in choosing to Φ may obligate others not to interfere with my choice but it need not obligate anyone to realize my choice. The exercise of my autonomy to smoke may obligate others to abstain from interfering with my choice, if it does not affect them adversely, but it does not obligate them to supply me with tobacco. One might argue, however, that a shopkeeper is obligated to supply me with tobacco products if I am prepared to pay for them. Yet the obligation of the shopkeeper and my right stem from considerations that have little to do with autonomy. The shopkeeper is obligated not to discriminate against me, and I have a right not to be discriminated against. However, if the shopkeeper chooses not to deal in tobacco products, the choice cannot be said to violate the exercise of my autonomy in choosing to smoke.

I believe the situation is similar, although more complicated, in cases where autonomy is exercised in relation to terminating a life. The autonomous choice of a person to terminate his/her own life need not necessarily by itself impose any obligation on or create any right for others to terminate this person's life. That one person's choice to terminate his/her own life does not by itself give anyone else the right to terminate this person's life is obvious. Otherwise, others would automatically have the right to kill, at the appropriate time or circumstances, anyone they knew to have made the autonomous decision to terminate his/her own life. This, of course, does not exclude the possibility that in some cases particular persons have such a right. Such cases, however, involve more than the mere exercise of autonomy in deciding to end one's own life. They may involve special relationships between the person who makes the choice to end his/her life and others who are to carry out the choice;[2] they may include agreements; and they must at least be cases in which the primary concern is the good of the person whose life is to be terminated.

Autonomy, at least as understood by most contemporary philosophers, does not play a prominent role in ancient Greek moral theory and, consequently, it does not figure prominently in discussions of termination of life. Plato, in particular, acknowledges it at times, but often speaks against recognizing any role for autonomy in the physician/patient relation, and the models he proposes for making practical decisions also leave no room for the exercise of autonomy.

Occasionally, I will refer to autonomy, although not everything the ancient Greeks say about the role of the physician and termination of life has a bearing on it. This, however, should not lead one to conclude that what these philosophers say is of no particular interest to us. That is, one should not draw the conclusion that the difference between the roles assigned to autonomy by the classical thinkers and us renders the study of their views on the question of termination of life of no relevance to us. Such a conclusion would be altogether hasty, considering how strongly similar the classical conception of medicine is to our own.

The Hippocratic Oath and the Physician's Role in Terminating Life

A striking fact about the Western medical tradition is its continuity from its origins in the ancient Greek world to the present. What is meant by this, of course, is not that contemporary medical treatments or procedures for certain ailments are the same as those ancient Greek physicians prescribed, although in some cases it is astounding how close they are. Rather, the claim about the continuity of medicine points to the essentially identical *conception* of medicine we and the ancient Greeks share. For them as well as for us, the activities classified under the terms *medicine (iatrike)* and their cognates are thought to be primarily of two types: (1) scientific investigation of diseases or various conditions of the body and of the means of treating them; and (2) practices with respect to diagnosis and treatment of bodily conditions—in short, theory and practice. The extant writings from the Hippocratic tradition include a number of short treatises on causal explanations of certain conditions from the perspective of a theoretical framework—for example, of epilepsy in terms of abnormalities of the brain.[3] They also include a considerable number of studies on procedures of diagnosis and treatment—for example, regimens of diet or activity, healing techniques, prescriptions, and so on.[4] Undoubtedly, these two elements of medicine are closely connected, with the one guiding the other and without a clear line separating the two.

The ancient Greek philosophical tradition is in complete agreement with what we find in the extant writings from the Hippocratic medical tradition. Plato and Aristotle see medicine as a practical/productive *science* that seeks to understand a certain subject matter as well as realize a certain end, i.e. health.[5] According to Plato, medicine "is the science of health" (*Charmides* 165d) or "the science of health and disease" (*Republic* iv 438e) and according to Aristotle "the science of things connected with health" (*Nicomachean Ethics* vi 10.1143a3) or "the science of producing health" (*Topics* ii 3.110b18–19). Both philosophers insist that medicine shares some of the basic features of the canonical sciences: it has a subject matter whose nature, principles, or causes it seeks to understand (Aristotle *Metaphysics* xi 7.1063b36–1064a1, *Physics* ii 2.194a23–24, 194b9–13; Plato *Gorgias* 465a, 501c, *Phaedrus* 270b, *Timaeus* 80a); as with the canonical sciences, medicine seeks to know general or universal truths about its subject matter (Aristotle *Metaphysics* i 1.981a16, *Nicomachean Ethics* x 9.1180b13–16) and even seeks to identify cures of general or universal application (*Rhetoric* i 2.1356b30–33, *Posterior Analytics* ii 13.97b26–28). Indeed, both philosophers distinguish between a mere medical practitioner, who might succeed in curing some on the basis of experience or by imitating others, and the physician who has a scientific understanding of diseases and their cures (Plato *Laws* iv 720a–723b, ix 857d; Aristotle *Metaphysics* i 1.981a16, *Nicomachean Ethics* x 9.1180b13–16).

This is an important fact about the conception of medicine in the ancient Greek philosophical tradition, a fact that has been obscured in some recent interpretations—especially in the case of Aristotle, who is often portrayed as holding the view that medicine, presumably like ethics, is not a serious scientific inquiry and cannot provide any scientific expertise.[6] For present purposes, the importance of this fact has another dimension: it is this conception of medicine as a practical science and of its practitioners as scientific experts on matters of health, disease, and its treatment that leads some of the classical thinkers, especially Plato, to grant considerable authority to the judgment of the physician concerning these matters. This is the same conception of medicine and of its practitioners that leads many in our own time to grant much say to the physician on matters of life or death since the physician is thought to have a scientific understanding of bodily conditions, to be able to offer explanations of the present state of health, and to be in a position to predict future developments. In agreement with Plato, most people today think that "There is one science of medicine which is concerned with the overseeing of health equally in all times, present, past and future" (*Laches* 198d). There is no doubt that we view medicine along the same lines—as consisting of a scientific understanding of certain bodily conditions and types of procedures for treating them.

The one feature that more than any other attests to the continuity between the classical and contemporary traditions of medicine is the professional ethical code that both share—the Hippocratic Oath. More than two millennia after the Hippocratic Oath became the professional code of the ancient Greek physicians it remains the same code embodied in the oath that physicians today swear to uphold, as physicians have done throughout the centuries. This is indeed an astonishing fact. Medicine has changed dramatically from the classical era to the present in terms of the *contents* of both its theoretical and practical components. Our understanding of epilepsy, for example, may share some common features with the understanding of this disease by the Hippocratic tradition—namely, that both see its cause in some condition of the brain. Yet our explanation of epilepsy has reached the neuronal level, and that of cancer the level of the gene and beyond. Similarly, the therapies we resort to in the case of epilepsy target the physics or chemistry of the minutest parts of the brain whereas those of the ancient Greeks consisted of some rather elementary regimens. Such differences should not be surprising, however, given the recent extraordinary advances in medical knowledge and their impact on the shaping of therapeutic techniques.

The Hippocratic Oath nonetheless continues to be the medical oath, despite the dramatic changes in both the theoretical and practical aspects of medicine. The reason for this may not be difficult to identify. The Oath is not centrally connected to either the theoretical or practical components of medicine and, as a consequence, the immense developments that have taken place in these two components have not had much impact on the Oath itself. Instead, the substance of the Oath is concerned with the goals of the medical discipline or art or with some broader ethical conceptions that perhaps are at the foundation of the goals of the medical profession. The acceptance, then, of the Oath throughout the centuries implies, at least prima facie, that our beliefs about the goals of the medical discipline, or perhaps the ethical foundations that underlie our conception of these goals, have remained on the whole unchanged (compare the discussion by Bartz in this volume). This implication of the continuity in the life of the Hippocratic Oath, if indeed a genuine continuity exists, is of some importance. As I shall argue, it casts doubt on some interpretations that seek to restrict the principles embodied in the Oath to the rather peculiar beliefs of a particular small society or group of thinkers of the ancient Greek world—beliefs that may have little or no relevance to us and perhaps had no relevance even to the general public of the ancient Greek world itself.

However, any continuity in the observance of the Oath may be in appearance only. The Hippocratic Oath quite explicitly enjoins against any act of euthanasia performed by a physician or even any act by a physician that consists of providing the means (for example, a pill or poison) by which a person could terminate his own or another's life. Actual medical practice in our times, however, does not necessarily abide by the restrictions on euthanasia found in the Oath. In addition, current prevalent public views with regard to euthanasia may not be consistent with those embodied in the Oath. Many contemporary writers on medical ethics and practices inform us that, although euthanasia is not legalized, hospitals and medical professionals practice it, often terminating lives. Strong support has also been prevalent in favor of giving a greater role to the physician in euthanasia. In the well-known words of Glanville Williams, decisions on cases of euthanasia should be made "by giving the medical practitioner a wide discretion and trusting to his good sense" (Williams 1958, 302).

The lack of relevance of the Oath to contemporary thought and practice concerning euthanasia is, according to some scholars of the ancient Greek medical tradition, nothing new. This view has always been with us because the Oath, and especially its injunctions against the physician's role in terminating life, were not of any relevance in the Greek world either.

The Oath did not reflect the views of the general public about these matters nor did it accurately represent the standard practice of the physicians.

Some interpreters of the Hippocratic Oath argue that the Oath is at odds with standard medical practices in the Greek world, where euthanasia seems to have been accepted and practiced by medical professionals. They point out that in a society where exposing children with defects to the inclement elements was common practice, euthanasia must have been a far lesser concern. Ludwig Edelstein in particular insists on the apparent discrepancy between the Hippocratic Oath and actual practice, at least as far as euthanasia is concerned, and offers an explanation of the alleged discrepancy (Edelstein 1989). He suggests the Hippocratic Oath reflects certain Pythagorean views that consider life sacred, something that must not be terminated. The Pythagorean origins of the Oath also explain its opposition to having the physician perform surgery since surgery involves handling and possibly spilling of blood—again proscribed by the Pythagoreans. The Oath's injunction against surgery is particularly problematic, since members of the Hippocratic medical tradition seem to have practiced surgery. One of the surviving treatises in the Hippocratic corpus is on surgery where numerous references to surgical incisions occur[7]—facts that lend some support to Edelstein's claim that the Oath does not reflect common medical practice but is imbued by the beliefs of a fringe group and is therefore not representative of the views of the mainstream medical practitioners in the ancient Greek world. Following Edelstein's line of argument, the Oath would be more accurately called the "Pythagorean Oath" instead of the "Hippocratic Oath."

The alleged connection between the Hippocratic Oath and Pythagoreanism sounds too simple to be true. The historical origins and intellectual or religious foundations of the Hippocratic Oath are shrouded in mystery and will possibly remain so, especially if they have anything to do with Pythagoreanism in its various forms. The first thing every student of Pythagoreanism comes to recognize is that the surviving fragments of some of the thinkers whom we take to have been Pythagoreans, or at least to have been influenced by Pythagoreanism (Alcmaeon, Empedocles, Hippasus, Philolaus, Plato) and the surviving testimony about Pythagoreanism comprise a perplexing set of evidence that does not straightforwardly support a consistent viewpoint about the matters under consideration here. This is true even of the surviving accounts of the Pythagoreans' most well-known practices—for example, prohibitions against blood spilling, meat eating, and sacrificing of animals. While Empedocles strongly supports such prohibitions, surviving testimony from Iamblichus and Gellius casts doubt on the hypothesis that Pythagoreans abided by any of them—including the sacrificing of animals and spilling of blood.[8] In any case, the alleged Pythagorean prohibition against blood spilling is not of great importance in relation to the termination of life since the latter can be done without spilling any blood—e.g., by administering a pill or drug, as the Oath itself makes clear.

The most reliable testimony about the views of Pythagoras himself is thought to be that of Porphyry, who puts us on notice that "What he [Pythagoras] said to his associates no one can say with certainty; for they preserved no ordinary silence" (Porphyry, *Life of Pythagoras* 19). Porphyry attributes to Pythagoras four primary theses: (1) the soul is immortal (the immortality thesis); (2) the soul migrates into different kinds of animals or bodies (the metempsychosis thesis); (3) at certain periods, whatever has happened happens again—nothing being absolutely new (the eternal-recurrence thesis); and (4) all living things should be considered as belonging to the same kind (the unity-of-the-living-world thesis). That any one of these four theses, either when taken by itself or conjoined with some others in the set, straightforwardly implies the wrongness of terminating a life is by no means obvious. Indeed, the immortality and metempsychosis theses seem to imply that the end of ordinary life is of no consequence—the soul will go on, moving from one animal to another. The soul, which, according to Empedocles, "is not of blood, nor blended breath"—these being the constituents of the body, which is earth-born and mortal—continues to exist and to retain its identity as it sequentially inhabits different bodies. Tradition attributes to Pythagoras himself, i.e., to his soul, a long journey through a number of bodies—from the time of the Trojan War, when he was Euphorbus and was killed by Menelaus, to the time when he was allegedly proving mathematical theorems or developing philosophical theories and founding a Pythagorean society several centuries later.[9]

These four primary theses nonetheless are not the only ones associated with Pythagoreanism. Many others, in some cases both a thesis and its negation, are reported as part of a system of Pythagorean beliefs. Some of these secondary theses seem to argue against terminating a life; others argue in favor of ending life; still others seem neutral in their implications with respect to the termination of life or cancel out when conjoined with other theses. One of the most important secondary theses, stated most clearly by Plato in the *Phaedo*, claims that the embodiment of the soul in any body is a kind of imprisonment and that liberation comes about by death, which is the freeing of the soul from the bonds of the body (*Phaedo* 66e, 81e, 82e). The imprisonment/liberation conception of life/death, respectively, is clearly stated by Empedocles also, who is thought to have been influenced by Pythagoras himself or at least his teachings.[10]

The imprisonment/liberation thesis itself, especially when understood in the extreme way that Empedocles, Plato, and other Pythagoreans seem to have understood it, argues clearly in favor of termination of life. According to them, life has no redeeming features. Even when taken without the immortality of the soul thesis, the imprisonment/liberation thesis implies that prolonging life is prolonging evil. When coupled with the immortality thesis, the implication in favor of the termination of life is even stronger: for some, the quicker the exit from life the sooner the soul will be free and able to enjoy the greatest goods.[11] Thus, elements of Pythagoreanism are not inconsistent with the termination of life; on the contrary, they strongly favor it. This consequence of Pythagoreanism was not lost on Plato, who in the *Phaedo* presents Socrates as being eager to depart from life and enjoy the benefits of the liberation of the soul from the body only to be confronted with the inevitable question—why not terminate one's own life as fast as one can? Plato's response to the question rests on another secondary assumption—the master/servant thesis.

The master/servant thesis, which raises some quite interesting questions about autonomy itself, is the most important secondary thesis for this discussion. Aiming to blunt the obvious consequence of the imprisonment/liberation thesis, especially when it is coupled with the immortality thesis—namely, that the earlier the departure from life the better—Plato argues that we are all servants, our masters being the gods. As servants, we have no right to end our lives since that would be interfering with the possessions of the gods, who have the authority to choose the time of departure from this life for each person (*Phaedo* 61d–63c). Some evidence exists that Plato's master/servant thesis was a part of Pythagoreanism, since others attribute it to Pythagoras's associates or followers.[12]

At the human level, the master/servant thesis seems to rule out both suicide and euthanasia—for the latter, both voluntary and involuntary. The thesis undercuts any autonomy humans might claim to have over their own lives and also neutralizes any authority some humans might claim to have over the lives of other humans, thus implying that one person has no authority over the life of another—even when one person consents to be under the authority of another person: the ultimate authority lies with the divinities, since every human is their possession. Even if in ordinary circumstances one is a servant or a slave of another, one remains the servant of the divinities, who have final authority over his life. This aspect of the master/servant thesis argues in favor of the inviolability of the life of a person as far as humans are concerned (and perhaps of the inviolability of the life of every animal). The implication, however, is not necessarily without some cost; the thesis implies that, regardless of how bad the condition of a particular person is or how great the suffering and how little hope for improvement, the authority to terminate the life of this person does not lie in any human hands but in the hands of the divinities. Thus, human life is not inviolable in relation to the gods but, presumably, they make, one hopes, the right choices.

The last point shows that, while the master/servant thesis by itself prohibits the practice of suicide and euthanasia among humans, it permits human euthanasia at the level of the gods. They have the right to make decisions about the life of humans, who are their possessions or servants. In the *Phaedo*, Socrates sees the imminent end of his life, which is not due to natural causes, as the outcome of divine decisions or choices. Indeed, if the master/servant thesis is to have any content, it must be assumed that the gods interfere with the natural order of things, at least with regard to the termination of life. Some, if not all, lives end not by the working out of natural causes—Socrates does not die of old age—but by a decision or act of the gods. It is also assumed by those who accept the master/servant thesis that the decisions and acts of the gods are based on complete knowledge, something that humans do not possess, and that the gods are motivated by beneficence—"The Gods, one and all, are our chiefest guardians, and the interests they guard are our chief interests" (Plato, *Laws* x 907).

In choosing to end, or to prolong, the life of someone, the gods are realizing the good, although it is not always clear that it is in every case the good of the person whose life is terminated or prolonged.[13] Thus, according to this view, some, if not all, human deaths are cases of euthanasia—they are brought about by divine decisions to terminate human lives, which otherwise might have continued, for the sake of the good.

This discussion shows that the views of the Pythagoreans with respect to terminating life, either one's own or that of others, are quite complicated. While some of their beliefs seem to be consistent with terminating life, others seem to oppose it. Even their most explicit statement on this issue, the master/servant thesis, while it unequivocally prohibits humans from committing suicide or practicing euthanasia, permits a kind of euthanasia that has its source in divine decisions and beneficent motives. Those who see the origins of the Hippocratic Oath in Pythagoreanism may argue that the Oath offers sufficient evidence to justify the claim that its injunction against any role by the physician in euthanasia or suicide is at bottom a reflection of some extreme Pythagorean views. The physician is, after all, a human and not a god, and the master/servant thesis makes clear that humans must not terminate any life, since they have no right to do so.

Yet the hypothesis of the alleged connection between Pythagoreanism and the Hippocratic Oath leaves too many things unexplained. To begin with, there is no explicit evidence of a Pythagorean connection in what the Oath says. Although the Oath begins by making reference to Apollo and Asclepios, not much can be inferred from this; these are simply the gods that the physicians as well as many others swear to.[14] The rest of the Oath is essentially about the code of conduct for a physician. Second, connecting the injunction against physician-assisted euthanasia found in the Hippocratic Oath to Pythagorianism does not help much with the question that must have been as important in classical times as it is in our own—namely, what role should the physician play in terminating human life? Perhaps the recognition of the urgency of this question by the Hippocratic physicians, whether Pythagorean or not in their beliefs, led them to address the matter of terminating human life in the physician's professional code. Third, if we assume that the Pythagorean-connection hypothesis is true, the question arises as to why the Oath has played the role it has played for so long. That the Oath has been considered for so many centuries the professional code of medical practitioners is truly amazing. Have physicians been swearing to uphold something that no one believes now and perhaps no one ever believed in the past, except possibly for some extreme Pythagoreans?

My guess is that what explains the continuity of the Oath, at least as an ideal for the physician to aspire to live by, is the fact that it reflects some fundamental moral beliefs shared by most and some basic views about the essential goals of medicine and those who practice it as a profession. The beliefs of the Pythagoreans in the inviolability of human life, as captured in the master/servant thesis, are not easily dismissed as belonging to some fringe group. Most people, rightly or wrongly, seem to accept something that comes very close to the Pythagorean thesis—namely, the sanctity of life. In addition, the Oath perhaps represents some views about how physicians should act that seem to most people to be, in principle, correct—views that capture the way medical practitioners should ideally behave in a world that is not riddled by the difficulties and contradictions that beset the world we all live in.

In particular, the Oath's injunction against a physician's participation in terminating a life stems from some very deep-seated convictions about the very nature or goals of medicine and the responsibilities of those who swear to realize them. Nothing in the Oath suggests that nonphysicians should also abstain from any participation in terminating life. Perhaps they should also abstain, if appropriate reasons are present. The prohibition in the Oath is exclusively directed at the physicians and, although the reasons for it are unstated, they are assumed to be self-evident. The Oath is a professional code of conduct, and the reasons for most of what it enjoins or recommends must have something to do with the goals of the profession. One of the reasons is found in some ideas expounded by both Plato and Aristotle. The way they conceive of the goals of medicine lends support to the injunction found in the Oath against any role of the physician in terminating life. I now turn to these ideas of Plato and Aristotle.

The Function and Goals of Medicine

One line of argument against assigning any role to the physician in the termination of life comes from what the ancient Greek philosophers understood as the end of medical knowledge and practice. They often referred to this end as the function of medicine. The function of something, characteristically what a thing alone can do or does better than other things, connects to the essential nature or the purpose of the thing. Thus the connection between seeing and the eye, hearing and the ear, or cutting and the knife is not, according to this view, an accidental or contingent, but an essential, one. In addition, both Plato and Aristotle argue that the excellences of a functional thing are determined in relation to its function, and therefore a functional thing is good of its kind if and only if it performs its function well. An eye is a good eye if and only if it sees well, and its excellences are just those conditions of the eye that are necessary and sufficient for seeing well.[15]

The ancient Greeks identified health as the end or function of medicine, meaning by this the restoration, improvement, or maintenance of health. The evidence in the philosophical tradition is unequivocal. According to Plato, the function of the art of the physician is to produce health (*Euthyphro* 13d, *Charmides* 165d, 174c, 175, *Euthydemus* 291e, *Gorgias* 477e, *Timaeus* 24c, *Laws* xii 962). According to Aristotle, health is the function, end, or good of medicine (*Eudemian Ethics* i 5.1216b1, i 8.1218b2–3, ii 1.1219a15, *Nicomachean Ethics* i 1.1094a8, i 7.1097a19). Also axiomatic for both philosophers is that health is a good thing and disease an evil or bad thing—sickness is an evil and health a good (*Lysis* 217b, 218e); health is the greatest blessing of mankind and among the arts concerned with the good is medicine (*Gorgias* 451e, 452, 500a); health, being desired for its own sake as well as its consequences, belongs to the class of highest goods (*Republic* ii 375c); Aristotle claims that "Nobody proves that health is a good (unless he is a sophist and not a physician)" (*Eudemian Ethics* i 8.1218b22–23), for all agree on this, and the physician does not deliberate whether he shall heal but assumes the end and considers how and by what means it is to be attained (*Nicomachean Ethics* iii 3.1112b12–13; also *Eudemian Ethics* ii 10.1227a18–20, 1227b25–31).

If the activities of restoring, improving, or maintaining health constitute the function, end, or goal of medicine, they cannot be incidentally related to it. On the contrary, for Plato and Aristotle, these activities have a special connection to medicine. Thus, the physician may be constrained by these ends not incidentally. A physician is not merely someone who has a capacity for applying a certain type of knowledge or technique. He must be aiming at the goals of medicine.

What exactly is this relationship between medicine and the physician, on the one hand, and the set of activities and goals that comprise the function of medicine and of the physician, on the other? What does this supposed relationship exclude or allow? One might be tempted to say that, given the supposed connection between the faculty, art, or science of medicine and health, one who possesses such faculty, art, or science (the physician) cannot aim at anything not conducive to health. Plato entertains such a possibility when in *Republic* (i 340d–341a) he discusses whether or not it is possible for the physician, acting as a physician, to err about medical matters. Although he seems to concede for the sake of the argument that the answer to this query may be "no," he elsewhere readily admits that physicians make mistakes (*Charmides* 164c). Aristotle also leaves room for error on the part of the physician: "in medicine it is possible to err in both ways (reasoning or perception)" (*Eudemian Ethics* ii 10.1226a37–38); "physicians do not always understand the nature of health, and also the means which they use may not effect the desired end" (*Politics* vii 13.1331b34–37); and "mistakes come to pass even in the operations of art: the grammarian makes a mistake in writing and the doctor pours out the wrong dose" (*Physics* ii 8.199a33–35).

Yet the possibility of the physician's error is not the interesting question in the present context since even in cases of error the physician could be aiming at health; he is just mistaken about how to bring it about. What is of interest is the possibility, discussed by both Plato and Aristotle, of the physician knowingly aiming at something that is not in agreement with the goals of medicine. Plato in *Republic* (i 340e) argues that the possession of a certain knowledge, art, or skill equips its possessor with the capacity to do either what is the normal end of such knowledge or skill or its opposite. One of the examples he gives is that of medical knowledge or art. The doctor, according to Socrates, is equipped with the knowledge either to make his patient healthy or to kill him. And he insists that the doctor can do the latter not because he makes a mistake but precisely because he has the knowledge or expertise for bringing it about—he can do it better than the nonphysician. He repeats the same observation in the

Statesman: "Every physician, you see, can preserve the life of any he wills among us, and can hurt any he wills by knife or cautery" (298a). Indeed, Plato seems intrigued by the ability of any art intentionally to produce the opposite of its end. At one point he affirms the superiority of the mind of the physician who knowingly aims at an end that is opposite to medicine's aims when compared to the mind of the physician who achieves the same end by mistake or ignorance; the former just knows his medicine better (*Hippias Minor* 375a–b).

Aristotle seems equally intrigued by this apparent ability of the arts to achieve ends that are opposite to their canonical ones, locates a "cause" for it, and shows that the relation of an art to the two opposite ends it is capable of achieving is not the same. In *Eudemian Ethics* (ii 10.1227a25–26) he observes that "a science does enable us to do a thing that is not the object of the science." In *Metaphysics* (ix 2.1046b4–10), he offers an explanation of this feature of the sciences and asserts once more that an art may be capable of producing two opposite ends but nonetheless its relation to one of the ends is a privileged one: "The hot is capable only of heating, but the medical art can produce both disease and health. The reason is that science is a rational formula, and the same rational formula explains a thing and its privation, only not in the same way; in a sense it applies to both, but in a sense it applies rather to the positive thing."

Aristotle's explanation in terms of the metaphysics of privation may not be transparent, but it points in a direction that is very different from that of recent commentators who have tried to interpret Plato's and Aristotle's remarks on any art's capacity to produce two opposite kinds of end. Commentators writing on this argument of Plato invariably point out that it is meant to show that the moral virtues are not skills or arts; they go on to suggest that what guarantees that the doctor will not use his medical skill to terminate the life of his patient, at least when he should not, is not another skill but the fact that the doctor has the required moral excellences—i.e., the dispositions or states of character of justice, temperance, and so on (Cross and Woozley 1964, 53–55). I do not wish to question the claim that Plato argues against the thesis that moral excellences are skills or arts. I think this is correct and is borne out by the discussion in the middle books of the *Republic* where Plato argues that the moral virtues are dispositions or states of character. However, I do wish to raise some questions about the claim that the requirements imposed on the doctor's behavior are only those stemming from the typical moral virtues.

Morality (moral virtue) imposes certain requirements on everyone, including the physician. But the requirement imposed on the physician to treat a patient and to aim at restoring or maintaining the patient's health is not merely a requirement of morality—for example, a requirement of justice or charity. If it were merely a requirement of morality, what is expected of the physician would be required of everyone. The physician as well is not to determine whether or not to bring about the health of a patient on the basis of considerations of justice. As Aristotle says, the physician does not deliberate whether or not he will try to restore the health of the patient but he does deliberate on the appropriate method or remedy of healing.

In addition, a physician is not evaluated on the basis of possessing the moral virtues but on possessing the excellence of the physician—i.e., the skills required to do well what the function of medicine is or what the profession requires—restoring or maintaining health. Thus, one can be a just person and a bad physician or a fine physician but not necessarily an exemplary human being. But one could not be a fine physician if one were unable to bring about or were not aiming at the goals of medicine. The physician is thus evaluated with reference both to his skills and his goals, which are determined by the nature of his discipline and not by something else—not even by morality. As Aristotle puts it, what is called perfect or complete of a certain kind is "That which in respect of excellence and goodness cannot be excelled in its kind; for example, we have a perfect [complete] doctor or flute-player, when they lack nothing in respect of the form of proper excellence" (*Metaphysics* v 16.1021b14–17). A bad doctor, according to him, is "one whom we should not call bad, simply" (*Nicomachean Ethics* vii 4.1148b8–9).

Aristotle's claim that medicine, despite its ability to bring about the opposite of health, has health as its end is repeated throughout his writings and is a part of his broad essentialist views and his account of causality. In *Topics* vi 5.143a2–5, for example, he admits that at times medicine is defined as that which "is concerned with the production of disease and health," but insists that "it [medicine] is said to do the latter [produce health] essentially, the former [produce disease] accidentally, since it is absolutely foreign to medicine to produce disease." The essential connection between medicine and health, which according to Aristotle accounts also for the necessary causal connection between the two, is defended throughout the *Metaphysics*: Aristotle argues that it is in the nature (*phusis*) of the doctor to produce health vi 2.1027a; that medicine is the form of health or, in a sense, health (vii 7.1032b11–14, claims he repeats at xii 4.1070b33 and xii 10.1075b10). Elsewhere in *Metaphysics* xii, Aristotle argues that medicine "is the formal cause of health" (3.1070a29–30) or "the moving cause [of health]" (4.1070b28) as well as in *Generatione et Corruptione* i 7.324b).

The Aristotelian position is quite clear—the relation between medicine and health (its end) is not accidental but essential,[16] and the goals of the discipline and its practitioners are not fixed by anything outside of this relationship. Thus both Plato and Aristotle insist that, although the practitioners of medicine benefit from their art, such benefits are not essential to its goals.[17] These and similar considerations (e.g., bribes[18]) should not determine the aim of the physician. Plato argues that medicine does not even benefit itself but seeks the benefit of the patient, a restriction that prohibits the physician from making decisions for the sake of the advancement of the medical discipline but at the expense of the aim of medicine, i.e., the health of the patient—a practice not undocumented in medical annals.[19] The essentialist conception of the goals of medicine that Plato and Aristotle expound does not allow for any considerations other than the health of the patient to determine physicians' actions. Aristotle insists that even friendship should not interfere with the goals of the physician as the medical art dictates, "For the physician does nothing contrary to rules from motives of friendship" (*Politics* iii 16.1287a35–36). The only consideration for the physician, when the matter is considered in the abstract, is the maximal realization of the goals of the medical art—"in the art of medicine there is no limit to the pursuit of health, and as in other arts there is no limit to their several ends, for they aim at accomplishing their ends to the uttermost" (*Politics* i 9.1257b25–27).

The considerations just described show that the injunction of the Hippocratic Oath against any role of the physician in the termination of life need not be an outlandish one—some strange belief of Pythagorean mystics. On the contrary, it appears to be consequent to a deeply held view about the nature of medicine and its goals. By placing an injunction on any role of the physician in terminating life, the Oath, aiming to codify the responsibilities of the ideal practitioners of the medical art, is in complete agreement with the implication of this deeply held view of medicine. This view of medicine and its goals, as well as its implications about the physician's role in ending life, does not necessarily exclude the possibility that in certain circumstances some lives must be terminated or be left to end. However, acts or decisions of this kind need not be a part of medical practice; the considerations that justify such acts or decisions might lie altogether outside of medicine. The injunction of the Oath against any role of the physician in terminating life and the Platonic/Aristotelian view it reflects set some ideal limits on what the purely professional goals of the medical practitioners must be.

Undoubtedly, the Platonic/Aristotelian essentialist view of medicine and its goals raises many questions. Although these questions cannot be discussed here, I wish to touch briefly on two issues likely to occur to anyone who thinks about these matters. First, one might raise the question of how the goals of medicine and its practitioners are fixed. This is a rather complicated issue for both Plato and Aristotle, and I only wish to point out that both philosophers treat this matter as having not much to do with the particular intentions, desires, or goals of any one individual. Rather, a social dimension, and at times even a natural one, exists in regard to this matter. Sometimes these philosophers treat certain arts as if they are constituents of the order of nature, just as some faculties are, because they satisfy a natural need. As Plato remarks, the body is not self-sufficient, "it has needs, and for this purpose the art of medicine exists and has now been discovered, because the body is defective, not self-sufficient. So to provide it with things advantageous to it the art of medicine has been developed" (*Republic* i 341e). At other times, however, all arts are seen as constituents of the social/political fabric, satisfying desires or needs of society and thus defined and regulated by something larger than any one individual, most often the *polis* itself. These two dimensions of the conception of medicine and its goals, the social/political and the natural, need not be at odds, and certainly Plato and Aristotle did not see any conflict between the two. After all, both try to base their political theories on a naturalistic foundation.

Second, one might object, regarding Plato and Aristotle, that the goals of medicine are less fixed than these philosophers presuppose: the goals of medicine are perhaps more flexible and vague than these thinkers construe them. In particular, one may argue that one way of understanding the goals of medicine is as the alleviation of pain. Understanding the goals in this way shows that one argument in favor of the physician's role in euthanasia is weighty as well as consistent with the goals of the discipline. The argument is a familiar one: In certain cases the physician is justified in terminating or in not extending a life in order to alleviate pain and suffering or not to prolong them.

Yet the goals of medicine cannot simply be the alleviating of pain or suffering, certainly not the alleviating of pain or suffering by any means or at all costs. In many cases, alleviation of pain or suffering could be achieved without improving or restoring health, that is, by certain drugs that mask pain and suffering. Such goals can be a part of the aim of medicine but not the only aim. The reason they are a part of medicine's aim is that a life without or with less pain or suffering is preferable to a life with or with more pain and suffering. In other words, in aiming to reduce pain or suffering the physician aims to improve a life; he aims to increase a good, namely life, and thus remains within the objectives of medicine. But when one terminates a life in order to alleviate pain, one is clearly not increasing the good of life. Rather, one eliminates it together with the evils of pain and suffering.

In addition, Aristotle and Plato claim that not all pains or sufferings justify alleviation by terminating life and not all pains or sufferings are necessarily bad. Aristotle, for instance, argues that to terminate one's life for pain or suffering that does not justify such a drastic act is to commit an act of vice, an act of cowardice or, at times, injustice—even though one might have exercised one's autonomy in doing so. In addition, some pains should not be eliminated at all, even by means far less drastic than ending life. To follow Aristotle's characterization of some acts of avoiding pain as acts of cowardice: some pains might be of such a nature that any effort to alleviate them might border on cowardice, since our acts signify that we are unable to face the smallest irritation (*Nicomachean Ethics* iii 7.1116a13). And some pains that should not be eliminated, at least not preemptively, are, for example, those that alert us to disease; they clearly are necessary for our survival and therefore beneficial. Plato, while examining particular conceptions of the good, at times points to the common belief that some pains are good, often necessary for our present and future well-being: for example, "physical training, military campaigns, doctors' treatment involving cautery or the knife or drugs or starvation diet ... [they are considered good] because in the future there result from them, health, bodily well-being, the safety of one's country, dominion over others, wealth" (*Protagoras* 354a–b; see also *Gorgias* 478b–c, 480c, *Laws* iii 684c–d).

Yet to try to deny that cases arise in which pain and suffering must be alleviated if life is to continue in any meaningful way would be foolish. The most difficult cases, in which continued existence, although at times without any pain or suffering, lacks altogether every kind of experience or activity associated with ordinary human life must also be considered. In these situations, a decision often must be made on whether the goodness of being alive outweighs the evil of suffering or on whether or not mere existence, which is devoid of all human experience, is a good any more. The decision process may very well lead us to the conclusion that either passive or active euthanasia is the right course in such cases.

Both Plato and Aristotle discuss cases which, in their judgment, justify either passive or active euthanasia—a view that seems, at least prima facie, to be at odds with the implication of the essentialist conception of medicine and its goals that both philosophers expound. Aristotle remarks that "without breathing or being awake or participating in movement we could not possess any good or any evil at all" (*Eudemian Ethics* i 2.1214b19–21). One might argue that the life Aristotle describes here, possessing neither any good nor any evil, provides us with no reason for trying to prolong it any more, or leaving it alone till it ends by itself, or terminating it. But this is not Aristotle's view; he goes on to ask "would anyone desire life for the pleasure of sleep; for what is the difference between slumbering without being awakened from the first day till the last of a thousand or any number of years, and living a vegetable existence?" (*Eudemian Ethics* i 5.1216a2–5). He even finds a life that contains experiences but is devoid of any pleasures or pains, or even one that only contains pleasures of an ignoble kind, to be such "that non-existence would be better than being alive" (1215b26). He adds that a life containing only the pleasure of food or sex alone, "with the other pleasures that knowledge or sight or any other of the senses provides for human beings abstracted, would not induce anybody to value life higher if he were not utterly slavish" (1215b30–35).

But Aristotle goes a step further by considering a life that may very well contain experiences or activities or even pleasures that need not necessarily be either ignoble or slavish but which nonetheless is a life that does not justify existence over nonexistence. He argues that a life that consisted of only instrumental ends, without anything in it that is pursued for its own sake, would be such a life—even if it were to last for an infinite time: "If one collected together the whole of the things that the whole of mankind do and experience yet do and experience unwillingly, because not for the sake of the things themselves, and if one added an infinite extent of time, these would not cause a man to choose to be alive rather than not alive" (1215b26–30). He further argues that many of the events of life lead people to throw away life, among which are diseases and sufferings (1215b19–20), and he strongly defends the practice of exposing deformed infants to the vicissitudes of weather (*Politics* vii 16.1335b19–26).

Plato also argues that occasions arise when life must be left to end without medical intervention or be terminated. In one of his early dialogues, he raises questions of whether those cases in which it would not be better for a man not to get up from an illness, whether in all cases to live is preferable, or whether in many cases it is not better to die (*Laches* 195d). His position on this matter is most forcefully presented in the *Republic* when he castigates a legendary trainer, Herodicus, who devised every means to cure an untreatable illness, thus managing to extend for a long time a life that was useless to himself and a burden to others (iii 406a–b). He applauds the carpenter who rejects the lengthy and cumbersome regimen prescribed by the physician because "he had no leisure to be ill and that life is no use to him if he has to neglect his work and always be concerned with his illness. After that he would bid good-bye to the doctor, resume his usual way of life, and either recover his health or, if his body could not withstand the illness, he would die and escape his troubles" (406c–e). Plato argues that the carpenter's choice should be a model for all, including for those who might not have a well-defined type of work as the carpenter does. Indeed, he goes so far as to argue that medicine was practiced and handed down by Asclepios primarily for those whose bodies are healthy in their natures and habits and have some specific disease. But for those whose bodies are riddled with disease, he did not prescribe anything to prolong a miserable life—"He [Asclepios] didn't think that he should treat someone who could not live a normal life, since such a person would be of no profit either to himself or to the city" (407e). He argues that people who are by nature sick and licentious should not be given medical care, since they are not profitable to themselves or to anyone else and since "medicine isn't intended for such people and they shouldn't be treated, not even if they are richer than Midas" (408b). According to legend, which Plato does not believe, Asclepios, the son of Apollo, was killed by his father for being bribed with gold to heal a rich man who was nearly dead (408b–c). As is well known, Plato also defends exposure of unfit children (v 460c).

Some of the passages just cited, especially those from Aristotle that do not make any reference to any role of the physician in terminating life, do not seem to be in conflict with the essentialist conception of medicine and its goals that, in principle, require practitioners of the medical art to aim at restoring or maintaining health. But the Platonic passages just cited expound a view that clearly places medicine and its practitioners right at the center of the practice of euthanasia. The kind of involvement by the practitioners of medicine in terminating life that this view reflects seems to be clearly in conflict with the implications of the essentialist conception of medicine and its goals that was discussed earlier. How real or deep is this conflict?

In the works of both Plato and Aristotle, we encounter a view that the physician is the sole arbiter on matters of health and possibly life itself on the grounds that authority lies in expertise or ability. The same conception of authority underlies the position of those in our times who also wish to strengthen the hand of medical practitioners in terminating life. Yet I contend that even if the Platonic/Aristotelian conception of authority as expertise were to be accepted, it would not necessarily follow that the physician is not bound by any of the constraints stemming from the essentialist conception of medicine and its goals and, consequently, should have a free hand in matters concerning the termination of life. At least the decision-making process about the termination of life does not fall within the authority of medicine and its practitioners, even if authority is understood in the way Plato and Aristotle understand it. Both philosophers saw clearly that the expertise of medicine, as well as the authority that presumably flows from it, have their limits; they do not extend to determining whether a life should continue or not. For them, such determinations primarily lie within the scope of different kinds of expertise—ethical or political. Thus the essentialist conception of medicine and its goals and the constraints they impose on the aims of the physician may be left mostly intact, even if one is willing to accept that the physician has sole authority on strictly medical matters. But first, we examine the conception of authority as expertise and its limits.

The Authority of Medicine and Its Practitioners

Given the ancient conception of medicine as a science, we can see how the physician might have come to be looked upon as an authority on all questions pertaining to life, including possibly those concerning its termination. Indeed, the dominant conception of authority in Plato and Aristotle and one type of authority recognized by us lend some support to the idea that the role of the physician in such matters should be a salient one.

Most commonly, we think that A has authority over B if A has the right to command B and B is required to obey. Philosophers often disagree as to the source or sources of A's right or claim to command and B's requirement to obey, thus disagreeing about the sources of authority, sometimes identifying several sources and therefore distinct types of authority. One such source, and therefore one type of authority, is ability or expertise. Our locution "X is an authority in such and such" reflects our recognition that X's pronouncements in a certain area, the area of X's expertise, have a certain weight; they command the right to be accepted.

Authority from ability may not be the paradigmatic kind of authority for us, but it assuredly was for Plato and Aristotle. In Plato's writings, the idea that in most cases authority stems from ability or expertise is one of the basic presuppositions of his thought, which need not be always explicitly stated. It is clearly presupposed as a fundamental principle in the political theory he develops in the *Republic* since the authority of the rulers of the ideal city he describes there derives primarily from their expertise or knowledge of the Forms. But at times Plato comes very close to stating the relation between expertise and authority as a general principle, although most often he illustrates the principle by reference to his favored examples—the sciences of ruling, medicine, and navigation. In the *Statesman* he remarks that "we must insist that in this disinterested scientific ability we see the distinguishing mark of true authority in medicine, and of true authority everywhere else" (293c). He repeats often that ability or expertise is a necessary condition for ruling over or commanding others (*Statesman* 292e, 293b, *Laws* xii 962b). More importantly, he argues that it is a sufficient condition for exercising authority over others—that the mere possession of the art of statesmanship or medicine makes one a ruler or physician, respectively, even though one may not be in power or an acknowledged practitioner of medicine (*Statesman* 259a–b; see also *Republic* i 341d on the example of the navigator and *Lysis* 210a–d for a general statement of the claim that expertise will give authority to anyone who has it). Elsewhere he defends the authority of the judgment in a particular field of those who have knowledge in that field as contrasted with the lack of authority of the opinions of those who lack expertise (*Crito* 47b–d, *Gorgias* 517e, 518a). And he often views the arts as ruling over persons on account of their expertise (*Republic* i 342c) and the physicians in particular as rulers and governors of bodies (342d).

Aristotle is in agreement with Plato on the relation between knowledge, expertise, or ability and authority. He argues that if a person wiser than all exists, that person is entitled to rule (*Politics* iii 13.1284a3ff.); the master has authority over the servant on account of his abilities (*Politics* i 13); some parts of the soul should rule over others because of their capacities (*Nicomachean Ethics* i 13). More specifically, he refers to medical science as a "ruling principle" (*Eudemian Ethics* viii 3.1249b12) and to the physician as someone who rules (or has authority) and gives orders or commands (*Rhetoric* i 15.1375b20–23, *Nicomachean Ethics* ii 4.1105b14–16). And he endorses Plato's view on the authority of the judgment of the medical expert: "With regard to the future, as Plato says, surely the opinion of the physician and that of the ignorant man are not equally authoritative, for instance, on the question whether a man will get well or not" (*Metaphysics* iv 5.1010b11–14).

What is the scope of the kind of authority from expertise that Plato and Aristotle attribute to medicine and its practitioners and what room, if any, does it leave for autonomy? Both philosophers concede at times something to consent or to the autonomous decision of those who are supposedly ruled by the various sciences, arts, or skills and their practitioners,[20] but the absence of consent or the denial of autonomy clearly would not alter the position of authority that some have over others. Elaborating his position on the source of the authority of rulers, Plato writes:

> And these men, whether they rule over willing or unwilling subjects, with or without written laws, and whether they are rich or poor, must, according to our present view, be supposed to exercise their rule in accordance with some art or science. And physicians offer a particularly good example of this position. Whether they cure us against our will or with our will, by cutting us or burning us or causing us pain in any other way, and whether they do it by written rules or without them, and whether they are rich or poor, we call them physicians just the same, so long as they exercise authority by art or science, purging us or reducing us in some other way, or even adding to our weight, provided only that they who treat their patients treat them for the benefit of their health and preserve them better than they were. (*Statesman* 293a–c)

In these remarks, Plato dismisses in a rather wholesale fashion the role or place of consent or of the exercise of autonomy on the part of the patient in medical treatment, giving unlimited authority to the physician to determine treatment and enforce it.

Most will likely question and object to Plato's total dismissal of consent or autonomy in medical matters. Yet we must not overlook the fact that Plato is talking strictly about medical treatment whose sole aim is to *restore* or *improve* health, an area where the physician's pronouncements *have* a claim to be heard and followed; they carry considerable authority. Here, one might say, the end to be attained is clearly recognized and beyond dispute as well as unequivocally within the explicit goals of medicine, and the physician's expertise or authoritative pronouncements concern the *means* for bringing about the undisputed end—for example, knife, cautery, or some other painful treatment (to use Plato's more or less equally unpalatable alternatives). As Plato's remarks make clear, physicians have the authority to enforce any or all of these unpleasant treatments "provided only that they who treat their patients treat them for the benefit of their health and preserve them by making them better than they were" (*Statesman* 293b). That is, their authority in matters of medical treatment that stems from their scientific expertise is constrained by the goals of medical practice as understood by the essentialist conception of medicine discussed earlier.

Those who urge that the physician should have a strong voice in cases in which the termination of life is at issue are to some extent treating cases of euthanasia and the kind of "difficult" case Plato discusses in the remarks above as being similar. Yet it is obvious that they are not. Whereas in Plato's case the end—i.e., health, its restoration, maintenance, or improvement—is clearly an undisputed good, the termination of life is really a means to something (i.e., death) that is not normally a good or it is so only in rare and extreme cases. Determining in which circumstances the termination of life is a greater good than continuation of life is not like determining whether the knife, cautery, or some other treatment will be used for the sake of restoring or improving health. In contrast to what Aristotle says when he insists that the physician does not deliberate about the end—i.e., whether or not to bring about health or whether or not health is a good—in cases where the termination of life is at stake, the only worthwhile deliberation is about the end; this kind of deliberation is clearly not about the means by which life is to be terminated, i.e., by injecting this into or withholding that from the patient. The deliberation in the context of euthanasia is, rather, about the *end* that is proper to aim at, either passively or actively; the questions facing us in such contexts are about the value of certain kinds of life or existence. These kinds of questions are not primarily medical ones, and the physician's expertise or ability commands no special authority. Medicine will be most useful in informing us of certain facts on which diagnosis and prognosis can be based; but the appropriate weight to place on the various alternatives open with respect to the continuation or the end of life—hence the assessment of value outcomes—is something that mostly falls under the scope of a type of deliberation, and possibly of expertise, that is not a part of the expertise of medicine.

Neither Plato nor Aristotle accepts the idea that deliberation and decision about termination of life lies within the expertise of medical knowledge despite the fact that they treat medicine as a science and are willing to grant considerable authority to those who possess such science in whatever concerns medical treatment aimed at what the essentialist conception of medicine requires. Both philosophers insist that decisions about terminating life fall within the scope of ethical or political deliberation and knowledge.

The Science of the Good of the Individual and Community

Even in his earliest writings (the Socratic Dialogues), Plato draws strict boundaries regarding the expertise and authority of the various sciences or arts and of those who possess and practice them. Each science or art is seen as having a well-defined subject matter, which also determines its expertise and authority. Plato argues that, while medicine is distinguished from other sciences by its subject matter (e.g., health and disease, *Charmides* 171a), "the physician understands nothing but health and disease" (170e). He claims that each of the sciences can do its work—medicine can produce health; cobbling produces shoes—without knowledge of good and evil, although they might not achieve their ends beneficially if the science of good is wanting (174c–d). Elsewhere he dismisses the opinion of those who think that the physician's knowledge of illness extends beyond that of the nature of health and disease by insisting that

the physician knows no more than this [health and disease]. Do you imagine, Laches, that he knows whether health or illness is the more terrible to a man?... And do you think that the same things are terrible to those who had better die and to those who had better live?... And do you suppose that the physician knows this, or indeed any other specialist, except the man who is skilled in the grounds of fear and hope? (*Laches* 195c–d).

The answer to the last question, as are the answers to the others, is negative: "whether the suffering or not suffering of these things will be best for a man is a question which is no more for a soothsayer than for anyone else" (*Laches* 196a). The knowledge required for answering such questions is not possessed by many, not even those possessing medical knowledge: "And not every man has this knowledge [of what is bad and to be feared or what is good and not to be feared]: the physician and the soothsayer have it not" (*Laches* 196d). The relevant knowledge for answering the most difficult and perplexing questions about the continuation or termination of life is, Socrates and Plato argue, that of the science of good and evil (*Laches* 199c) or of the science of what is beneficial (*Charmides* 174c).

The idea that knowledge of the good is required for as well as giving authority to those possessing it in making most of the important decisions about life or death is one of the key elements of Plato's *Republic*, *Statesman*, and *Laws*. This knowledge is seen not merely as the understanding of what is beneficial for the individual, but as the understanding of the good of the community and how it can be realized. The rulers in Plato's ideal city are those few who have access to knowledge of the Forms, including that of the Forms of the Good and of justice—the latter as it relates to the city (political community or *polis*) and the individual. And these experts of the science of ruling make all the critical decisions in almost every sphere of life. The rest of the particular sciences or arts and their practitioners, although they have expertise within their own specific domains, are under the rule or authority of the science of ruling or those who possess it—i.e., the science of justice. Thus, according to this view, deliberation about many things falls outside the specific arts; it belongs in the sphere of the ruling art and its knowledge of the good and justice both of the individual and the community.

In the *Republic*, Plato explicitly construes deliberations about ending life, or even about typical medical treatment, as possessing a political dimension, since the good of the city is involved along with that of the individual. Indeed, he goes as far as attributing this political dimension of medicine even to the very invention of the discipline by Asclepios.

In the passages from the *Republic* quoted earlier, Plato applauds the carpenter who does not let his disease and the regimen the physician prescribes interfere with his allotted function in the city. A lengthy healing process is good for neither the carpenter nor the city. According to Plato, it was not because he was ignorant that "Asclepios failed to teach this type of medicine [one that aims to cure ailments that should be left alone] to his sons, but because he knew that everyone in a well-regulated city has his own work to do and that no one has the leisure to be ill and be under treatment all his life" (iii 407c). Asclepios did not treat those who were of no profit to themselves or to the city, a practice which, according to Plato, reveals the political ingenuity of Asclepios and his sons as well as their full understanding of the political dimension of some of their decisions (407e, 408b). Plato himself proposes that in his ideal city, the founders will legislate for the kind of medicine that "will look after those who are naturally well endowed in body and soul. But as for the ones whose bodies are naturally sickly or whose souls are incurably evil, won't they [medicine and justice] let the former die of their own accord and put the latter to death?" (410a). The degree to which Plato makes medicine political and the drastic measures he proposes against those who do not contribute any more to the good of the city raise serious questions. Whatever the answers to such questions might be, the important point is that he understood that decisions to terminate life have an ethical/political dimension and fall under the scope of ethical/political expertise, assuming that such a thing exists.

Aristotle's views on these matters echo those of Plato. He also thinks that deliberation about terminating life is primarily an ethical and political deliberation. Ending life, according to him, may violate the virtues of courage or justice, something that will be revealed only by the proper kind of deliberation that weighs the good and evils of the situation.[21] He also argues that a certain expertise is required if one is to deliberate correctly on these matters and hit the truth, and that not all the opinions about matters of conduct are equally valid.[22] He also agrees with Plato on the political dimension of decisions regarding the termination of life. His defense of exposing of children is based on political considerations, the good of the community (*Politics* vii 16.1335b19–25). More importantly, he sees the political art or science having authority over the particular arts since its good or end (the political end or good of the community) is the highest and greatest among the ends pursued, and therefore deliberations on important things are inevitably about the good of the community and its relation to individual ends.[23]

This discussion shows that Plato's and Aristotle's essentialist conception of medicine and its goals need not be altogether inconsistent with their position that at times life must be left to expire on its own or even be terminated. Both philosophers limit the influence medicine and its practitioners are allowed to exercise in deliberating on and deciding whether or not life should be left to expire or terminated. In their view, an expertise, distinct from that of medicine and of the physician, operates, and within the scope of this expertise matters of life and death must be deliberated and decided on.

Plato's and Aristotle's appeal to an expertise outside of technical medical knowledge for addressing the question of the role of the physician in terminating life, no doubt, has its problems and will not satisfy everyone. The Platonic/Aristotelian model of ethical and political expertise includes at least the following theses or assumptions: (a) goodness or the good is objective, and deliberations about terminating life therefore reach either a correct or incorrect conclusion; (b) an ethical and political expertise exists and at least some agents possess it; and (c) this kind of expertise, if properly applied, can answer questions about terminating life in the particular and concrete circumstances within which they arise.

Thesis or assumption (a) will be problematic to those who place much weight on the autonomy of the individual in deciding questions of life or death or to those who see the good or goodness in terms of desire or preference satisfaction—that is, those who hold a subjective conception of the good or goodness. In both instances, primacy is given to the desires of the preferences of an agent in reaching a decision about matters of death. However prepared we might be to respect autonomy and preference, the idea that these determine the rightness or goodness of choices seems to be problematic. One need not go so far as Plato, when he rejects autonomy completely, in order to see that the position of Plato and Aristotle on the question regarding the objectivity of any choice about ending life must be taken seriously. Autonomy might be respected for a variety of reasons, for example, as a political right, which need not determine the ethical character of the decision that results from its exercise: A person might autonomously make the wrong choice. One should therefore be cautious in granting absolute primacy to autonomy or preferences, if what is meant by doing so is that no objectivity of any kind obtains in deliberations about what is beneficial or right and what is not. And there is much room for going wrong on these matters, as Plato argues when he raises questions about the ability of those who are in certain extreme circumstances to deliberate correctly. Aristotle also remarks that "doubtless there is some element of value contained even in the mere state of being alive," but he is quick to add "provided there is not too great an excess on the side of hardships of life." But he goes on further to add that "it is clear that most people cling to life at the cost of enduring much suffering, which shows that life contains some measure of well-being and of sweetness in its essential nature" (*Politics* iii 6.1278b25–30).

Aristotle does not suppose that determining whether or not there is some sweetness or value in a life is easy. He clearly recognizes that fixing the threshold at which life loses all value will be difficult. But he also seems to say that such threshold is rather low, since life naturally contains some well-being and sweetness, and it cannot be fixed or specified in any way one likes. Whether or not a certain life has still some element of value seems to be an objective fact, something to be decided by weighing the hardships against the joys, the evil against the good. Clearly, one could go wrong and end a life that, on balance, still contains enough well-being and sweetness worth having. And going wrong in such cases is going wrong irreversibly. As Philippa Foot forcefully argues in defending the objectivity of decisions about terminating life, we can go drastically wrong in cases when, for a variety of reasons, we decide in favor of terminating the life of mentally retarded people who seem capable of experiencing some of the sweetness of life (Foot 1983).

Theses or assumptions (b) and (c) have also been questioned, even before Plato and Aristotle formulated them in the way I have discussed. Protagoras at least is reputed to have objected to Socrates's claim that some are experts on matters of conduct while others are not (Plato *Protagoras* 322). His position that, unlike the other arts, knowledge or expertise of matters of conduct has been given to all alike seems to imply that there is ethical expertise and it is possessed by all. In the recent years, many have questioned whether there is any expertise on these matters, especially of the kind that Plato assumes in terms of possessing a rigorous and fully articulated theory of ethics and politics. And, of course, some have raised doubts as to whether the possession of the kind of theoretical expertise in ethical/political matters favored by Plato will be of any use in answering any of the questions about life and death that are likely to confront us in concrete circumstances. According to them, theory of the kind Plato, and to some extent Aristotle, envisage will not be of much use, and it does not seem to play a role in the way decisions are actually made.[24]

Despite the many objections that may be raised against the views of Plato and Aristotle, there seems to be a point that even those who do not share their views about objectivity in decisions about terminating a life or on the importance of autonomy or on the extend to which the good of the community should influence deliberations about ending individual life will agree—that is, deliberation about matters of life and death lies mostly outside technical medical knowledge and is ethical in character. This conclusion reached by the ancient philosophers was as important for their time as it is for ours. Plato and Aristotle tried to set some limits on the authority of the physician and to identify its proper boundaries. For our time the influence of technical expertise is, of course, much greater. The extraordinary advances in technology and the enormous increase in scientific/technical expertise often threaten to make all deliberation, including whether or not to terminate or initiate life, a matter of technical expertise. If the ancient Greek philosophers are right, deliberations about such matters raise questions that require a kind of expertise that is not merely of the scientific/technical kind.

In addition, the views of the classical philosophers remind us that deliberating about ending life is no ordinary deliberation. It seems to be one of those awesome problems that push against the limits of practical rationality—that is, the very thing that underlies practical reasoning and deliberation in ordinary circumstances. Life, as Aristotle observes, is such a good that it is almost always assumed as an implicit end or good in all deliberation, at least as a conditional end or good of all the other ends whose means we seek to identify in our deliberations and to implement in our actions. It is the background of all of our ends, including the highest one. But when we deliberate about terminating life, the role the good of life normally plays in deliberation cannot be the same. Here we seek to identify another end in order to justify the elimination of the good in relation to which we normally tend to see almost all other goods. Such deliberation is not trivial. And, as Aristotle observes, it is not easy either. Fixing the threshold below which life ceases to be a good is a most difficult task, especially if life contains in its nature the kind of sweetness and well-being that Aristotle attributes to it.[25]

Notes

1. Of course, this is an oversimplification of the complex nature of euthanasia. It seems to pass over the distinction between active and passive euthanasia, the latter being a way of ending a life that may not involve any interference with the natural course of events. Even passive euthanasia may, however, be construed as involving an interference with the normal course of events, since it could be argued that the normal course is to try to prolong life. Some have raised doubts about the validity of the distinction between active and passive euthanasia (see Rachels 1983) while others have defended it (see, e.g., Foot 1983). I shall not take sides on

this issue, although the ancient Greek philosophers speak of terminations of human life that fall under both kinds of euthanasia.

2. Of course, obligations stemming from relations may point in different directions. In Sophocles' *The Women of Trachis*, Heracles claims that his son, Hyllus, has the obligation to start the pyre and put him on it to end his misery. But Hyllus convinces his father that he only has an obligation to start the pyre but not to place him on it. To do the latter, Hyllus argues, would be killing his own father and polluting himself (1157–1215).

3. See *The Sacred Disease* and *The Science of Medicine* in the Hippocratic corpus (W. H. S. Jones trans.).

4. See, for example, the treatises *Diseases*, *Regimen on Acute Diseases*, and *Regimen in Health* in the Hippocratic corpus (W. H. S. Jones trans.).

5. Both Plato and Aristotle divide sciences into theoretical, productive, and practical. The first group (e.g., mathematics or physics) consists of the disciplines that have no end beyond knowledge of their respective subject matters. The second and third groups consist of those disciplines that have an end beyond knowledge of their subject matter, the end for the sake of which the cognitive activity itself is pursued—e.g., health in the case of medicine and action in the case of ethics (see Polansky in this volume).

6. For a statement of this position, see Nussbaum 1986. Aristotle at times speaks in ways that suggest that medical phenomena, and presumably also ethical phenomena, do not fall under a science (*Nicomachean Ethics* ii 2.1104a3–5) or that medicine is concerned with the health of some individual only and not with the general phenomena of health and disease (i 6.1097a10–13). In these instances, however, Aristotle is talking about the physician's concern with some individual case of disease or the care of some particular individual, the treatment of which requires not only knowledge about the general or universal that the science of medicine provides but also an assessment of the particular circumstances of the case.

7. See the Hippocratic treatise on fractures (LCL, Jones, Vol. III); references to surgical incisions and instruments are to be found throughout the Hippocratic writings.

8. See Empedocles, B 128.8, B 137, B 139; Iamblichus, *On the Pythagorean Way of Life* 81–87; and Aulus Gellius, *Attic Nights* iv 11.1–13.

9. Diogenes Laertius, *Lives of the Philosophers* viii 4–5 and Diodorus, *Universal History* x 6.1–3.

10. "These, then, he [Empedocles] says must wander and 'become in time all sorts of mortals, changing the painful paths of life' [B 115], for the souls change from body to body, altered and punished by strife and not allowed to remain a unity" (Hippolytus, *Refutations of All Heresies* v 30); life in this world is like being enclosed in a cave—"we have come to this roofed cave" [B 120], from which liberation comes after the end of a cycle of reincarnations [B 147].

11. "A soul in this state [pure and free of the body] makes its way to the invisible, which is like itself, the immortal and wise, and arriving there it can be happy,

having rid itself of confusion, ignorance, fear, violent desires and the other human ills and, as is said of the initiates, truly spend the rest of time with the gods" (*Phaedo* 81a).

12. According to Iamblichus, *On the Pythagorean Way of Life* (81ff.), the Pythagoreans urged that "you must have children in order to leave behind another servant of the gods in your place."

13. "It is not logical that the wisest of men should not resent leaving this service in which they are governed by the best of masters, the gods, for a wise man cannot believe that he will look after himself better when he is free" (*Phaedo* 62d). In *Laws* (907a) Plato insists that the gods guard the noblest of things and are supremely skillful. According to Iamblichus, the Pythagoreans think that "[it] is absurd for men to look for the good from any source other that the gods; it is as if you were living in a monarchy and paid service to some subordinate among citizens, ignoring the ruler of all.... For since god exists and is sovereign over everything, it is clear that one must ask for the good from the sovereign" (*On the Pythagorean Way of Life* 87).

14. Plato in the *Cratylus* claims that Apollo is the founder of medicine (405; see also *Symposium* 197a) and his name means "the purifier." Some have connected purification in medicine with Pythagoreanism, but the notions of purification, purging, or cleansing are basic to the Hippocratic medical tradition as well.

15. See on this matter Plato, *Republic*, end of book 1 and Aristotle, *Nicomachean Ethics* i 7.

16. B. Williams has argued that, given this essentialist conception of medicine and its goals, certain consequences about rights to medical treatment as well as limits on earning money by practicing medicine follow (see B. Williams 1969). R. Nozick is critical of Williams's position, arguing that the latter's essentialist claims can be avoided by making the goal of earning money a part or the whole of the essence of medicine (see Nozick 1974). Plato and Aristotle do not deny that the physician benefits from the practice of his art, and they do not wish to eliminate such benefits. They only insist that profit is not a necessary part of the goals of medicine, a position that differs from those of Williams and Nozick.

17. Plato argues that the physician who cures a patient may do good to the patient and to himself also (*Charmides* 164b), but the physician's benefits are not essential to the goals of his art. Plato expresses this often by saying that the physician qua physician is not an earner of fees but a healer (*Republic* i 341c). The physician "precisely speaking" aims at the good of the patient (342d–e); the receiving of wages does not result from the practice of the medical but of some other kind of art (346d). Aristotle remarks that "The arts are exercised for the good of the governed, as we see to be the case in medicine, gymnastics, and the arts in general, which are only accidentally concerned with the good of the artists themselves" (*Politics* iii 6.1278b39–1279a2; see also i 9.1258a10–12 where Aristotle argues that the goal of medicine is health and not wealth).

18. See Plato's *Statesman* (298) and Aristotle's *Politics* (iii 16.1287a38–40) for a discussion of the failure of physicians to aim at what medicine requires when they receive bribes, especially from the patient's enemy.

19. Plato in the *Republic* argues that the art of medicine does not exist for its own advantage or benefit (i 342a–c). This is an important constraint on the aim of medicine because in some cases decisions on medical treatment have been influenced by the interest in improving medical knowledge or, to use Plato's and Aristotle's language, to perfect the art of medicine. For a study of using patients for medical experimentation, see Jones 1993.

20. Plato argues in the *Republic* (vi 489c) that the natural course of events is for the sick person to go to the physician and request treatment. In the *Laws*, he distinguishes a treatment that gives explanations to and persuades the patient from treatments that do not (iv 720a–d); he extends the requirement of persuasion to the area of political ruling and legislating (iv 723a, ix 857c–e). Aristotle also distinguishes treatments that proceed on the basis of persuasion from those that do not (*Politics* iii 11.1282a1–7); at one point he asserts that the physician is not expected to coerce but in the same breath seems to be saying that the physician is not expected to persuade either (vii 2.1324b29–31).

21. In his discussion of courage in *Nicomachean Ethics*, Aristotle argues that to terminate one's own life in order to escape from pain, sorrow, and some other types of suffering is an act of cowardice (iii 7.1116a12–14). In his discussion of justice, he argues that in some cases taking one's own life is a form of injustice and therefore forbidden by law (v 11.1138a5–11).

22. For Aristotle's views on the opinions of the many and of those who are considered experts on matters of conduct, see *Eudemian Ethics* i 3.1214b28–31 and *Nicomachean Ethics* i 4.1095a28–30, b19–23.

23. On the authoritative nature of the political art or science and the priority of the good it aims at, see *Nicomachean Ethics* i 2. For a general discussion of Aristotle and communitarianism, see Miller 1995; and for an application of communitarian ethics that echo some Aristotelian themes in medical ethics, see Kuczewski 1998.

24. For a recent discussion of some of these issues, see Hannay 1998.

25. A version of this paper was read at the meeting of the Society for Bioethics and Classical Philosophy at the Central Division Meetings of the American Philosophical Association, May 1998. I am grateful to Ron Polansky and Mark Kuczewski for inviting me to take part in this meeting. Most of all, I wish to thank them for their patience and perseverence that made it possible for me to prepare the final version.

References

Batin, M., R. Rhodes, and A. Silvers, eds. 1998. *Physician-Assisted Suicide: Expanding the Debate*. New York: Routledge.

Beauchamp, T., and S. Perlin, eds. 1978. *Ethical Issues in Death and Dying*. Englewood Cliffs, N.J.: Prentice Hall.

Beauchamp, T., and J. Childress. 1994. *The Principles of Biomedical Ethics*. New York: Oxford University Press.

Cross, R. C. and A. D. Woozley. 1964. *Plato's "Republic": A Philosophical Commentary*. New York: St. Martins Press.

Dworkin, R., T. Nagel, R. Nozik, J. Rawls, T. Scanlon, J. J. Thomson. 1998. The Philosophers' Brief, 431–441 in *Physician-Assisted Suicide: Expanding the Debate*, ed. R. Batin, R. Rhodes, and A. Silvers. New York: Routledge.

Edelstein, L. 1989. The Hippocratic Oath: Text, Translation, and Interpretation, 6–24 in *Cross Cultural Perspectives in Medical Ethics*, ed. R. Veatch. Boston: Jones and Bartlett.

Foot, P. 1983. "Euthanasia," 7–28 in *Moral Issues*, ed. J. Narveson. New York: Oxford University Press.

Hannay, A. 1998. "What can philosophers contribute to social ethics?" *Topoi* 17: 127–136.

Johnston, D. 1994. *The Idea of a Liberal Theory*. Princeton, N.J.: Princeton University Press.

Jones, J. H. 1993. *Bad Blood: The Tuskegee Syphilis Experiment*. New York: The Free Press.

Jones, W. H. S., trans. 1923. *Hippocrates*, vols. 1–4, LCL. Cambridge, Mass.: Harvard University Press.

Kamisar, Y. 1978. "Euthanasia Legislation: Some Nonreligious Objections." 220–231, in *Ethical Issues in Death and Dying*, eds. T. Beauchamp and S. Perlin. Englewood Cliffs, NJ: Prentice Hall.

Kuczewski, M. G. 1998. "Physician-assisted death: Can philosophical bioethics aid social policy?" *Cambridge Quarterly of Healthcare Ethics* 7(4): 339–347.

Kuhse, H. 1998. "From Intention to Consent," 252–266 in Batin, Rhodes, and Silvers 1998.

Miller, F., Jr. 1995. *Nature, Justice and Rights in Aristotle's* Politics. Oxford: Clarendon Press.

Narveson, J., ed. 1983. *Moral Issues*. New York: Oxford University Press.

Nozick, R. 1974. *Anarchy, State, and Utopia*. New York: Basic Books.

Nussbaum, M. C. 1986. *The Fragility of Goodness*. Cambridge: Cambridge University Press.

Rachels, J. 1983. "Active and Passive Euthanasia," 1–6 in *Moral Issues*, ed. J. Narveson. New York: Oxford University Press.

Rawls, J. 1993. *Political Liberalism*. New York: Columbia University Press.

Williams, B. 1969. "The Idea of Equality," 153–171 in J. Feinberg ed. *Moral Concepts*. New York: Oxford University Press.

Williams, G. 1958. *The Sanctity of Life and the Criminal Law*. London: Faber and Faber.

Williams, G. 1978. "Euthanasia Legislation: A Rejoinder to the Nonreligious Objection," 232–239 in *the Principles of Biomedical Ethics*, eds. T. Beauchamp and S. Perlin. New York: Oxford University Press.

Contributors

Georgios Anagnostopoulos is Professor of Philosophy at the University of California at San Diego, where he was department chair from 1982 to 1986 and 1998 to 2000. He is currently Acting Dean of Arts and Humanities. His major research interests are in ancient Greek philosophy and ethics. He is the author of *Aristotle on the Goals and Exactness of Ethics* (University of California Press, 1994) and of a number of articles in ancient philosophy.

Julia E. Annas studied Classics at Oxford University and has a doctorate from Harvard. She was a Fellow of St. Hugh's College Oxford from 1972 to 1986, and since then has taught at the University of Arizona, apart from a year at Columbia University. She was the founding editor of *Oxford Studies in Ancient Philosophy* for ten years, a Fellow of the American Academy of Arts and Sciences, and for five years was a Senior Fellow of the Center for Hellenic Studies. She has written five books and co-written three, and has published about sixty articles on numerous aspects of ancient philosophy.

Robert Bartz is a family physician in the Department of Family and Community Medicine and a doctoral candidate in the history of medicine at the University of California, San Francisco. His research interests include the history of patient-doctor relationships and the history of medical ethics.

Tod Chambers is Assistant Professor of Medical Ethics and Humanities and of Medicine at Northwestern University Medical School. His recently published book, *The Fiction of Bioethics* (Routledge 1999), examines how the case, which is the primary data of medical ethics, is constructed to support particular philosophical perspectives. His current research focuses on the general rhetoric of the field of medical ethics.

Christopher E. Cosans has a doctorate in the Conceptual Foundations of Science from the University of Chicago. He teaches in the Department of Philosophy at the George Washington University. He does research on the history and philosophy of science and bioethics. His publications include "Aristotle's Anatomical Philosophy of Nature" (*Biology & Philosophy*, 1998) and "Experimental Foundations of Galen's Teleology" (*Studies in History and Philosophy of Science*, 1998).

Mark G. Kuczewski is the Director of the Institute for Bioethics and Health Policy at the Stritch School of Medicine, Loyola University Chicago. He has published extensively on the relationship of ethical theory and clinical practice. This work includes the books *Fragmentation and Consensus: Communitarian and Casuist Bioethics* (Georgetown University Press, 1997) and (with Rosa Lynn Pinkus) *An Ethics Casebook for Hospitals: Practical Approaches to Everyday Cases* (Georgetown University Press, 1999). He is also the co-founder of the Society for Bioethics and Classical Philosophy.

Alex John London is Assistant Professor of Philosophy at Carnegie Mellon University. His research interests include the ethics and moral psychology of Plato and Aristotle, ethical issues in cross-cultural medical research, and the use of enhancement technologies. He is currently working on a book manuscript tentatively titled "Aristotelian Practical Ethics" and editing a special issue of the journal *Theoretical Medicine and Bioethics* dealing with the role of theory in practical ethics.

Chris Megone studied classics at Oxford, where he also did his doctorate in philosophy on practical reason. He is now Senior Lecturer in the School of Philosophy at the University of Leeds. Recent publications include "Aristotle's Function Argument and the Concept of Mental Illness" (*Philosophy, Psychiatry, and Psychology*, 1998) and "Aristotelian Ethics" in the *Encyclopaedia of Applied Ethics* (Academic Press, San Diego, 1997).

Kathryn Montgomery is Professor of Medical Ethics and Humanities and of Medicine at Northwestern University Medical School and Director of its Medical Ethics and Humanities Program. Her book, *Doctors' Stories: The Narrative Structure of Medical Knowledge* (Princeton University Press, 1991), describes the narrative epistemology of clinical medicine. Fascinated by the curious process that turns students of science into physicians, she is currently writing about the inculcation of clinical judgment.

Ronald Polansky is professor of philosophy at Duquesne University and editor of the journal *Ancient Philosophy*. He is the co-founder of the Society for Bioethics and Classical Philosophy. He has published numerous articles on ancient philosophy and dabbled in modern political thought. His book, *Philosophy and Knowledge: A Commentary on Plato's Theaetetus* (Bucknell University Press), appeared in 1992 and he is working on a commentary on Aristotle's *De Anima*.

David C. Thomasma is the Fr. Michael I. English Professor of Medical Ethics and Director of the Medical Humanities Program at Loyola University Chicago Medical Center. He is the author or co-author of twenty-two books and more than three hundred articles. He is the editor-in-chief of *Theoretical Medicine and Bioethics*, founding co-editor of *Cambridge Quarterly of Healthcare Ethics*, and co-editor of the International Library of Ethics, Law, and the New Medicine book series from Kluwer Academic Publishers.

Daryl McGowan Tress is Associate Professor of Philosophy at Fordham University. Her recent publications include "Aristotle Against the Hippocratics on Sexual Generation: A Reply to Coles" (*Phronesis*, 1999), "The Metaphysical Science of Aristotle's *Generation of Animals* and its Feminist Critics" (*Aristotle: Critical Assessments*, Routledge, 1999), and "Aristotle's Child: Formation through *Genesis, Oikos* and *Polis*" (*Ancient Philosophy*, 1997).

Index

A prioris
  existential, 69, 85, 86
  experiential, 84, 86
Abortion, ix, xii, 123, 155–175, 179,
  186, 190
Abscess, 6, 8
Absolutism, 82
Abstraction in mathematics, 50n6
Academic prose, 109
Account, 49n4
Achilles, 20n13
Action (*praxis*), xi, 38, 39, 46, 51n13,
  51n14, 51n15, 51n16, 73, 194, 197,
  217, 222, 237, 252
Activity (*energeia*), 51n13
Actuality and potentiality, 157
Aeschylus, 20n8
Aetius, 125n8
Affirmative action, 190n2
AIDS, 25n38
Albania, 84
Alcmaeon, 43, 113, 125n8, 261
Aleshire, S., 19n5
Altruism, 72
American Medical Association (AMA),
  67
American Medical Consumers, 151n2
Anagnostopoulos, G., xiii
Angiostatin, 58, 60
Animals, 156, 174
Annas, J., xii, 53n26, 120, 126n18,
  137, 151n7, 151n8, 236
Antibiotic, 111, 115, 116, 125n12, 243

Antifoundationalism, 68, 69, 73, 79,
  85, 86
Antigone, 217
Apollo, 4, 20n8, 20n13, 265
Appetite, 78
Apprentices, 4, 17
Aquinas, St. Thomas, 76, 77, 78, 87,
  190
Architecture, 52n21
Aristo of Chios, 247n3
Aristotle, ix, 18, 31–42, 62, 64, 67,
  73, 77, 79, 81, 83, 86, 97, 134, 145,
  151n4, 151n6, 153n16, 153n17,
  155–175, 179, 188, 190, 196, 205,
  207, 208, 214, 217, 221, 223,
  224n15, 226n30, 251, 252, 254,
  258, 266–286
  De Anima, 170
  Eudemian Ethics, 267, 268, 269,
  274–275, 278, 289n22
  Generatione et Corruptione, 271
  Metaphysics, 32, 33, 34, 35, 37, 38,
  49n4, 59, 64, 158, 160, 161, 164,
  258, 269, 270, 271, 278
  Nicomachean Ethics, 37, 39, 40, 41,
  42, 47, 49n3, 50n12, 51n16, 53n25,
  53n27, 54n31, 60, 151n5, 151n6,
  153n16, 205, 206, 216, 220, 258,
  267, 270, 273, 278, 287n6, 288n15,
  289n21, 289n22, 289n23
  *On Youth, Old Age, Life and Death,
  and Respiration*, 41
  Organon, 49n5

Aristotle (cont.)
  Parts of Animals, 35, 36
  Physics, 35, 49n4, 157, 158, 159,
    258, 268
  Poetics, 215, 216, 219
  Politics, 50n9, 51n16, 52n16,
    152n17, 225n26, 254, 268, 271,
    275, 278, 283, 284, 288n17,
    288n18, 289n20
  Posterior Analytics, 33, 49n3, 49n4,
    50n8, 50n10, 258
  Rhetoric, 258, 278
  Sense and Sensibilia, 41
  Topics, 38, 50n10, 52n18, 270
Arithmetic, 34
Arius Didymus, 126n18
Arrian, Flavius, 230, 237
Arrows, 4
Art (*techne*), craft, xi, xii, 9, 11–12,
    13, 14, 16, 20n7, 24n37, 31, 35–38,
    40, 41, 42, 44, 46, 48, 53n23, 59,
    61, 62, 64, 132, 133, 134, 136, 138,
    139, 141, 142, 144, 151n4, 151n10,
    152n11
  hierarchy of arts, 37
  morally neutral, 37
  using and making, 35, 41
Asclepius, Asclepiads, 214, 265, 276,
    282
Asia Minor, 15
Aulisio, M., 88
Authority, 277–281, 282, 286
Autonomy, 95, 96, 195, 196, 199,
    200, 210, 218, 223, 252, 253–257,
    263, 264, 279, 284
Axiomatic presentation of science, 33,
    34

"Baby Doe" rules, 199
Barnes, J., 125n8
Bartz, R., xi, 19n1, 21n16, 54n33,
    55n34, 260
Battle, 4
Beauchamp, T., 19n1, 94, 95, 199,
    254
Beiser, F. C., 88
Belmont Report, 68

Beneficence, 199, 264
Bentham, J., 166
Beresford, E., 68, 202, 207, 224n9,
    224n10
Berlin, I., 80
Bernardin, J. Cardinal, 67
Best-interests-of-the-child guideline,
    195, 197–202
Bioethics, 95, 105
  consultation standards, 71
  postmodern, 67
Biology, x
Biomedical ethics, ix
  bioethics, xi
Bleeding, blood, 115, 261, 262
Bloom, A., 152n11
Blundell, M., 23n29, 241
Bonhöffer, A., 236, 246n1, 247n9,
    247n10
Bosk, C., 65n8, 79, 103
Bosnia, 84
Brightman, E. S., 94
Brody, H., 193, 208, 209–211, 223n1,
    223n2, 224n5, 224n6, 224n14,
    225n27, 225n28
Bruner, J., 64n3
Buddhists, 104, 105
Bulger, R., 19n1
Burke, K., 101
Burkert, W., 19n5, 20n7, 20n9,
    20n11, 24n33
Burnett, D. G., 64n1
Bursztajn, H., 63
Bye, C. R., 20n6

Calchas, 4, 20n13
Callahan, D., 153n16, 180
Cancer, 61
Capitation, 142, 144
Care perspective (on ethics), 104
Carnevale, F. A., 85, 86, 223n1
Carrick, P., 225n20
Cartesianism, 58, 72, 73, 79
Case-by-case, xii
Cassell, E., 61
Casuistry, 68, 94, 104, 185, 203,
    224n10

Catholic, Orthodox, 97
Cato, 230
Causes, x, 31, 49n4
Cavities of the body, 10
Certitude, xi
Chad, 84
Chambers, T., xi, 209
Chance, 36
Change, 157–159, 162
Changeable things, 33, 42
Character, 16, 39, 40, 46, 47, 51n14,
  53n27, 112, 193, 197, 220–222,
  243, 269–270
Charmides, 44
Charvet, J., 76
Chemistry, x
Children, xii, 155, 157, 193–223, 234
Childress, J., 19n1, 94, 95, 199, 254
China, 71, 101
Chisholm, R., 79
Choice (*proairesis*), 37, 38, 39, 46,
  51n15, 194, 200, 203, 220, 221,
  238–241, 242–243, 246, 247n9,
  253, 255, 256, 264, 284
Christianity, 93
Chrysippus, 109
City (*polis*), 15, 23n29
Cleitophon, 135, 136
Clinic, x
Clinical medical practice, xiii, 18
Clinton, H., 179
Clinton, President, 179
Codes, 3, 266
Cognition, 51n13
Coma victim, 173
Common good, 96
Common understanding, shared, 181
Commonweal, 70
Communitarian, 96, 180, 181, 185,
  186, 187, 190n1
 cultures, 71
 view of the person, 186
Communitarianism, ix, xii, 98, 104,
  105, 179, 180, 188, 189, 289n23
Community Health Plan (CHP), 96,
  182, 183

Community, 77, 83, 84, 85, 95, 97,
  145, 146, 182, 189
Competition, competing views. *See*
  Marketplace
Computer science, 65
Confidentiality, 17
Connor, S., 69
Conquest, 51n16
Consensus, xi, 68, 190, 202, 205
Consent, 279
Consequentialism, 193, 195, 199–202,
  206, 218–219
Constitution (*politeia*), 51n14
Contagion, 53n28
Contemplation, 221
Contextualism, 104
Contraries, 37, 39, 48
Coolidge, F. P., 53n26
Cooper, J., 158, 159, 209, 225n23
Cornford, F. M., 85
Correspondence theory, 83
Cosans, C., xii, 45
Cosmos, 232, 245, 246
Counseling, 45
Courage, 76, 243, 251
Craft. *See* Art
Critchley, S., 70
Cross, R. C., 269
Crosscultural standards, 71, 86
Crossexamination, 49n4
Crowley, S., 94
Cultures, 217

Daniels, N., 153n16
Davis, F. D., 79, 223n1
De Lacy, P., 124n1
Dean-Jones, L., 19n5
Death and dying, xiii, 156, 167, 173,
  230, 245, 246
Deliberation, 39, 46, 220, 221, 222,
  223, 252, 256, 270, 280–281, 283,
  284, 285–286
 communal, 186–188
Democracy, 100, 137
Democritus, 116
Demonstration, 33, 34

Denmark, 84
Deontology, 193, 195, 199–202, 206, 218–219
Descartes, R., 50n7
Desire, 39, 40, 219
deWachter, M. A., 71
Diagnosis, 46, 257, 258, 280
Diet, 6, 44, 115, 119, 125n11
Dignity, 17
Diodorus, 287n9
Diogenes Laertius, 230, 231, 247n3, 287n9
Disagreement, fundamental, 183
Disease, 3, 114, 229, 258, 273
Disposition, 78
Dissection, 53n23
Division of the sciences, 31–42
Dobbin, R., 238, 239
Doctor-patient relationship (physician-patient relationship), 131
Dodds, E. R., 20n11
Doing. *See* Action
Dostoyevsky, F., 210
Downie, R. S., 224n7
Dreyfus, H. L., 59
Dreyfus, S. E., 59
Duty, role-specific, 83
Dworkin, R., 253

Economy, 23n26
Edelstein, E., 19n5
Edelstein, L., 19n5, 21n14, 22n23, 23n28, 24n37, 125n3, 261
Egoism, 76
Eleatic visitor, 113, 115
Emanuel, E., 97, 148, 181, 182, 183, 186, 188
Emotions, passions, 112, 115, 169, 207, 219, 237, 241
Empedocles, 6, 125n9, 261, 262, 263, 287n8, 287n10
Empiricist school of medicine, 52n22, 111, 124
Encyclopedia of Religion, 94
Endoxa, 34, 50n10
Engel, G., 65n5

Engelhardt, H. T., 77, 87n2, 95, 96, 97, 98, 229
Englert, W., 230, 239, 246n1
Enlightenment, 70, 72, 81, 82, 181, 185, 188
Enos, R. L., 106
Entitlement programs, 190n2
Environment, 3
Epictetus, xii, 229–246
Epicureans, 52n18, 110, 121
Epidemic, 24n33
Equal opportunity, 190n2
Essence, essentialist, 158–162, 195, 267, 270–272, 274, 276–277, 280–281, 283, 288n16
Ethical particularism, 194, 196, 197
Ethical theory, x, 69
Ethics
    applied, 67
    citizen based, 15
    clinical, 67, 79, 83, 85
Ethos, 3, 15
Euclid, 33
Eudaemonism, 193
Euthanasia, xii, 155, 174, 251–286
    active and passive, 274, 280, 286n1
Everson, S., 49n4
Exercise, 44, 115, 117, 119
Experience vs. science, 258
Experiment and the relation of medicine research and practice, 42
Expertise, ability, 277–281, 282, 283–286
Exposure of children, 223, 283
Externals, 239–240, 242, 244, 246

Facts, 188
False belief, 112, 115, 121
Fee, 4
Fee-for-service, 142, 144
Fetus, xii, 155–157, 163–164
Fevers, 21n18
Finley, M. I., 20n6, 23n26
Finnis, J., 164
Fischer, M. M. J., 99
Fish, S., 102, 103

Fletcher, J., 88n3
Flux, 6
Folk healers, 4, 13
Foot, P., 252, 285, 287n1
Ford, N. M., 175n4
Foregoing medical treatment, 244
Form, 35, 37, 51n13, 51n15, 158, 161, 196, 217, 221, 282
Forschner, M., 239
Fortune, 230
Foss, S., 94
Foundationalism, ix, 73, 79
Foundations of Bioethics, 95, 97
Fox, R., 65n8, 103, 104
Frede, M., 49n4, 52n20, 52n22, 53n26
Free will, free choice, 51n15, 239
Friendship, 18, 23n29, 75, 271
Function (*ergon*), 136, 139, 152n13, 267, 270

Gadamer, H.-G., 45, 49n2, 54n30, 65n9
Galen, 53n24, 109, 124n1, 124n3, 247n9
Galison, P., 64n1
Garland, R., 19n5
Geertz, C., 102
Gellius, A., 262, 287n8
Gender selection, 180
Genome, 61
Geometry, 33, 34
Germany, 84
Germs, 114
Gill, M. L., 161, 164, 170, 176n6
Glaucon, 152n12
Glendon, M. A., 104
God, goddess, 4–5, 7, 20n13, 25n37, 44, 195, 212, 216, 221, 234, 235, 239, 241, 243, 244, 245, 263–265
Godel's theorem, 80
Good life, 181, 185, 189
Good, public and private, 39
Good, the, 72, 76, 77, 80, 82, 96, 103
  shared concept of, 181
Gorgias (the sophist), 101

Government commissions, x
Graber, G., 78
Grahame, K., 67
Great Britain, 152n14
Griffith, R. D., 212, 225n16
Grmek, M., 21n18
Guthrie, W. K. C., 99
Gymnastics, 113
Gynecology, 44, 53n23

Habermas, J., 79
Habits, 45, 46, 116, 120, 122
Habituation, 40
Hankinson, R., 113–114
Hannay, A., 289n24
Hanson, A. E., 19n5
Hanson, V. D., 225n21
Happiness (*eudaimonia*), 34, 40, 193, 205, 206, 208, 217, 219–220, 222, 230, 237, 238
Hare, R. M., 84, 175n1
Harris, J., 84, 155, 156, 176n5
Havelock, E., 98
Headache, 44, 111
Health, 6, 41, 42, 43, 113, 114, 124
  overall-balance model, 116–118
Health maintenance organization (HMO), 142, 143
Heart-related ailments, 44, 115–116
Heath, J., 225n21
Heavens, 6
Hellen, 112
Hellenistic period, 110
Help friends, harm enemies, 23n29
Help or do no harm, 16, 18
Help ourselves, 123–124
Hepatoscopy, 4, 20n9
Hermeneutic, 62
Herodicus, 275
Hierarchy of goods, shared, 181
Hippasus, 261
Hippocrates, 3, 19n3
Hippocratic corpus, 4, 15, 19n4, 52n20, 53n26, 110, 125n4, 125n11, 132, 151n3
Affections, 16

Hippocratic corpus (cont.)
Airs Waters Places, 23n30
Ancient Medicine, 52n20
Art, 8, 9, 10, 11
Decorum, 52n19
Diseases, 15, 16, 23n31
Epidemics, 7, 8, 14, 16, 18, 21n18,
    23n30, 24n34
Law, 52n19
Nature of Man, 53n24, 125n9
On Fractures, 287n7
Prognostic, 4, 5, 7, 21n19, 21n20
Regimen, 24n36, 126n13
Regimen in Acute Diseases, 21n15,
    21n20, 287n3
Sacred Disease, 21n15, 225n20
Hippocratic Oath, 3, 17, 24n37,
    225n25, 252, 257–266, 271–272
Hippolytus, 287n10
Hirshorn, M. W., 142
Historicism, xi, 33
Holder, A., 223n3
Holistic method, 112
Holladay, A. J., 225n17
Holocaust, 76
Homer, 4, 20n6, 20n7, 20n10, 20n13,
    231
Homocide, 251
Horgan, T., 70
Hospital, x, 201, 209, 218, 260
House building, 35
Household, 17, 23n29, 38
Hoy, D. C., 69
Hubris, 62
Human being vs. person, 155–156,
    165–168
Humanities, 49n2
Humility, 76, 187, 189
Humor, 6, 8, 53n24, 113, 125n9,
    125n12
Humphreys, S. C., 23n29
Huntington, S. P., 71
Hursthouse, R., 167–173
Husserl, E., 88n4
Hussey, E., 20n7

Iamblichus, 262, 287n8, 287n12,
    287n13
Idealism, 32
Idealization of medical practice, 111,
    119
Identity conditions, 163, 172
Impressions (*phantasiai*), 237
Impulses, 231
Incubation, 214
Independence, freedom, 230, 238
Indifferents, preferred and not pre-
    ferred, 230, 231, 234, 239, 243,
    244
Individual, the, 181, 182
Individualism, 96
Infection, 53n28, 111, 114, 116,
    213
Injury, 45, 229
Intellect, 78
Intellectual treatment of the medical
    art, 41
Interests of humans, 167, 173–174,
    176n9, 181, 199, 200, 201, 209,
    219
Interpretation, xii, 201, 240
Irwin, T., 23n26, 152n11, 175n3
Islam, 71
Isonomia, 43, 113

James, C., 82
James, W., 64n3
Jarrett, S. C., 94, 98, 101, 102
Jaundice, 114
Johnston, D., 255
Joly, R., 19n3
Jones, C. A., 64n1
Jones, J. H., 28919
Jones, W. H. S., 19n4, 151n3
Jonsen, A., 68, 69, 193, 224n10
Jouanna, J., 19n3
Judaism, Orthodox, 183
Judgment, clinical, xii, 60, 64, 67,
    259, 278
Justice, 43, 48, 104, 135, 138, 144,
    199, 208, 241, 251, 269, 270, 282

Kairos, 100, 102, 105
Kamisar, Y., 254
Kant, I., 52n18, 72, 80, 97, 167, 181, 253
Kekes, J., 76
Keonig, B., 104
Kerferd, G. B., 23n26
King, H., 19n5, 21n16
Kingsley, P., 21n17, 225n19
Kirk, G. S., 21n17
Kleinman, A., 104
Knowing, 31
Knowledge (*episteme*), 15
  antifoundationalist, x
  applied, x
  capable of contraries, 37, 268–269
  ethical, x, xi
  of the good, 282
  medical, x, xi
Konstan, D., 23n29
Koop, C. E., 199–200
Kopelman, L. M., 197, 198, 200, 223n3, 223n4, 224n5, 224n7
Kornblith, H., 81
Kraut, R., 224n13
Kuczewski, M., xii, 94, 187, 188, 289n23
Kudlien, F., 20n8
Kuhse, H., 254

Larson, E., 151n2
Law, 126n14, 217
Layperson, 16
Levinsky, N., 146
Liberal tradition, 96
Liberalism, 98, 253
Lloyd, G. E. R., 19n3, 19n5, 20n12, 21n22, 22n25, 225n18, 225n20
Lo, B., 25n38
Location, 6
Loewy, E., 77
Logic, 52n18, 120
Logical positivism, 73
London, A., xii, 65n10, 151n10, 152n11

Long, A. A., 52n18, 232, 237, 238, 239, 240, 247n2, 247n6
Longrigg, J., 125n3, 125n9, 125n11, 225n20

Machaon, 4
MacIntyre, A., 67, 69, 74, 97, 104, 105, 179, 182, 185, 190n1, 190n2, 193, 203–205, 208, 210, 218
Maclean, A., 74, 84, 85
Madness, 247n9
Magic, magicians, 4, 225n20
Making (*poiesis*), 38
Malaria, 21n18
Mallon, T., 70
Managed care, xii, 25n38, 131
Managed-care organizations (MCO), 131, 142, 143, 149, 150, 152n15
Mansfeld, J., 19n3
Marcus Aurelius, 238
Marcus, G. E., 99
Marketplace (competitive environment), 15, 17, 18, 23n28, 111, 121–123
Marshall, P., 104
Marta, J., 209
Mathematics, 32, 33, 34, 36, 195
Matter, 34, 35, 36, 42, 158, 164
McCarthy, T., 69
McGee, G., 79
Mean, 40, 196, 217
Medical education, 43, 209
Medical schools in antiquity, rationalist, empiricist, methodist, 111, 122
Medical theory in relation to medical practice, 52n22
Medicare, 148
Megone, C., xii, 157, 158
Menelaus, 112, 262
Mental retardation, 285
Metaphysics, 120, 205
Metempsychosis, 262
Methodist school of medicine, 111, 122
Michaels, W. B., 71
Microbes, 115, 125n12

Midwives, 4
Miller, F., 289n23
Millican, P., 175n1
Mistake, 268
Monarchia, 43, 113
Montgomery, K., xi, 58, 61, 65, 87n1
Moore, G. E., 73
Moral significance, 166–167, 170, 171, 173–175, 219, 233
Moral virtue. *See* Virtue
Morreim, H., 147, 153n18
Mortality, 229, 242
Motion (*kinesis*), 51n13
Motives for action, 51n15
Mourelatos, A., 158
Multiculturalism, 70, 71, 77

Narrative, narrative methods, xi, 9, 16, 59, 62, 85, 187, 194, 196, 197, 202, 203, 206–211, 216, 218–219, 221
National Commission for the Protection of Human Subjects of Biomedical and Behavioral Research, 68
Natural law, 70, 185, 209
Natural substances, 157–162, 164, 166, 172
Naturalistic thought, 195, 207, 214, 272
Naturalists, 70
Nature, 35–36, 45–46, 82, 158–162, 165
Navigation, 54n32, 117, 278
Nazis, 77
Nelson, H. L., 206, 224n14
Nestor, 4
Netherlands, 101
Nicholson, P., 151n8
Nielson, K., 70
Nominalism, 32
Nomos, 100, 101, 102, 103, 104, 105, 106
Noncognitivism, 75
Nonmaleficence, 199
Nonmedical considerations, 23n28

Norris, C., 71
Nozick, R., 288n16
Nursing homes, x
Nussbaum, M. C., 22n23, 50n10, 110, 193, 203–205, 207–208, 218, 224n12, 245, 287n6
Nutton, V., 25n39

Objective morality, 70
Objective truth, 83
Objectivity, 63, 284–285
Oedipus, 211–216, 222
Oldfather, W., 238, 247n4
Orentlicher, D., 143, 152n14
Owen, G. E. L., 50n10

Page, C., 224n11
Pain, 12, 13, 46, 155, 230, 239, 242, 254, 273–274, 289n21
Pantel, P. S., 20n11, 225n19
Parker, R., 19n5, 20n10
Parry, A., 213
Particulars, particularism, xi, 196, 202, 203–204, 208, 211, 216, 218–219, 221, 287n6
Pascal, 94
Patients, x, 195
Pediatric medical ethics, 193, 195
Pediatric medicine, 44
Pellegrino, E., 19n1, 67, 79, 83, 87n1, 225n22
Perfectionism, 198
Persuasion vs. compulsion, 117–119, 289n20
Pharmacology, 52n20
Phase I trial, 58
Phillips, E. D., 53n24, 54n34, 125n6, 125n12
Philo of Larissa, 118–122, 126n16, 126n18
Philolaus, 261
Philosophers, x
  as doctor of the soul, 109–110, 124
Philosophy and medicine, 18, 22n23, 54n34, 109–124
Physician-assisted suicide, 93, 103

Physician-healer, 3
Physics, x, 41, 52n18
Plague, 4, 20n13, 212, 215
Planned Parenthood of Southeastern Pennsylvania v. Casey, 180
Plants, 167, 170–171, 174
Plato, xii, 11, 18, 31, 33, 34, 41, 50n11, 51n15, 53n24, 94, 98, 100, 101, 102, 131, 132, 133, 145, 151n1, 151n4, 153n16, 187, 196, 204, 205, 207, 217, 219, 221, 224n15, 251, 252, 257, 258, 259, 261, 266–286
  Apology, 235
  Charmides, 43–44, 50n11, 53n26, 111–112, 258, 267, 268, 281, 288n17
  Cratylus, 288n14
  Crito, 187, 278
  Euthydemus, 151n5, 267
  Euthyphro, 267
  Gorgias, 12, 37, 94, 151, 258, 267, 274, 278
  Laches, 12, 37, 49n4, 259, 275, 281
  Laws, 117, 120, 126n15, 126n19, 258, 264, 267, 274, 278, 282, 288n13, 289n20
  Lesser Hippias, 37, 269
  Lysis, 13, 267, 278
  Meno, 151n5
  Phaedo, 34, 49n4, 263, 264, 288n11, 288n13
  Phaedrus, 52n20, 125n6, 258
  Protagoras, 13, 274, 285
  Republic, 34, 36, 37, 38, 43, 45, 50n12, 54n32, 54n35, 113, 117, 126n14, 126n19, 131, 132, 141, 151n5, 152n12, 219, 258, 267, 268, 269–270, 275–276, 277, 278, 282–283, 288n15, 288n17, 289n19, 289n20
  Rival Lovers, 36
  Sophist, 113, 115
  Statesman, 50n12, 117, 126n14, 126n19, 269, 278, 279–280, 282, 288n18

Symposium, 288n14
Theaetetus, 50n9
Timaeus, 52n20, 54n29, 225n26, 258, 267
Pleasure, 39, 41
Pleonexia, 140
Pluralism, xii, 49n1, 70, 71, 74, 100, 195, 204, 210, 214
Plutarch, 213, 230
Pneumonia, 114
Podalirius, 4
Pogroms, 77
Polansky, R., xi, 51n13, 52n17, 65n10, 87n1, 287n5
Political philosophy, 75
Pollution, 114
Pomeroy, S., 23n29
Poole, J. C. F., 225n17
Porphyry, 262
Porter, R., 49n1
Postmodernism, 68, 69, 70, 71, 72, 76, 77, 79, 81, 84
Potentiality, power, 133, 136, 155–175
  active and passive, 160
  essential, material, and state potentialities, 157, 163–165, 168, 170–175
Potter, P., 19n4, 24n32
Poulakos, J., 94, 98, 101
Practical syllogism, 76
Practical wisdom (*phronesis*, practical reason, prudence), ix, xi, 31, 39, 40, 45, 46, 47, 51n16, 61, 62, 64, 65, 67, 68, 69, 75, 76, 77, 78, 79, 80, 81, 82, 84, 86, 87, 202, 203–205, 221, 223
Practice, 57, 64, 131, 143, 145, 150. *See also* Art
Practices vs. theory, 206
Pragmatism, 74
Pragmatists, 70
Precision, xi, 34, 40, 52n17, 54n31, 126n14
Prediction, 8, 21n14, 259
Presocratics, 34, 43, 52n20, 113
Preterm neonate, 173

Preventable death, 24n35
Priests, 13, 211–212
Principle of permission, 96
Principles, transcendent and universal, 51n16
Principlism, 104
Pritzl, K., 50n10
Probabilism, 185
Prognosis, 6, 8, 16, 21n14, 198, 280
Prognostics, 5, 7, 15, 16, 21n18, n22
Prophets, prophesy, 13, 215, 225n19
Protagoras, 94, 98, 100, 285
Psychiatry, 44
Psychology, 75
Public policy recommendations, x
Purgation, purgatives, 8, 219, 287n14
Purification, 115
Pythagoreans, 24n37, 261–266, 271

Quality-of-life considerations, 196
Quine, W. V. O., 73

Rabies, 247n9
Rachels, J., 84, 253, 286n1
Racism, 166
Rand, A., 76
Randall, F., 224n7
Rational medicine, 214, 225n20
Rationalism, 52n22
Rationalist school of medicine, 111, 122
Rationality, 155, 166, 168, 171, 173, 222, 286
Raven, J. E., 21n17
Rawls, J., 253
Realism, 175n3, 217–218
Reeve, C. D. C., 151n1, 151n8, 151n9, 151n10, 224n13
Regimen, 9, 16–17, 24n36, 53n26, 115, 116, 117, 125n11, 259
Reich, W., 104
Relationships, 44
Relativism, 99, 102, 219
Religion, 4, 24n37, 49n1, 225n20
Reputation, 5, 15, 21n14, 24n37
Responsibilities, 189

Responsibility for health and disease, 45, 115–116
Rhetoric, 12, 16, 23n31, 35, 36, 99, 121, 234, 235–236, 246
Ricciardi, V., 151n2
Riddle, J., 19n5
Right, xii, 95, 96, 104, 156, 167, 179, 180, 189, 190, 195, 196, 197, 210, 218, 219, 254, 277, 284
Risse, G., 21n18, 25n39
Rist, J., 231, 236
Rockmore, T., 73
Roe (*v. Wade*), 180
Roman Catholic tradition, 87
Roman Empire, 70
Roman law, 70
Romantics, 70
Roochnik, D., 50n11, 152n11
Rorty, R., 73, 74
Ross, W. D., 75
Rules, 203
Russell, B., 73

Sallares, R., 21n18
Sanctity of human life, 71, 181, 266
Sarpedon, 231
Scarborough, J., 19n5
Schofield, M., 21n17
Schultz, D. S., 85, 86, 223n1
Schwartz, M. A., 65n5
Science, 57, 58, 61, 62, 63, 64, 72, 138
  aim or work, 31, 32, 35, 36
  applied, x, 49n2
  of good and evil, 281
  method, 31, 36
  natural, 31, 32, 34, 41, 42, 49n2, 52n22
  practical, 35, 38–41, 42–48, 258
  precision, 31, 32, 34, 40, 52n17
  productive, 35–38, 258
  pure, 49n2, 53n23
  social, 49n2
  subject matter, 32, 36
  theoretical, 32–34, 36, 40, 41–42, 48, 51n16

Scientific knowledge (*episteme*) 62, 79, 133, 136
Scientism, 73
Scott, P. A., 223n1
Secular, secularism, xii, 49n1, 204, 210, 218, 225n22
Sedley, D., 52n18, 232, 239, 247n2
Seers, 4, 5, 20n7
Segal, C., 216
Self, unencumbered, 182
Self-consciousness, 166, 171, 173
Self-discovery, mutual, 187
Self-understanding, xi
Seneca, 230, 236, 244, 245
Sexism, 166
Sexual acts, 17, 24n37
Sexuality, 53n29
Sheep, shepherds, 38–39
Ship building, 35
Siegler, M., 88n3
Sifakis, G. M., 212
Sigerist, H., 21n16
Signs, 5, 6, 7, 10, 14, 18
Silverman, W., 224n4
Singer, P., 84, 155, 166–168, 171–172, 174, 175n1, 176n4, 176n9
Skepticism, xi, 52n22, 65, 74, 110, 118, 121, 206
Skill, xi, 41
  trivial skills, 36
Slaves, 126n15
Smith, W., 19n3
Snow, C. P., 213
Social/political conception of medicine, 272
Society for Bioethics Consultation, 88
Society for Health and Human Values, 88
Society, 95
Sociology, 98
Socrates, xii, 4, 94, 102, 112, 131, 132, 135, 137, 138, 139, 140, 141, 142, 151n10, 152n13, 187, 190n3, 204, 217, 223, 235, 236, 237, 241, 264, 268

Sophistry, sophist, xi, 14, 23n26, 94, 99, 100, 102, 217, 267
Sophocles, 23n29, 196, 211–216, 222, 229, 287n2
Sorabji, R., 124n2
Soul, 37, 43–45, 47, 51n13, 53n25, 54n29, 112, 242, 262, 263, 278
Sourvinou-Inwood, C., 20n11
Speculation, 52n20, 52n22, 54n34, 204, 205, 221
Spells, 111–112
Standards, 35, 37, 48, 195, 198, 217
Starr, C. G., 23n26
Statesmanship, 43
Stephens, W. O., 237, 241, 244, 247n7
Stobaeus, 126n18
Stockdale, J., 240
Stoics, 52n18, 109, 110, 112, 115, 121, 124n2, 229–246
Strand, M., 202
Subjectivism, subjectivity, 32, 284
Suffering, xii, 18, 166–167, 174, 198, 213, 214, 254, 264, 273–274, 289n21
Suicide, xii, 229–246, 251, 254, 264, 265
Surgery, 52n20, 53n23, 261
Swazey, J., 103, 104
Systemic ailments, 44

Taylor, C., 65n7, 179
Teaching, 34, 40
Technological development, 33, 53n23, 193, 214, 286
Teiresias, 215
Teleological explanation, teleology, 159, 206, 217
Telfer, E., 85
Telos, 181
Temperance (*sophrosune*), 44, 269
Temple priests, 4
Theorizing, 34
Therapeutic process, 16, 259
Therapy, xii, 119
  model of, 110
  philosophy as, 109–124

Thick ethical concepts, 83
Thin nonanthropocentric concept of a
    person, 168–169, 172–173
Thing in Itself (*Das Ding an Sich*), 80
Thinking for oneself, 110, 124
Thomas, L., 65n4
Thomas, R., 21n21
Thomasma, D., xi, 19n1, 68, 71, 78,
    83, 225n22
Thornton, T. P., 70
Thought, 39, 230
Thrasymachus, xii, 131, 132, 135,
    137, 139, 140, 141, 142, 143, 144,
    149, 151n6, 152n12, 152n13
Thucydides, 212–213
Tienson, J., 70
Tollefson, C., 79
Tolstoy, L., 244, 247n8
Tool, 43, 46, 239, 243, 244
Tooley, M., 167, 175n1, 176n5
Toulmin, S., 68, 69, 72, 73, 193,
    202–205, 208, 209, 218, 224n9,
    224n10
Traditions, 99, 185, 203, 205, 214
Transcendent factors, 194–195, 197,
    207, 219, 221, 224n12
Tress, D., xii, 52n16
Troy, Trojan War, 4, 262
Trust, 13, 14–15, 17
Truth, 12, 33

U.S. President's Commission, 201
University, 186
Untersteiner, M., 99, 101
Utilitarian considerations, 167, 199
Utilitarianism, 74, 84, 86

Values, 181, 183, 188
Van der Eijyk, P. J., 21n15
Veatch, R. M., 19n1, 72
Venesection, 8
Versenyi, L., 99
Vico, G., 65n9
Vietnam, 190n2, 240
Virtue (*arete*), xi, xii, 34, 39, 40, 41,
    44, 45, 51n15, 53n27, 61, 67, 75,

81, 137, 194–197, 205, 207, 220,
    222, 223, 230, 236, 245, 246, 251,
    267, 269–270
analogous to health in body, 113
Virtue ethics, 193–195, 202, 222
Virus, 115, 125n12
Vitruvius, 52n21
Von Staden, H., 24n37

Wallace, J. D., 78
Waller, B. N., 75
Walzer, M., 144, 145
*Webster v. Reproductive Health
    Services*, 180
Welton, W., 52n17
White, N. P., 125n10
Whiting, J., 176n8
Wiggins, O., 65n5
Will, 78
Willett, S. J., 217
Williams, B., 110, 287n16
Williams, G., 260
Wisdom, 76
Women, 19n5, 24n37
Woozley, A. D., 269
Work satisfaction, 44
World War II, 69
Wounds, 4, 53n23
Writing, 7

Xenakis, I., 233, 235, 236, 238
Xenocrates, 52n18
Xenophanes, 50n9

Zaidman, L. B., 20n11, 225n19
Zalmoxis, 44
Zaner, R., 59, 60, 65n6
Zeno, 109, 230, 241, 247n3
Zeus, 100
Zussman, R., 103